CHART SMART

The A-to-Z Guide to Better Nursing Documentation

SECOND EDITION

CHART SMART

The A-to-Z Guide to Better Nursing Documentation

SECOND EDITION

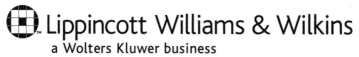

Lippincott Williams & Wilkins
a Wolters Kluwer business
Philadelphia • Baltimore • New York • London
Buenos Aires • Hong Kong • Sydney • Tokyo

STAFF

Executive Publisher
Judith A. Schilling McCann, RN, MSN

Editorial Director
David Moreau

Clinical Director
Joan M. Robinson, RN, MSN

Senior Art Director
Arlene Putterman

Editorial Project Manager
Coleen M.F. Stern

Clinical Project Manager
Beverly Ann Tscheschlog, RN, BS

Editor
Diane M. Labus

Clinical Editor
Marcy S. Caplin, RN, MSN

Copy Editors
Kimberly Bilotta (supervisor),
Karen C. Comerford, Pamela Wingrod

Designers
Debra Moloshok (book design),
Donna S. Morris (project manager)

Digital Composition Services
Diane Paluba (manager), Joyce Rossi Biletz,
Donna S. Morris

Manufacturing
Patricia K. Dorshaw (director), Beth J. Welsh

Editorial Assistants
Megan L. Aldinger, Karen J. Kirk,
Linda K. Ruhf

Indexer
Karen C. Comerford

CSAZ010106–030307

FOCUS CHARTING is a registered trademark of Creative Healthcare Management, Inc.

Library of Congress Cataloging-in-Publication Data
ChartSmart : the A-to-Z guide to better nursing documentation.–2nd ed.
    p. ; cm.
Includes bibliographical references and index.
1. Nursing records–Handbooks, manuals, etc. I. Lippincott Williams & Wilkins.
    [DNLM: 1. Nursing Records. WY 100.5 C4867 2007]
RT50.C487 2007
610.73–dc22
ISBN13 978-1-58255-987-2
ISBN10 1-58255-987-2 (alk. paper)   2005029063

Contents

Advisory board

Contributors and consultants

Adrianne E. Avillion, RN, DEd
President
AEA Consulting
York, Pa.

Peggy Bozarth, RN, MSN
Professor
Hopkinsville (Ky.) Community College

Cheryl L. Brady, RN, MSN
Nurse Educator
Canfield, Ohio

Virginia L. Branson, RN, MA, CBCS
Program Director — Medical Office
   Management
Virginia College
Birmingham, Ala.

Linda Carman Copel, RN, PhD,
   CGP, CS, DAPA
Associate Professor
Villanova (Pa.) University

Christine Greenidge, RN, MSN, BC
Director of Nursing Professional Practice
Montefiore Medical Center
Bronx, N.Y.

Merita Konstantacos, RN, MSN
Consultant
Clinton, Ohio

Theresa Pulvano, RN, BSN
Nursing Educator for LPNs
Ocean County Vocational Technical
   School
Lakehurst, N.J.

Roseanne Hanlon Rafter, MSN,
   APRN, BC
Director of Nursing Professional Practice
Pottstown (Pa.) Memorial Medical
   Center

Elsa Nicklas Sanchez, RN, BSN, BA
Staff Development
Meadowview Nursing Home Atlantic
   County
Northfield, N.J.

Rita M. Wick, RN, BSN
Education Specialist
Berkshire Health Systems
Pittsfield, Mass.

Foreword

Documentation is one of the most important responsibilities of all health care providers. It's a means of communicating among health care team members and the primary way by which nurses record factual information about a patient's status and the care provided – from the time of admission to follow-up after discharge. To allow for timely and accurate assessment of the patient's needs and ensure the continuity of quality patient care, all nursing documentation must be complete, concise, and up to date.

Hospital risk managers and accreditation agencies such as the Joint Commission on Accreditation of Healthcare Organizations (JCAHO) use nursing documentation to evaluate the quality of patient care. Therefore, it must be an accurate reflection of the care provided. Also, insurance companies, including Medicare and Medicaid, review such documentation to determine which procedures the patient received. If your documentation is incomplete, both the hospital and the patient may be denied reimbursement for care that was actually provided.

Additionally, the courts may scrutinize nursing documentation in the event of a lawsuit that questions the quality or level of care a patient did or didn't receive. In such cases, what you document and how you describe the patient care provided are equally important and speak to your credibility as a professional health care provider. If a patient is injured and brings a nursing malpractice lawsuit against you, your documentation may be the most critical evidence of the standard of care you provide to the patient. Consequently, your notes must include a record that traces your total involvement in patient care – beginning with assessment of the patient's needs and following through with care provided in collaboration with other members of the health care team.

Because documentation is so critical to patient care and professional practice, nurses need a comprehensive source that explains not only what to document, but also how and when to document. This second edition of *ChartSmart: The A-to-Z Guide to Better Nursing Documentation* serves just that purpose. This handy reference covers the documentation of common nursing care activities as well as some of the most challenging and high-risk scenarios encountered by nurses. Its easy A-to-Z format allows for quick retrieval of information, and the inclusion of real-life charting scenarios in each entry makes it an indispensable tool for everyday use.

ChartSmart includes discussions on many sensitive topics, including suspected child or elder abuse, advance directives and living wills, and documenting questionable doctor's orders. The book also covers various technical nursing procedures that require careful documentation, such as blood transfusion reactions, adverse reactions resulting from drug administration, and allergy testing.

Besides the documentation of common nursing procedures and professional issues, this new edition also tackles many of the current "hot topics" in health care – for example, reporting of critical test values, cultural needs identification, end-of-life care, falls precautions, and the Health Insurance Portability and Accountability Act.

In the Appendices, you'll find a comprehensive discussion of various recognized nursing documentation systems with examples and forms that allow you to evaluate and compare the different options for documenting care. Advocacy is an important aspect of nursing, and having a thorough understanding of these options will enable you to advocate for your professional practice when your hospital or agency is exploring the most effective form of nursing documentation to use. In addition, there's a section on the electronic health record, which increases your efficiency and accuracy in documenting patient care. You'll also find JCAHO's National Patient Safety Goals and its list of abbreviations to avoid as well as the newest NANDA nursing diagnoses.

Whether working in a hospital or community agency or in an urban or rural setting, nurses will find *ChartSmart: The A-to-Z Guide to Better Documentation* to be a helpful hands-on tool. Learning what to document and how to do so efficiently and professionally will enhance your competency and credibility and help ensure that the high standards of nursing care are being met in every health care setting.

Penny S. Brooke, APRN, MS, JD
Professor and Director of Outreach
University of Utah College of Nursing
Salt Lake City

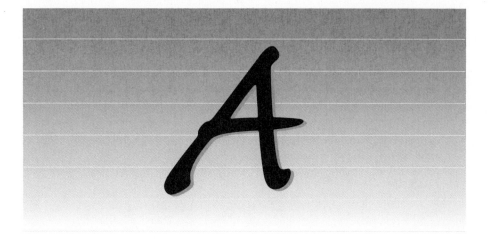

ABUSE, SUSPECTED

Abuse may be suspected in any age-group, cultural setting, or environment. The patient may readily report being abused or may fear reporting the abuser. Types of suspected abuse include neglect and physical, sexual, emotional, and psychological abuse.

In most states, a nurse is required by law to report signs of abuse in children, the elderly, and the disabled. (See *Common signs of neglect and abuse,* page 2.) Use appropriate channels for your facility and report your suspicions to the appropriate administrator and agency. Document suspicions on the appropriate form for your facility or in your nurse's notes. If the patient is a child, interview the child alone and try to interview caregivers separately to note inconsistencies with histories. An injunction can be obtained to separate the abuser and the abused, ensuring the patient's safety until the circumstances can be investigated.

Remember, certain cultural practices that produce bruises or burns, such as coin rubbing in Vietnamese groups, may be mistaken for child maltreatment. Regardless of cultural practices, the judgment of child maltreatment is decided by the department of social services and the health care team. (See *Your role in reporting abuse,* page 3.)

ESSENTIAL DOCUMENTATION

When documenting, record only the facts and be sure to leave out personal opinions and judgments. Record the time and date of the entry. Provide a comprehensive history, noting inconsistencies in histories, eva-

COMMON SIGNS OF NEGLECT AND ABUSE

If your assessment reveals any of the following signs, consider neglect or abuse as a possible cause and document your findings. Be sure to notify the appropriate people and agencies.

NEGLECT

- Failure to thrive in infants
- Malnutrition
- Dehydration
- Poor personal hygiene
- Inadequate clothing
- Severe diaper rash
- Injuries from falls
- Failure of wounds to heal
- Periodontal disease
- Infestations, such as scabies, lice, or maggots in a wound

ABUSE

- Recurrent injuries
- Multiple injuries or fractures in various stages of healing
- Unexplained bruises, abrasions, burns, bites, damaged or missing teeth, strap or rope marks
- Head injuries or bald spots from pulling out hair
- Bleeding from body orifices
- Genital trauma
- Sexually transmitted diseases in children
- Pregnancy in young girls or women with physical or mental handicaps
- Verbalized accounts of being beaten, slapped, kicked, or involved in sexual activities
- Precocious sexual behaviors
- Exposure to inappropriately harsh discipline
- Exposure to verbal abuse and belittlement
- Extreme fear or anxiety

ADDITIONAL SIGNS

- Mistrust of others
- Blunted or flat affect
- Depression or mood changes
- Social withdrawal
- Lack of appropriate peer relationships
- Sudden school difficulties, such as poor grades, truancy, or fighting with peers
- Nonspecific headaches, stomachaches, or eating and sleeping problems
- Clinging behavior directed toward health care providers
- Aggressive speech or behavior toward adults
- Abusive behavior toward younger children and pets
- Runaway behavior

YOUR ROLE IN REPORTING ABUSE

As a nurse, you play a crucial role in recognizing and reporting incidents of suspected abuse. While caring for patients, you can readily note evidence of apparent abuse. When you do, you must pass the information along to the appropriate authorities. In many states, failure to report actual or suspected abuse constitutes a crime.

If you've ever hesitated to file an abuse report because you fear repercussions, remember that the Child Abuse Prevention and Treatment Act protects you against liability. If your report is bona fide (that is, if you file it in good faith), the law protects you from any suit filed by an alleged abuser.

sive answers, delays in treatment, medical attention sought at other hospitals, and the person caring for the individual during the incident. Document your physical assessment findings using illustrations and photographs as necessary (per police department and social service guidelines). Describe the patient's response to treatments given. Record the names and departments of people notified within the facility. Provide the names of people notified, such as social services, the police department, and welfare agencies. Record any visits by these agencies. Include any teaching or support given.

06/08/05	1700	Circular burns 2 cm in diameter noted on lower ® and
		ⓛ scapulae in various stages of healing while
		auscultating breath sounds. Pt. states these injuries
		occurred while playing with cigarettes he found at his
		babysitter's home. When parents were questioned
		separately as to the cause of injuries on child's back,
		mother stated the child told her he fell off a swing
		and received a rope burn. Father stated he had no idea
		of the child's injuries. Parents stated the child is being
		watched after school until they get home by the
		teenager next door, Sally Johnson. Parents stated that
		their son doesn't like being watched by her anymore, but
		they don't know why. Parents state they're looking into
		alternative care suggestions. Dr. Gordon notified of
		injuries and examined pt. at 1645. Social worker, Nancy
		Stiller, and nursing supervisor, Nancy Taylor, RN,
		notified at 1650. ——————— Joanne M. Allen, RN

ACTIVITIES OF DAILY LIVING

Activities of daily living (ADLs) checklists are standard forms completed on each shift by the nursing staff and, in some cases, the patient performing the activities. After completion, you review and sign them. These forms tell the health care team members about the patient's abilities, degree of independence, and special needs so they can determine the type of assistance each patient requires. Tools that are useful in assessing and documenting ADLs include the Katz index, Lawton scale, and Barthel index and scale.

ESSENTIAL DOCUMENTATION

Be sure to include the patient's name, the date and time of the evaluation, and your name and credentials.

On the Katz index, rank your patient's ability in six areas:
- bathing
- dressing
- toileting
- moving from wheelchair to bed and returning
- continence
- feeding.

For each ADL, check whether your patient can perform the task independently, needs some help to perform the task, or can't perform the task without significant help. (See *Katz index*.)

The Lawton scale evaluates your patient's ability to perform complex personal care activities necessary for independent living, such as:
- using the telephone
- cooking or preparing meals
- shopping
- doing laundry
- managing finances
- taking medications
- doing housework.

Rate your patient's ability to perform these activities using a three-point scale: (1) completely unable to perform task, (2) needs some help, or (3) performs activity without help. (See *Lawton scale,* page 6.)

(Text continues on page 9.)

AccuChart

KATZ INDEX

Below you'll find a sample of the Katz index, which is used to assess six basic activities of daily living.

Evaluation Form   Name *Harold Kaufmann*   Date *6/1/05*

For each area of functioning listed below, check the description that applies.

Indicates independence	Indicates assistance needed	Indicates dependence
Bathing: Sponge bath, tub bath, or shower. ☑ Receives no assistance; gets into and out of tub, if tub is usual means of bathing.	☐ Receives assistance in bathing only one part of the body, such as the back or leg.	☐ Receives assistance in bathing more than one part of the body or can't bathe.
Dressing: Gets outer garments and underwear from closets and drawers and uses fasteners, including suspenders, if worn. ☑ Gets clothes and gets completely dressed without assistance.	☐ Gets clothes and gets dressed without assistance except for tying shoes.	☐ Receives assistance in getting clothes or in getting dressed or stays partly or completely undressed.
Toileting: Goes to the room termed "toilet" for bowel movement and urination, cleans self afterward, and arranges clothes. ☑ Goes to toilet room, cleans self, and arranges clothes without assistance. May use object for support, such as cane, walker, or wheelchair, and may manage night bedpan or commode, emptying it in the morning.	☐ Receives assistance in going to toilet room or in cleaning self or arranging clothes after elimination or in use of night bedpan or commode.	☐ Doesn't go to toilet room for the elimination process.
Transfer ☑ Moves into and out of bed and chair without assistance. May use object, such as cane or walker, for support.	☐ Moves into or out of bed or chair with assistance.	☐ Doesn't get out of bed.
Continence ☑ Controls urination and bowel movement completely by self.	☐ Has occasional accidents.	☐ Supervision helps keep control of urination or bowel movement, or catheter is used, or is incontinent.
Feeding ☐ Feeds self without assistance.	☑ Feeds self except for assistance in cutting meat or buttering bread.	☐ Receives assistance in feeding or is fed partly or completely through tubes or by I.V. fluids.

Evaluator: *Holly Sebastain, RN*

Overall evaluation: *B*

A: Independent in all six functions.
B: Independent in all but one of these functions.
C: Independent in all but bathing and one additional function.
D: Independent in all but bathing, dressing, and one additional function.
E: Independent in all but bathing, dressing, toileting, and one additional function.

F: Independent in all but bathing, dressing, toileting, transferring, and one additional function.
G: Dependent in all six functions.
Other: Dependent in at least two functions but not classifiable as C, D, E, or F.

© Adapted with permission from Katz, S., et al. "Studies of Illness in the Aged: The Index of ADL-A Standardized Measure of Biological and Psychosocial Function," *JAMA* 185:914-19, 1963.

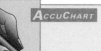

LAWTON SCALE

The Lawton scale evaluates more sophisticated functions—known as instrumental activities of daily living—than the Katz index. Patients or caregivers can complete the form in a few minutes. The first answer in each case—except for 8a—indicates independence; the second indicates capability with assistance; and the third, dependence. In this version, the maximum score is 29, although scores have meaning only for a particular patient, as when declining scores over time reveal deterioration. Questions 4 to 7 may be gender specific; modify them as necessary.

Name *Martha Lutz* **Rated by** *Nancy Kline, RN* **Date** *February 13, 2005*

1. Can you use the telephone?
   Without help . . . . .③
   With some help 2
   Completely unable 1

2. Can you get to places beyond walking distance?
   Without help . . . . .③
   With some help 2
   Completely unable 1

3. Can you go shopping for groceries?
   Without help . . . . .③
   With some help 2
   Completely unable 1

4. Can you prepare your own meals?
   Without help . . . . .③
   With some help 2
   Completely unable 1

5. Can you do your own housework?
   Without help 3
   With some help . . . . .②
   Completely unable 1

6. Can you do your own handyman work?
   Without help 3
   With some help . . . . .②
   Completely unable 1

7. Can you do your own laundry?
   Without help . . . . .③
   With some help 2
   Completely unable 1

8a. Do you take medicines or use any medications?
   Yes (If yes, answer Question 8b.) . . . . .①
   No (If no, answer Question 8c.) 2

8b. Do you take your own medicine?
   Without help (in the right doses at the
   right times) . . . . .③
   With some help (if someone prepares it for you
   and reminds you to take it) 2
   Completely unable 1

8c. If you had to take medicine, could you do it?
   Without help (in the right doses at the
   right times) 3
   With some help (if someone prepares it for you
   and reminds you to take it) 2
   Completely unable 1

9. Can you manage your own money?
   Without help . . . . .③
   With some help 2
   Completely unable 1

   Total Score _26_

BARTHEL INDEX

The Barthel index, shown below, is used to assess the patient's ability to perform 10 activities of daily living, document findings for other health care team members, and reveal improvement or decline.

Date *December 14, 2005*

Patient's name *Joseph Amity*

Evaluator *John Kaiser, RN*

Action	With help	Independent
Feeding (if food needs to be cut = help)	5	(10)
Moving from wheelchair to bed and return (includes sitting up in bed)	5 to (10)	15
Personal toilet (wash face, comb hair, shave, clean teeth)	0	(5)
Getting on and off toilet (handling clothes, wipe, flush)	(5)	10
Bathing self	0	(5)
Walking on level surface (or, if unable to walk, propelling wheelchair)	0	(5) or 15
Ascending and descending stairs	(5)	10
Dressing (includes tying shoes, fastening fasteners)	(5)	10
Controlling bowels	5	(10)
Controlling bladder	(5)	10

Definition and Discussion of Scoring
A person scoring 100 is continent, feeds himself, dresses himself, gets up out of bed and chairs, bathes himself, walks at least a block, and can ascend and descend stairs. This doesn't mean that he's able to live alone; he may not be able to cook, keep house, or meet the public, but he's able to get along without attendant care.

Feeding
10 = Independent. The person can feed himself a meal from a tray or table when someone puts the food within his reach. He must be able to put on an assistive device, if needed, cut the food, use salt and pepper, spread butter, and so forth. Also, he must accomplish these tasks in a reasonable time.
5 = The person needs some help with cutting food and other tasks, as listed above.

Moving from wheelchair to bed and return
15 = The person operates independently in all phases of this activity. He can safely approach the bed in his wheelchair, lock brakes, lift footrests, move safely from bed, lie down, come to a sitting position on the side of the bed, change the position of the wheelchair, if necessary, to transfer back into it safely, and return to the wheelchair.
10 = Either the person needs some minimal help in some step of this activity, or needs to be reminded or supervised for safety in one or more parts of this activity.
5 = The person can come to a sitting position without the help of a second person but needs to be lifted out of bed, or needs a great deal of help with transfers.

Handling personal toilet
5 = The person can wash hands and face, comb hair, clean teeth, and shave. He may use any kind of razor but he must be able to get it from the drawer or cabinet and plug it in or put in a blade without help. A woman must put on her own makeup, if she uses any, but need not braid or style her hair.

(continued)

BARTHEL INDEX *(continued)*

Getting on and off toilet
10 = The person is able to get on and off the toilet, unfasten and refasten clothes, prevent soiling of clothes, and use toilet paper without help. He may use a wall bar or other stable object for support, if needed. If he needs to use a bed pan instead of toilet, he must be able to place it on a chair, use it competently, and empty and clean it.
5 = The person needs help to overcome imbalance, handle clothes, or use toilet paper.

Bathing self
5 = The person may use a bath tub or shower or give himself a complete sponge bath. Regardless of method, he must be able to complete all the steps involved without another person's presence.

Walking on a level surface
15 = The person can walk at least 50 yards without help or supervision. He may wear braces or prostheses and use crutches, canes, or a walkerette, but not a rolling walker. He must be able to lock and unlock braces, if used, get the necessary mechanical aids into position for use, stand up and sit down, and dispose of the aids when he sits. (Putting on, fastening, and taking off braces is scored under Dressing).
5 = If the person can't ambulate but can propel a wheelchair independently, he must be able to go around corners, turn around, maneuver the chair to table, bed, toilet, and other locations. He must be able to push a chair at least 150' (45.7 m). Don't score this item if the person receives a score for walking.
0 = Unable to walk.

Ascending and descending stairs
10 = The person can go up and down a flight of stairs safely without help or supervision. He may and should use handrails, canes, or crutches when needed, and he must be able to carry canes or crutches as he ascends or descends.
5 = The person needs help with or supervision of any one of the above items.

Dressing and undressing
10 = The person can put on, fasten, and remove all clothing (including any prescribed corset or braces) and tie shoe laces (unless he requires adaptations for this). Such special clothing as suspenders, loafers, and dresses that open down the front may be used when necessary.
5 = The person needs help in putting on, fastening, or removing any clothing. He must do at least half the work himself and must accomplish the task in a reasonable time. Women need not be scored on use of a brassiere or girdle unless these are prescribed garments.

Controlling bowels
10 = The person can control his bowels without accidents. He can use a suppository or take an enema when necessary (as in spinal cord injury patients who have had bowel training).
5 = The person needs help in using a suppository or taking an enema or has occasional accidents.

Controlling bladder
10 = The person can control his bladder day and night. Spinal cord injury patients who wear an external device and leg bag must put them on independently, clean and empty the bag, and stay dry, day and night.
5 = The person has occasional accidents, can't wait for the bed pan or get to the toilet in time, or needs help with an external device.

The total score is less significant or meaningful than the individual items because these indicate where the deficiencies lie. Any applicant to a long-term care facility who scores 100 should be evaluated carefully before admission to see whether admission is indicated. Discharged patients with scores of 100 shouldn't require further physical therapy but may benefit from a home visit to see whether any environmental adjustments are needed.

© Adapted with permission from Mahoney, F.I. and Barthel, D.W. "Functional Evaluation: The Barthel Index," *Maryland State Medical Journal* 14:62, 1965.

The Barthel index and scale is used to evaluate:

- feeding
- moving from wheelchair to bed and returning
- performing personal hygiene
- getting on and off the toilet
- bathing
- walking on a level surface or propelling a wheelchair
- going up and down stairs
- dressing and undressing
- maintaining bowel continence
- controlling the bladder.

Score each ADL according to the amount of assistance the patient needs. Over time, results reveal improvement or decline. Another scale, the Barthel self-care rating scale, evaluates function in more detail. (See *Barthel index,* pages 7 and 8.)

ADVANCE DIRECTIVE

An advance directive is a legal document used as a guideline for life-sustaining medical care of a patient with an advanced disease or disability who is no longer able to indicate his own wishes. Advance directives also include living wills (which instruct the doctor regarding life-sustaining treatment) and durable powers of attorney for health care (which names another person to act on the patient's behalf for medical decisions in the event that the patient can't act for himself).

Because laws vary from state to state, be sure to find out how your state's laws apply to your practice and to the medical record.

If a patient has previously executed an advance directive, request a copy for the chart and make sure the doctor is aware of it. Some health care facilities routinely make this request a part of admission procedures. (See *Advance directive checklist,* page 10.)

ESSENTIAL DOCUMENTATION

Document the presence of an advance directive, and notify the doctor. Include the name, address, and telephone number of the person entrusted with decision-making power. Indicate that you've read the advance directive and have forwarded it to risk management (or the appropriate de-

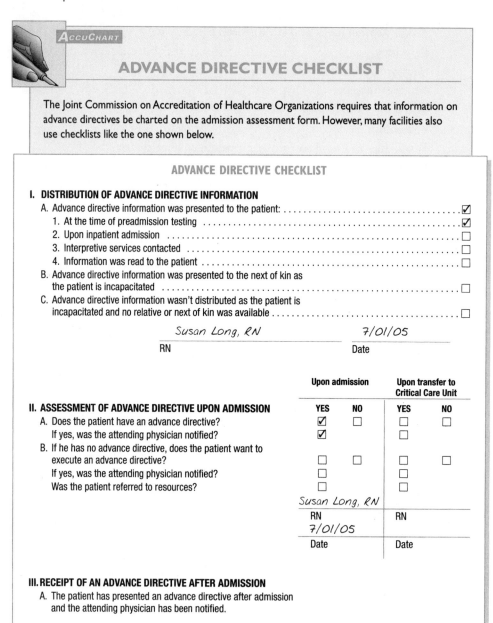

ADVANCE DIRECTIVE CHECKLIST

The Joint Commission on Accreditation of Healthcare Organizations requires that information on advance directives be charted on the admission assessment form. However, many facilities also use checklists like the one shown below.

ADVANCE DIRECTIVE CHECKLIST

I. DISTRIBUTION OF ADVANCE DIRECTIVE INFORMATION

A. Advance directive information was presented to the patient: ....☑
   1. At the time of preadmission testing ....☑
   2. Upon inpatient admission ....☐
   3. Interpretive services contacted ....☐
   4. Information was read to the patient ....☐
B. Advance directive information was presented to the next of kin as the patient is incapacitated ....☐
C. Advance directive information wasn't distributed as the patient is incapacitated and no relative or next of kin was available ....☐

Susan Long, RN	*7/01/05*
RN	Date

II. ASSESSMENT OF ADVANCE DIRECTIVE UPON ADMISSION	Upon admission		Upon transfer to Critical Care Unit	
	YES	NO	YES	NO
A. Does the patient have an advance directive?	☑	☐	☐	☐
If yes, was the attending physician notified?	☑		☐	
B. If he has no advance directive, does the patient want to execute an advance directive?	☐	☐	☐	☐
If yes, was the attending physician notified?	☐		☐	
Was the patient referred to resources?	☐		☐	

Susan Long, RN	
RN	RN
7/01/05	
Date	Date

III. RECEIPT OF AN ADVANCE DIRECTIVE AFTER ADMISSION

A. The patient has presented an advance directive after admission and the attending physician has been notified.

RN	Date

partment at your institution) for review. If the patient's wishes differ from those of his family or doctor, make sure that the discrepancies are thoroughly documented in the chart.

If a patient doesn't have an advance directive, document that he was given written information concerning his rights under state law to make decisions regarding his health care. If the patient refuses information on an advance directive, document this refusal using the patient's own words, in quotes, if possible. Record any conversations with the patient regarding his decision making. Document that proof of competence was obtained (usually the responsibility of the medical, legal, social services, or risk management department).

7/28/05	1000	Pt. admitted with an advance directive. Dr. Wellington notified at 0950 about advance directive in chart. Copy of advance directive read and placed in medical record, and copy forwarded to Melissa Edwards in Risk Management. Mary Gordon, pt.'s daughter, has durable power of attorney for health care (123 Livingston Drive, Newton, VT, phone: 123-456-7890). ————— Carol Edwards, RN

ADVANCE DIRECTIVE, FAMILY CONTESTS PATIENT'S WISHES FOR

In most states, the advance directive is a legal document formulated by the patient while he's of sound mind that dictates the patient's wishes should he become incapacitated and unable to make decisions. Ideally, the patient should discuss his feelings and desires with his family members, and they should agree to the patient's desires. However, there may be occasions when the family doesn't agree with the advance directive or want it activated. Should this occur, the legality of the situation dictates that the living will is upheld. The family's rights are superseded by the living will.

Should the family members express opposition to the advance directive, notify the patient's attending physician, the nursing supervisor, and the risk manager. The family members can be encouraged to discuss their feelings with the patient and these individuals, or they may be referred for counseling that may help them in their situation.

ESSENTIAL DOCUMENTATION

Document your conversation with the family members, recording their exact words in quotes. Record your assessment of the family situation. Document the name and department of any person notified. Chart the names of the notified doctor, nursing supervisor, and risk manager and the time they were contacted. Include any visits by these individuals and any counseling offered.

| 10/8/05 | 1500 | Sally Jones, 20 y.o. daughter of Mr. Jones, in to visit this evening and stated, "I don't want my father's advance directive carried out. I want everything possible done for my father." Father and daughter live together since death of mother and brother in a car accident 3 years ago. Daughter informed of necessity to follow her father's legal wishes. Daughter encouraged to talk to father about his feelings. Notified Dr. Brown; Carol Deed, RN, nursing supervisor; and Mrs. Smitch, risk manager. Dr. Brown stated he'll call daughter at her home at 2100. Mrs. Smitch will meet with daughter at 1600 to discuss the situation. Name and number of risk manager given to daughter to assist in follow-up. ———————————————————————————Jane Dolan, RN |

ADVANCE DIRECTIVE, NURSE WITNESS OF

Many patients wait until they're hospitalized to consider an advance directive or to make significant legal decisions. If a patient wants to execute a living will during his hospital stay, you aren't required, or even allowed in some states, to sign as a witness. Check with your state's laws about whether you can sign as a witness. In many facilities, the social services or risk management department oversees this process. Find out which is the responsible department in your facility. The person who acts as witness can be held accountable for the patient's competence. Keep in mind that only a competent adult can execute a legally binding document. To prevent a patient's relatives from later raising questions about his competence, the record should include documented proof of competence (usually the responsibility of the medical, legal, social services, or risk management department).

ESSENTIAL DOCUMENTATION

Record the patient's desire to institute an advance directive. If social services and risk management are involved, document the time you notified them and the name of the person with whom you spoke. Record any visits from social services, risk management, or the patient's own lawyer. Note that proof of competence was obtained, and record the name of the person who obtained it. If an advance directive is instituted, the health care team should be notified of its existence. Chart that the doctor was notified of the presence of an advance directive. Place the signed and witnessed document in the medical record.

9/20/05	2000	Pt. stated he wanted to execute an advance directive. He has read the written information on advance directives given to him on admission. Risk management notified at 1930. Pt. visited by his lawyer, Mr. Jones, and risk manager, Lisa Deed, RN. Proof of competence obtained by Ms. Deed. Copy of living will placed in chart, and Dr. Brown, pt.'s doctor, was notified. ———— Joan Stevens, RN

ADVANCE DIRECTIVE REVOCATION

At the time of admission, the patient should be asked if he has an advance directive and if it reflects his wishes. Ideally, the advance directive should be reviewed yearly and updated as necessary. An advance directive becomes active only if the conditions under which the patient has defined the document to be activated have occurred, such as a permanent unconscious state or a terminal condition. The patient may revoke his advance directive at any time. For example, the patient may revoke his directive if he changes his mind about his previous decision or if his condition mandates that he revise his directive (his diagnosis changes for the better or worse). Legally, the patient can revoke an advance directive at any time either orally or in writing.

ESSENTIAL DOCUMENTATION

Place a copy of the patient's written revocation in the medical record, or sign and date a statement in the patient's own words explaining that the patient made the request orally. Include the names of witnesses who heard the patient revoke his advance directive. Record that the doctor, risk manager, and nursing supervisor were notified of the revocation. Consult your facility's policy and your state's laws pertaining to living wills and advance directives; revocation statements may need to be countersigned.

7/21/05	2000	Pt. stated, "I don't want my advance directive to be
		activated, because it doesn't meet my present situation
		or desires at this time." Pt.'s wife, Mary Blank, present
		when pt. made this statement. Wife verbalized support
		of pt.'s decision. Notified Dr. Brown; Tamara Hardy, RN,
		nursing supervisor; and Kathy Day, RN, risk manager, of
		the revocation. Note placed on front of pt.'s chart
		alerting staff to revocation of advance directive by pt.
		———————————————————— May Stewart, RN

ADVICE TO PATIENT BY TELEPHONE

Nurses, especially those working in hospital emergency departments (ED), frequently get requests to give advice to patients by telephone. A hospital has no legal duty to provide a telephone advice service, and you have no legal duty to give advice to anyone who calls. Check your facility's policy and procedure manual to determine whether nurses are allowed to give telephone advice.

The best response to a telephone request for medical advice is to tell the caller to come to the hospital because you can't assess his condition or treat him over the phone. One exception is a life-threatening situation, in which someone needs immediate care, treatment, or referral.

If you do dispense advice over the phone, keep in mind that a legal duty arises the minute you say, "OK, let me tell you what to do." You now have a nurse-patient relationship, and you're responsible for any advice you give. When you start to give advice by telephone, you can't decide midway through that you're in over your head and simply hang up; that could be considered abandonment. You must give appropriate advice or a referral.

ESSENTIAL DOCUMENTATION

If your hospital allows telephone advice, there should be a system of documenting such calls; for example, by using a telephone log. The log should include:

- date and time of the call
- caller's name, if he'll give it
- caller's address
- caller's request or reason for seeking care

LOGGING CALLS
FOR TELEPHONE ADVICE

Some nurses hesitate to use a log to record advice given by telephone because they assume that if they don't document, they won't be responsible for the advice they give. This assumption is faulty. A patient may make only one call to the hospital, usually about something important to him. He'll remember that; you may not.

The telephone log can provide evidence and refresh your recollection of the event. It may remind you that you didn't tell the patient to take two acetaminophen tablets to lower his fever of 105° F (40.6° C). Instead you told him to come to the emergency department (ED). Or maybe you told a young athlete to come to the ED for an X-ray of his injured ankle.

When you log such information, the law presumes that it's true because you wrote it in the course of ordinary business.

- disposition of the call, such as giving the caller a poison-control number or suggesting that he come to the ED for evaluation
- name of the person who made that disposition.

Document whatever information you give. (See *Logging calls for telephone advice.*)

| 11/6/05 | 1615 | Louis Chapman of 123 Elm St., New City, VT, 123-456-7890, phoned asking how big a cut has to be to require stitches. I asked him to describe the injury. He described a 4" gash in his ℚ arm from a fall. I recommended that he apply pressure to the cut and come into the ED to be assessed. ———————————— Claire Bowen, RN |

AGAINST MEDICAL ADVICE, DISCHARGE

A patient usually leaves a health care facility against medical advice (AMA) because he doesn't understand his condition or treatment, has pressing personal problems, wants to exert control over his health care, or has religious or cultural objections to his care.

Although a patient can choose to leave a health care facility AMA at any time, the law requires clear evidence that he's mentally competent to make that choice. In most facilities, an AMA form (also known as a *responsibility release form*) serves as a legal document to protect you, the doctors, and the facility if any problems arise from a patient's unapproved discharge. (See *Patient discharge against medical advice,* page 16.)

PATIENT DISCHARGE AGAINST MEDICAL ADVICE

The patient's bill of rights and the laws and regulations based on it give a competent adult the right to refuse treatment for any reason without being punished or having his liberty restricted. Some states have turned these rights into law, and the courts have cited the bills of rights in their decisions. The right to refuse treatment includes the right to leave the hospital against medical advice (AMA) any time, for any reason. All you can do is try to talk the patient out of it.

If your patient still insists on leaving AMA and your hospital has a policy on managing the patient who wants to leave, follow it exactly. Adhering to policy will help to protect the hospital, your coworkers, and you from charges of unlawful restraint or false imprisonment.

Provide routine discharge care. Even though your patient is leaving AMA, his rights to discharge planning and care are the same as those of a patient who's signed out with medical advice. Therefore, if the patient agrees, escort him to the door (in a wheelchair, if necessary), arrange for medical or nursing follow-up care, and offer other routine health care measures. These procedures will protect the hospital as well as the patient.

ESSENTIAL DOCUMENTATION

Have the patient sign the AMA form, and in your notes clearly document:

- patient's reason for leaving AMA
- that the patient knows he's leaving AMA
- names of relatives or others notified of the patient's decision and the dates and times of the notifications
- notification of the doctor, doctor's visit, and any instructions or orders given
- explanation of the risks and consequences of the AMA discharge, as told to the patient, including the name of the person who provided the explanation
- instructions regarding alternative sources of follow-up care given to the patient
- list of those accompanying the patient at discharge and the instructions given to them
- patient's destination after discharge. (See *Responsibility release form.*)

ACCUCHART

RESPONSIBILITY RELEASE FORM

An against medical advice (AMA) form is a medical record as well as a legal document. It's designed to protect you, your coworkers, and your institution from liability resulting from the patient's unapproved discharge.

RESPONSIBILITY RELEASE

This is to certify that I, _Robert Brown_

a patient in _Jefferson Memorial Hospital_

am being discharged against the advice of my doctor and the hospital administration. I acknowledge that I have been informed of the risk involved and hereby release my doctor and the hospital from all responsibility for any ill effects that may result from such a discharge. I also understand that I may return to the hospital at any time and have treatment resumed.

Robert Brown	_11/4/05_
[Patient's signature]	[Date]
Carl Giordano, MD	_11/4/05_
[Witness' signature]	[Date]

RE: _Robert Brown_   Patient identification # _123456_
[Name of patient]

Document any statements and actions reflecting the patient's mental state at the time he chose to leave the facility. This will help protect you, the doctors, and the facility against a charge of negligence. The patient may later claim that his discharge occurred while he was mentally incompetent and that he was improperly supervised while he was in that state.

Also check your facility's policy regarding incident reports. If the patient leaves without anyone's knowledge or if he refuses to sign the AMA form, you'll probably be required to complete an incident report.

If a patient refuses to sign the AMA form, document this refusal on the AMA form, and enter it in his chart. Use the patient's own words to describe his refusal.

| 11/4/05 | 1500 | Pt. found in room packing his clothes. When asked why he was dressed and packing, he stated, "I'm tired of all these tests. They keep doing tests, but they still don't know what's wrong with me. I can't take anymore. I'm going home." Dr. Giordano notified and came to speak with pt. Doctor told pt. of possible risks and consequences of his leaving the hospital with headaches and hypertension. Pt. agrees to see Dr. Giordano in his office in 2 days. Prescriptions given to pt. Pt.'s wife notified, and she came to the hospital. She was unable to persuade husband to stay. Pt. signed AMA form. Discussed low Na diet, meds, and appt. with pt. and wife. Gave pt. drug information sheets. Pt. states he's going home after discharge. Accompanied pt. in wheelchair to main lobby with wife. Pt. left at 1445. — Lynn Nakashima, RN |
| | | |

AGAINST MEDICAL ADVICE, OUT OF BED

Even after you've told a patient that he must not get out of bed alone and that he must call you for help, you may go to his room and find him climbing out of bed, or you may discover relatives helping him to the bathroom because they don't want to disturb you. Either scenario puts the patient at risk for a fall and you at risk for a lawsuit. Proper documentation in this situation can protect you in a lawsuit. Some facilities also require you to complete an incident report for a near miss even though no injury has occurred.

ESSENTIAL DOCUMENTATION

Record the date and time of your entry. Clearly document your instructions and anything that the patient does in spite of them. Record the names of any visitors or family members present at the time of your instruction. Be sure to include any devices being used to ensure patient safety, such as bed alarms or leg alarms. This shows that you recognized the potential for a fall and that you tried to prevent it.

2/10/05	0300	Assisted pt. to bathroom. Weak, unsteady on feet. States
		she gets dizzy when she stands. Instructed pt. to call
		for assistance to get OOB. Call bell within reach. Pt.
		demonstrated proper use of the call bell and verbalized
		that she will call for help when she needs to get OOB.
		———————— Joseph Romano, RN
2/10/05	0430	Found pt. walking to bathroom on own. Stated she
		didn't want to bother anyone. Reminded her to call for
		assistance. Told her nurse would check with her every
		1½ hr to see if she needed to go to bathroom. Pt.
		agreed she would wait for nurse. Care plan amended to
		reflect q 1½-hr checks. ———————— Joseph Romano, RN

ALCOHOL FOUND AT BEDSIDE

Alcohol at a patient's bedside could pose a threat to the patient, other patients, visitors, or staff members. If you observe that your patient has alcohol in his possession, you must inform him that it can't be left at the bedside and can't be consumed without an order from his doctor. Further explain that the alcohol must be sent home or locked up and returned to the patient at discharge.

If the doctor writes an order for alcohol, it may be poured by the nurse and consumed by the patient at the times specified and in the amount prescribed. If you receive an order for alcohol, tell the patient you must start from an unopened bottle or can. Explain that you must dispose of already opened bottles. Have another nurse witness the disposal of the liquid contents. If your patient refuses to comply with facility regulations, notify the nursing supervisor, security, and the patient's doctor. Follow your facility's policy for dealing with a patient with alcohol in his possession.

ESSENTIAL DOCUMENTATION

If you discover alcohol in your patient's room or on his person, document the circumstances of the discovery. Describe the appearance of the container, the information on the label, and the smell and color of the liquid. Document that you told the patient about the facility's policy on alcohol, and record the patient's response (such as sending the alcohol home, pouring it out under your observation, or locking it up in a designated hospital storage area). If the alcohol is locked up, then record in the chart the:

- number of bottles
- description on the labels
- color of the liquid
- amount left
- names and departments of the people you notified, any instructions given, and your actions.

Fill out an incident report according to your facility's policy.

If the doctor writes an order for alcohol, document this in your nurse's note, and transcribe the order to the medication record. Record that you explained the alcohol order to the patient as well as when he can drink the alcohol and the amount prescribed. Document that you've started from an unopened bottle, and record the information from the bottle's label.

4/25/05	1000	While reaching into bedside table at 0930 to retrieve
		basin to assist with a.m. care, observed clear bottle filled
		with clear liquid with label saying "vodka." Bottle was
		unopened. When questioned, pt. stated, "That's vodka. I
		brought it to the hospital because I enjoy an occasional
		drink before bed." Explained that alcohol couldn't be kept
		at the bedside and that he would need to send it home
		or keep it locked up at the nurses' desk. In answer to
		pt.'s questions, explained that I would contact his doctor
		to obtain an order for a nightly drink. Dr. Smith called
		at 0940 and situation explained. T.O. given for 1 1/2 oz
		of vodka at bedtime, one drink each night, as requested
		by pt. Order transcribed on medication Kardex. Pharmacy
		and dietary notified. Vodka bottle locked in medication
		cart. Also alerted nursing supervisor, Tricia Hamilton,
		RN, who confirmed that this was within hospital policy.
		———————————— Kelly Norton, RN

ALLERGY TESTING

Allergy testing may be performed on an individual experiencing allergy-type symptoms related to an unidentified cause. Radioallergosorbent test, or RAST, is a blood test performed to identify immunoglobulin E reactions to a specific allergy causing rash, asthma, hay fever, drug reactions, and other atopic complaints. Skin testing is performed to determine specificity and degree of reactions to allergic agents. In this test, the patient is injected or scratched with various allergens. Identification of the allergic agent will help specify modality of treatment, such as medications or injections.

A consent form may be required before skin testing, delineating possible adverse effects and benefits. If required, check to see that it's signed before testing and that the patient understands the procedure.

ESSENTIAL DOCUMENTATION

Record the type of test given and the date, time, and route of testing. If required, document that the patient has signed a consent form. If venipuncture is performed, document the site and note whether a hematoma is present. Many facilities have a special form on which this information can be documented and diagrammed.

If skin testing is performed, document the following:

- type of allergen
- strength of solution
- location of injections
- size and type of skin reaction
- frequency and length of time monitored
- signs and symptoms of complications (such as tachycardia, wheezing, and difficulty breathing), treatments given, and response.

4/23/05	1200	Allergy testing performed for bee, wasp, and yellow
		jacket venom for previous allergic reaction to a
		"bee sting." Solutions of 1/10,000 dilution injected
		subcutaneously on Ⓡ lower forearm (bee), Ⓡ upper
		forearm (yellow jacket), and Ⓛ lower forearm (wasp).
		2-cm erythematous area noted on Ⓡ upper forearm
		15 sec. after injection. No reactions noted on Ⓡ lower
		forearm and Ⓛ lower forearm. Pt. denies difficulty
		breathing. P 72, BP 120/82, RR 16, oral T 97.6° F. No
		facial edema noted. Pt. c/o intense itching and burning
		of erythematous site on Ⓡ upper forearm. Dr. Brown
		notified of pt.'s reaction to injections. Hydrocortisone
		cream 1% ordered and applied to erythematous area.
		Will recheck pt. in 15 min. ———— Jane Gordon, RN

ANAPHYLAXIS

A severe reaction to an allergen after reexposure to the substance, anaphylaxis is a potentially fatal response requiring emergency intervention. Quickly assess the patient for airway, breathing, and circulation, and begin cardiopulmonary resuscitation as necessary. Remain with the patient, and monitor vital signs frequently, as indicated. If the cause is immediately evident (a blood transfusion, for example), stop the infusion and keep the I.V. line open with a normal saline solution infusion. Contact the doctor immediately and anticipate orders such as administering an epinephrine injection. When the patient is stable, perform a thorough assessment to identify the cause of the anaphylactic reaction.

ESSENTIAL DOCUMENTATION

Document the date and time that the anaphylactic reaction started. Record the events leading up to the anaphylactic response. Document the patient's signs and symptoms, such as anxiety, agitation, flushing, palpitations, itching, chest tightness, light-headedness, throat tightness or swelling, throbbing in the ears, or abdominal cramping. Also, document how soon after allergen exposure these findings started. Include your assessment findings, such as arrhythmias, rash, wheals or welts, wheezing, decreased level of consciousness, unresponsiveness, angioedema, decreased blood pressure, weak or rapid pulse, edema, and diaphoresis.

Note the name of the doctor notified, the time of notification, emergency treatments and supportive care given, and the patient's response. If the allergen is identified, note the allergen on the medical record, medication administration record, nursing care plan, patient identification bracelet, doctor's orders, and dietary and pharmacy profiles. Document that appropriate departments and individuals were notified, including pharmacy, dietary, risk management, and the nursing supervisor. In addition, you may need to fill out an incident report form.

9/1/05	1545	Pt. received Demerol 50 mg I.M. for abdominal incision
		pain. At 1520 pt. was SOB, diaphoretic, and c/o intense
		itching "everywhere." Injection site on Ⓛ buttock has 4-cm
		erythematous area. Skin is blotchy and upper anterior
		torso and face are covered with hives. BP 90/50, P 140
		and regular, RR 44 in semi-Fowler's position. I.V. of D₅
		½ NSS infusing at 125 ml/hr in Ⓛ hand. Exp. wheezes
		heard bilaterally. O₂ sat. 94% via pulse oximetry on room
		air. O₂ at 2 L/min via NC started with no change in O₂
		sat. Alert and oriented to time, place, and person. Pt.
		anxious and restless. Dr. Brown notified of pt.'s condition
		at 1525 and orders noted. Fluid challenge of 500 ml
		NSS over 60 min via Ⓛ antecubital began at 1535. O₂
		changed to 50% humidified face mask with O₂ sat.
		increasing to 99%. After 15 min of fluid challenge, BP
		110/70, P 104, RR 28. Benadryl 25 mg P.O. given for
		discomfort after fluid challenge absorbed. Allergy band
		placed on pt.'s Ⓛ hand for possible Demerol allergy.
		Chart, MAR, nursing care plan, and doctor's orders
		labeled with allergy information. Pharmacy, dietary, and
		nursing supervisor, Barbara Jones, RN, notified. Pt. told
		he had what appeared to be an allergic reaction to
		Demerol, that he shouldn't receive it in the future, and
		that he should notify all health care providers and
		pharmacies of this reaction. Recommended that pt. wear a
		medical ID bracelet noting his allergic reaction to
		Demerol. Medical ID bracelet order form given to pt.'s
		wife. ————————————————— Pat Sloan, RN

ARRHYTHMIAS

Arrhythmias occur when abnormal electrical conduction or automaticity changes heart rate or rhythm, or both. They vary in severity from mild, asymptomatic disturbances requiring no treatment to catastrophic ventricular fibrillation, which requires immediate resuscitation. Arrhythmias are classified according to their origin (ventricular or supraventricular). Their clinical significance depends on their effect on cardiac output and blood pressure. Your prompt detection and response to your patient's arrhythmia can mean the difference between life and death.

ESSENTIAL DOCUMENTATION

Record the date and time of the arrhythmia. Document events before and at the time of the arrhythmia. Record the patient's symptoms and the findings of your cardiovascular assessment, such as pallor, cold and clammy skin, shortness of breath, palpitations, weakness, chest pain, dizziness, syncope, and decreased urine output. Include the patient's vital signs and heart rhythm (if the patient is on a cardiac monitor, place a rhythm strip in the chart). Note the name of the doctor notified and time of notification. If ordered, obtain a 12-lead ECG and report the results. Document your interventions and the patient's response. Include any emotional support and education given.

5/24/05	1700	While assisting pt. with ambulation in the hallway at 1640,
		pt. c/o feeling weak and dizzy. Pt. said he was "feeling my
		heart hammering in my chest." Pt. stated he never felt
		like this before. Apical rate 170, BP 90/50, RR 24,
		peripheral pulses weak, skin cool, clammy, and diaphor-
		etic. Denies chest pain or SOB. Breath sounds clear
		bilaterally. Pt. placed in wheelchair and assisted back to
		bed without incident. O₂ via NC started at 2 L/min. Dr.
		Brown notified at 1645 and orders noted. Lab called to
		draw stat serum electrolyte and digoxin levels. Stat ECG
		revealed PSVT at a rate of 180. I.V. infusion of D₅W
		started in Ⓛ hand at 30 ml/hr with 18G cannula. Placed
		pt. on continuous cardiac monitoring with portable
		monitor from crash cart. At 1650 apical rate 180, BP
		92/52, and pulses weakened all 4 extremities, lungs
		clear, skin cool and clammy. Still c/o weakness and
		dizziness. Patient transferred to telemetry unit. Report
		given to Nancy Powell, RN. Nursing supervisor, Carol
		Jones, RN, notified. ———————————— Cathy Doll, RN

ARTERIAL BLOOD SAMPLING

An arterial blood sample must be collected when arterial blood gas (ABG) analysis is ordered. The sample may be obtained from the brachial, radial, or femoral arteries or withdrawn from an arterial line. Before attempting a radial puncture, Allen's test should be performed. Most ABG samples can be collected by a respiratory therapist or specially trained nurse. However, a doctor usually performs collection from the femoral artery.

ABG analysis evaluates lung ventilation by measuring arterial blood pH and the partial pressure of arterial oxygen and carbon dioxide. ABG samples can also be analyzed for oxygen content and saturation and for bicarbonate values.

ESSENTIAL DOCUMENTATION

Document what you teach the patient about the procedure and why it's being performed as well as his response to the teaching. Record the site of the arterial puncture. If the radial artery is used, record the results of Allen's test. Include the time that the procedure was performed; the patient's temperature, pulse, blood pressure, and respiratory rate; the amount of time pressure was applied to control bleeding; and the type and amount of oxygen therapy the patient was receiving. If the patient is receiving mechanical ventilation, indicate ventilator settings. Record any circulatory impairment, such as swelling, discoloration, pain, numbness, or tingling, in the affected limb and bleeding at the puncture site.

After obtaining an arterial blood sample, fill out a laboratory request for ABG analysis, including the patient's current temperature and respiratory rate, his most recent hemoglobin level, and the fraction of inspired oxygen and tidal volume if he's receiving mechanical ventilation. In most facilities, this is entered as a computerized order.

Document the results of the ABG analysis when they become available. Indicate that the doctor was notified and whether any change in therapy was required.

3/12/05	1010	Procedure and reasons for obtaining arterial blood
		sample for ABG analysis explained to pt. Pt. indicated
		that he has undergone this procedure before and had
		no questions. Blood drawn from ® radial artery after +
		Allen's test with capillary refill less than 3 sec. Pressure
		applied to site for 5 min and pressure dressing applied.
		No discoloration, bleeding, hematoma, or swelling noted.
		No c/o pain, numbness, or tingling by pt. ® hand pink,
		warm with 2-sec. capillary refill. Sample for ABGs sent
		to the lab. Patient on 4L O_2 by NC. T 99.2° F, P 82, BP
		122/74, RR 18, Hgb 10.2. ————————— Pat Toricelli, RN
3/12/05	1030	ABG results Pao_2 88 mm Hg, $Paco_2$ 40 mm Hg, pH 7.40,
		O_2 sat. 94%, HCO_3 24 mEq/L. Results reported to Dr.
		Smith. Oxygen therapy discontinued per dr.'s order. ——
		————————————————————— Pat Toricelli, RN

ARTERIAL LINE INSERTION

An arterial line permits continuous measurement of systolic, diastolic, and mean pressures as well as arterial blood sampling.

After obtaining informed consent, the doctor uses a preassembled preparation kit to prepare and anesthetize the insertion site. Under sterile technique, he then inserts the catheter into the artery and attaches the catheter to a fluid-filled pressure tubing.

Direct arterial monitoring is indicated when highly accurate or frequent blood pressure measurements are required.

ESSENTIAL DOCUMENTATION

When assisting with the insertion of an arterial line, record the doctor's name; time and date of insertion; insertion site; type, gauge, and length of the catheter; and whether the catheter is sutured in place. Document systolic, diastolic, and mean pressure readings upon insertion, and include a monitor strip of the waveform. Indicate the position of the patient each time a blood pressure reading is obtained. Record circulation in the extremity distal to the insertion site by assessing color, pulses, and sensation. Include the amount of flush solution infused every shift. Document emotional support and patient teaching.

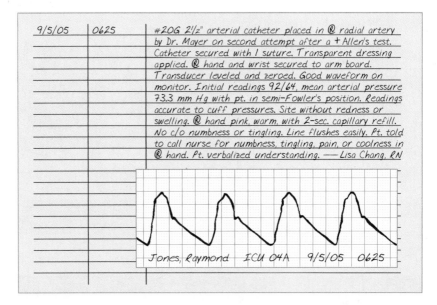

9/5/05	0625	#20G 2½" arterial catheter placed in Ⓡ radial artery
		by Dr. Mayer on second attempt after a + Allen's test.
		Catheter secured with 1 suture. Transparent dressing
		applied. Ⓡ hand and wrist secured to arm board.
		Transducer leveled and zeroed. Good waveform on
		monitor. Initial readings 92/64, mean arterial pressure
		73.3 mm Hg with pt. in semi-Fowler's position. Readings
		accurate to cuff pressures. Site without redness or
		swelling. Ⓡ hand pink, warm, with 2-sec. capillary refill.
		No c/o numbness or tingling. Line flushes easily. Pt. told
		to call nurse for numbness, tingling, pain, or coolness in
		Ⓡ hand. Pt. verbalized understanding. — Lisa Chang, RN

Jones, Raymond   ICU 04A   9/5/05   0625

ARTERIAL LINE REMOVAL

An arterial line is removed when it's no longer necessary or the insertion site needs to be changed. Consult your facility's policy and procedures to determine whether registered nurses with specialized training are permitted to perform this procedure. Explain the procedure to the patient, and assemble the necessary equipment. Observe standard precautions, and turn off the monitor alarms. Carefully remove the dressing and sutures. Withdraw the catheter using a gentle, steady motion. Apply pressure to the removal site for at least 10 minutes, and cover the site with an appropriate dressing.

ESSENTIAL DOCUMENTATION

When the arterial catheter is removed, record the time and date, name of the person removing the catheter, length of the catheter, condition of the insertion site, and the reason why the catheter is being removed. If any catheter specimens were obtained for culture, be sure to document that also. Record how long pressure was maintained to control bleeding. Include the type of dressing applied. Document circulation in the extremity distal to the insertion site, including color, pulses, and sensation, and compare findings to the opposite extremity. Continue to document circulation in the distal extremity every 15 minutes for the first 4 hours, every 30 minutes for the next 2 hours, and then hourly for the next 6 hours.

3/7/05	1200	Arterial catheter removed from ® radial site by the RN.
		Insertion site without bruising, swelling, or hematoma.
		No drainage noted on dressing. BP 102/74, P 84, RR 16,
		oral T 99.7° F. Catheter tip sent to laboratory for
		culture and sensitivity. Pressure applied for 10 min.
		Sterile gauze dressing with povidone-iodine ointment
		applied. ® and Ⓛ hands warm, pink. Radial pulse strong.
		No c/o numbness, tingling, or pain in ® or Ⓛ hand. Will
		continue to check circulation to ® hand according to
		orders. ———————————————— Lisa Chang, RN

ARTERIAL OCCLUSION, ACUTE

A potentially life-threatening condition that usually develops abruptly, acute arterial occlusion reduces blood flow and oxygen delivery, leading to ischemia and infarction in distal tissues and organs. The most common cause of acute arterial occlusion is obstruction of a major artery by a clot. The occlusive mechanism may be endogenous, resulting from emboli formation, thrombosis, or plaques, or may be exogenous, resulting from trauma or fracture.

After you recognize the manifestations of acute arterial occlusion, you'll need to act quickly to save the limb or life of your patient. Immediately notify the doctor, and place the patient on complete bed rest. Anticipate orders for heparin to inhibit thrombus growth and reduce the risk of embolization, thrombolytic drugs to dissolve a thrombus, or both. If indicated, prepare your patient for procedures, such as embolectomy or thrombectomy.

ESSENTIAL DOCUMENTATION

Document the patient's signs and symptoms of acute arterial occlusion. Record the presence of any complaints of pain; include location, intensity, quality, and duration. If the occlusion involves an extremity, document any limb pain, the absence or presence of pulses and their strength, paresthesia, skin color and temperature, capillary refill, and any motor deficits. Assess both limbs, and note any differences. Record whether pulses were present by palpation or Doppler ultrasound. If the occlusion involves a cerebral artery, record signs and symptoms of stroke. For a coronary artery occlusion, include manifestations of acute myocardial infarction. For renal involvement, document urine output.

Record the name of the doctor you notified, the time of notification, and note whether any orders were given. Include any treatments or interventions performed and the patient's response. If the patient requires surgery or other invasive procedures, document your patient teaching as well as the patient's response.

11/13/05	1250	At 1230 pt. c/o pain in Ⓛ leg, rated as 7 on scale of 0
		to 10, w/ 10 being the worst pain imaginable. Femoral
		artery insertion site from cardiac catheterization this
		morning without hematoma or bruising. Moderate swelling
		noted in Ⓛ foot and Ⓛ lower leg up to knee. Femoral,
		popliteal, dorsalis pedis, and posterior tibial pulses not
		palpable on Ⓛ leg. Strong pulses palpable on Ⓡ leg and
		foot. Faint pulses heard by Doppler on Ⓛ lower extremity.
		Pt. reports numbness in Ⓛ foot with decreased sensation
		to light touch. Normal sensation noted in Ⓡ leg and foot.
		Ⓛ leg and foot cool and pale, with sluggish capillary refill.
		Ⓡ leg and foot warm, pink, with capillary refill less than
		3 sec. Normal strength and ROM to Ⓡ leg, reduced
		strength and normal ROM to Ⓛ leg. Dr. Hampton notified
		of possible arterial occlusion at Ⓛ femoral cath site at
		1235 and came to assess pt. at 1240. Pt. to undergo
		embolectomy. Reviewed procedure with pt. and answered
		his questions. (See pt. education flow sheet for details.)
		Pt. states he's anxious but understands the need for the
		procedure. Procedure explained by surgeon, Dr. Thomas,
		including the risks, complications, and alternatives.
		Informed consent signed and in chart. Pt. left for
		procedure at 1250. ———————— Mary Donahue, RN

ARTERIAL PRESSURE MONITORING

Used for direct arterial pressure monitoring, an arterial line permits continuous measurement of systolic, diastolic, and mean pressures. It also permits arterial blood sampling.

Direct arterial monitoring is indicated when highly accurate or frequent blood pressure measurements are required, such as for patients with low cardiac output and high systemic vascular resistance or patients who receive titrated vasoactive drugs. Patients who need frequent blood sampling may also benefit from arterial line insertion.

ESSENTIAL DOCUMENTATION

Document systolic, diastolic, and mean arterial pressure readings as indicated for the patient's condition or per unit protocol. Some facilities may use a frequent vital signs assessment sheet for this purpose. Make sure the patient's position is documented when each blood pressure reading is obtained. Describe the appearance of the waveform, and include a monitor strip showing it. A comparison with an auscultated blood pressure should also be included.

Record circulation in the extremity distal to the site by assessing and noting color, warmth, capillary refill, pulses, pain, movement, and sensation. Describe the appearance of the insertion site, noting any evidence of infection or bleeding. If you change the tubing or flush solution, perform a dressing change and site care, or recalibrate the equipment, you'll also need to document these procedures. Include the amount of flush solution infused. Infused flush solution will also need to be recorded on the intake and output record. (See "Intake and output," page 230.)

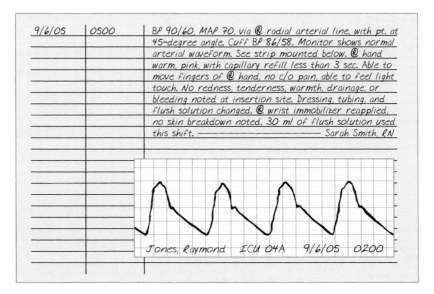

9/6/05	0500	BP 90/60, MAP 70, via ® radial arterial line, with pt. at
		45-degree angle. Cuff BP 86/58. Monitor shows normal
		arterial waveform. See strip mounted below. ® hand
		warm, pink, with capillary refill less than 3 sec. Able to
		move fingers of ® hand, no c/o pain, able to feel light
		touch. No redness, tenderness, warmth, drainage, or
		bleeding noted at insertion site. Dressing, tubing, and
		flush solution changed. ® wrist immobilizer reapplied,
		no skin breakdown noted. 30 ml of flush solution used
		this shift. ———————————————— Sarah Smith, RN

Jones, Raymond   ICU 04A   9/6/05   0200

ARTHROPLASTY CARE

Care of the patient after arthroplasty – the rebuilding of joints or the surgical replacement of all or part of a joint – helps restore mobility and normal use of the affected extremity and prevents complications, such as infection, phlebitis, and respiratory problems. Arthroplasty care includes maintaining alignment of the affected joint, assisting with exercises, and providing routine postoperative care. An equally important nursing responsibility is teaching home care and exercises that may continue for several years, depending on the type of arthroplasty performed and the patient's condition. The two most common arthroplastic procedures include knee and hip joint rebuilding or replacement. Other joints, such as the shoulders, elbows, and knuckles, may also be replaced.

ESSENTIAL DOCUMENTATION

Record the neurovascular status of the affected limb, maintenance of traction (for cup arthroplasty and hip replacement), or knee immobilization (for knee replacement). Describe the patient's position, especially the position of the affected leg; use of positioning devices such as an abducter pillow; skin care and condition; respiratory care and condition; and the use of elastic stockings. Document all exercises performed and their effect, and the use of continuous passive motion devices. Also, record ambulatory efforts, the type of support used, and the amount of traction weight.

Record vital signs and fluid intake and output on the appropriate flow sheets. (See "Vital signs, frequent," page 442, and "Intake and output," page 230.) Note turning and skin care schedules and the current exercise and ambulation program. Also, include the doctor's orders for the amount of traction and the degree of flexion permitted. Record discharge instructions and how well the patient understands them. Some facilities may use a flow chart to record this data.

11/12/05	1000	Dsg to Ⓛ hip dry and intact. Hemovac drained 30 ml of
		serosanguineous fluid over last 2 hr. See I/O flowsheet
		for shift totals. Ⓛ pedal pulses strong; foot warm, pink,
		capillary refill less than 3 sec. Able to move toes, ankle,
		and knee of Ⓛ leg and to feel light touch. P 84, BP 140/88,
		RR 118, oral T 99.4° F. Pt. reports tenderness at incision
		but no pain elsewhere on Ⓛ leg or foot. No evidence of
		warmth, swelling, tenderness, or Homans' sign in either leg.
		Abductor pillow in place, HOB at 45-degree angle. Pt. using
		trapeze to shift weight in bed q2hr. Back massage given
		and lotion applied to back and buttocks; no evidence of
		skin breakdown noted. Understands importance of not
		bending more than 90 degrees at the hip. Pt. encouraged
		to C&DB q1hr while awake. Assisted pt. with incentive
		spirometer. Able to exhale 850 ml. Lungs clear, cough
		nonproductive. Elastic hose on Ⓡ leg removed to wash and
		lubricate leg; skin intact. Elastic hose reapplied. Reinforced
		teaching of physical therapist to perform dorsiflexion,
		plantar flexion, and quadriceps setting exercises. Call bell
		within reach. Pt. ambulated 25 feet in room with walker
		and assist of nurse and physical therapist. Pt. showed
		proper use of walker. Needed reinforcement not to bend
		hip more than 90 degrees on transfers. ————————
		———————————— Thomas Bates, RN

ASPIRATION, FOREIGN BODY

Aspiration of a foreign body may cause sudden airway obstruction if the foreign body lodges in the throat or bronchus. An obstructed airway causes anoxia, which in turn leads to brain damage and death in 4 to 6 minutes. The Heimlich maneuver is used in conscious adults; if the patient is unconscious, use an abdominal thrust. However, the abdominal thrust is contraindicated in pregnant women, markedly obese patients, and patients who have recently undergone abdominal surgery. For such patients, use a chest thrust, which forces air out of the lungs to create an artificial cough. If you see an object in the mouth or throat, remove it using a finger sweep.

These maneuvers are contraindicated in a patient with incomplete or partial airway obstruction or when the patient can maintain adequate ventilation to dislodge the foreign body by effective coughing. However, the patient's inability to speak, cough, or breathe demands immediate action to dislodge the obstruction.

ESSENTIAL DOCUMENTATION

After the emergency has passed, record the date and time of the procedure, the patient's actions before aspirating the foreign body, signs and symptoms of airway compromise, the approximate length of time it took to clear the airway, and the type and size of the object removed. Also, note the patient's vital signs after the procedure, any complications that occurred and nursing actions taken, and his tolerance of the procedure. Include any emotional support and education provided after the event. Document the name of the doctor notified, the time of notification, and any orders given.

12/26/05	1410	After taking 2 acetaminophen tabs for headache at 1350,
		pt. started to choke but was able to speak and cough.
		Encouraged pt. to continue to cough forcefully. Pt. then
		became unable to speak or cough. Performed Heimlich
		maneuver X2 and pt. expelled both tablets intact. Pt.
		remained awake and alert. P 82, BP 138/84, RR 24, oral
		T 97.2° F. Total episode lasted approximately 90 sec. Pt.
		states "I've always had difficulty swallowing pills." Dr.
		Compton notified at 1400. Medications changed to liquid
		form, and pharmacy notified. Speech therapist to see pt.
		to evaluate swallowing. Pt. upset about incident, reassur-
		ances given. Pt. told to tell all health care providers that
		she has difficulty swallowing pills and to request an
		alternative form, if available. ———— Todd Smith, RN

ASPIRATION, TUBE FEEDING

Tube feedings involve the delivery of a liquid feeding formula directly into the stomach, duodenum, or jejunum. Tube feeding that has been accidentally aspirated into the lungs may result in respiratory compromise, such as pneumonia or acute respiratory distress syndrome. Causes of aspiration include incorrect tube placement, gastroesophageal reflux when the head of the bed isn't elevated, and vomiting caused by the patient's inability to absorb or digest the formula.

If you suspect tube-feeding aspiration, immediately stop the feeding. Then elevate the head of the bed, and perform tracheal suctioning. Notify the doctor, and anticipate orders for a chest X-ray and chest physiotherapy. If aspiration pneumonia is suspected, the doctor may order sputum cultures and antibiotics.

ESSENTIAL DOCUMENTATION

Record the date and time of the aspiration. Include evidence of aspiration, such as vomiting of tube-feeding formula or suctioning of tube feeding from the trachea. Describe the color, odor, and amount of suctioned secretions. Report your immediate actions, including stopping the feeding and performing tracheal suctioning, and the patient's response. Document your assessment of the patient's airway, breathing, circulation, and any other noted signs and symptoms. Check the position of the patient and the placement of the feeding tube, and record your findings. Note the time and name of the doctor you notified, and record new orders and actions, such as removing the feeding tube, obtaining a chest X-ray, administering oxygen, or starting antibiotics. Document emotional support and patient education.

1/2/06	1400	Called by pt. at 1340. Pt. reported she had just
		vomited. Found pt. sitting upright in bed with large
		amount of blue-colored vomitus on gown and noisy
		respirations. Immediately stopped tube feeding and
		suctioned small amount of thin, blue-tinged fluid from
		trachea. P 110, BP 98/64, RR 32, rectal T 102° F. Basilar
		crackles auscultated bilaterally. Skin diaphoretic and
		pink. O_2 sat. 89% by pulse oximetry on room air. Started
		O_2 at 4L by NC. Able to hear rush of air over stomach
		after injecting 5 ml of air through feeding tube but
		unable to aspirate any stomach contents. Dr. Hampton
		notified at 1350 and orders received. Tube feedings
		on hold. NG tube placed to low intermittent suction.
		I.V. infusion of D_5W ½ NSS with 20 mEq of KCL at
		125 ml/hr started in ℚ antecubital with 18G needle.
		Radiology called for stat portable CXR. Urine, blood, and
		sputum cultures obtained and sent to lab. Explained
		procedures to pt. and answered her questions. ———
		——————————————————— Joanne Wilder, RN

ASSESSMENT, INITIAL

Also known as a nursing database, the nursing admission assessment form contains your initial patient assessment data. Completing the form itself involves collecting information from various sources and analyzing it to assemble a complete picture of the patient. Information obtained can assist with forming nursing diagnoses and creating patient problem lists. The nursing admission form may be configured in a variety of ways, which may differ among facilities and even among departments in the facility.

ESSENTIAL DOCUMENTATION

On the nursing admission assessment form, record your nursing observations, the patient's perception of his health problems, the patient's health history, and your physical examination findings. Include data on the patient's current use of prescription and over-the-counter drugs; allergies to foods, drugs, and other substances; ability to perform activities of daily living; support systems; cultural and religious information; the patient's expectations of treatment; and documentation of the patient's advance directive, if he has one. Depending on the form, you may fill in blanks, check off boxes, or write narrative notes.

For an example of a completed initial assessment, see *Completing the nursing admission assessment*.

ASTHMA

Asthma is a chronic inflammatory airway disorder characterized by airflow obstruction and airway hyperresponsiveness to various stimuli. It's a type of chronic obstructive pulmonary disease marked by increased airflow resistance. The widespread but variable airflow obstruction seen in asthma is caused by bronchospasm, edema of the airway mucosa, and increased mucus production.

The best treatment for asthma is prevention by identifying and avoiding precipitating factors, such as environmental allergens or irritants, and taking drugs to block the acute obstructive effects of antigen exposure. Usually, such stimuli can't be removed entirely, so desensitization to specific antigens may be helpful, especially in children. If your patient is having an acute asthma attack, your prompt recognition of respiratory distress is essential to reversing the airway obstruction and possibly preventing death. Expect to administer low-flow humidified oxygen and drugs to decrease bronchoconstriction, reduce bronchial airway edema and inflammation, and increase pulmonary ventilation.

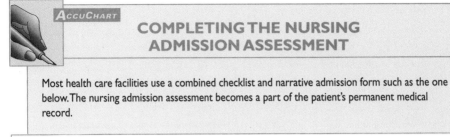

COMPLETING THE NURSING ADMISSION ASSESSMENT

Most health care facilities use a combined checklist and narrative admission form such as the one below. The nursing admission assessment becomes a part of the patient's permanent medical record.

ADMISSION DOCUMENT
(To be completed on or before admission by admitting RN)

Name: David Connors
Age: 74
Birth date: 4/15/31
Address: 3401 Elmhurst Ave.
Jenkintown, PA
Hospital I.D. No.: 4227
Insurer: Aetna
Policy No.: 605310P
Physician: Joseph Milstein
Admission date: 1/28/06

Preoperative teaching according to standard?
☑ Yes   ☐ No
Preoperative teaching completed on 1/28/06
If no, ☐ Surgery not planned
☐ Emergency surgery
Signature Kate McCauley, RN

T 101° F P 120 R 24
BP (Lying/sitting) Left: 124/66
Right: 120/68
Height 5'7"
Weight 160
Pulses:
L: P Radial P DP P PT
R: P Radial P DP P PT
Apical pulse 120
☑ Regular ☐ Irregular
P = Palpable   D = Doppler   O = Absent

Admitted from:
☐ Emergency department
☐ Home
☑ Doctor's office
☐ Transfer from_____

Mode:
☐ Ambulatory
☑ Wheelchair
☐ Stretcher
Accompanied by: wife

Signature Kate McCauley, RN

Medical and surgical history

Check (P) if patient or (R) if a blood relative has had any of the following. Check (H) if patient has ever been hospitalized. If it isn't appropriate to question patient because of age or sex, cross out option, for example, ~~infertility~~.

	(R) (P) (H) comments		(R) (P) (H) comments		(R) (P) (H) comments
Addictions (e.g.,alcohol, drugs)	☐☐☐	Fainting	☐☐☐	Myocardial infarction	☐☐☐
Angina	☐☐☐	Fractures	☐☐☐	Prostate problems	☐☐☐
Arthritis	☐☐☐	Genetic condition	☐☐☐	Rheumatic fever	☐☐☐
Asthma	☐☑☑ lungs clear	Glaucoma	☐☐☐	Sexually trans. disease	☐☐☐
Bleeding problems	☐☐☐	Gout	☐☐☐	Thyroid problems	☐☐☐
Blood clot	☐☐☐	Headaches	☐☐☐	TB or positive test	☐☐☐
Cancer	☐☐☐	Hepatitis	☐☐☐	Other	☐☐☐
Counseling	☐☐☐	High cholesterol	☐☑☐		
CVA	☐☐☐	Hypertension	☐☐☐	List any surgeries the patient has had:
Depression	☐☐☐	~~Infertility~~	☐☐☐	Date Type of surgery
Diabetes	☑☐☐	Kidney disease/ stones	☐☐☐	
Eating disorders	☐☐☐	Leukemia	☐☐☐	Has the patient ever had a blood
Epilepsy	☐☐☐	Memory loss	☐☐☐	transfusion: ☐ Y ☑ N
Eye problems (not glasses)	☐☐☐	Mood swings	☐☐☐	reaction: ☐ Y ☐ N

(continued)

COMPLETING THE NURSING
ADMISSION ASSESSMENT *(continued)*

UNIT INTRODUCTION

Patient rights given to patient:	☑ Y	☐ N	Patient valuables:	Patient meds:
Patient verbalizes understanding:	☑ Y	☐ N	☑ Sent home	☑ Sent home
☑ Patient ☑ Family oriented to:			☐ Placed in safe	☐ Placed in pharmacy
Nurse call system/unit policies:	☑ Y	☐ N	☐ None on admission	☐ None on admission
Smoking/visiting policy/intercom/				
siderails/TV channels:	☑ Y	☐ N		

Allergies or reactions

Medications/dyes	☑ Y	☐ N	*PCN*
Anesthesia drugs	☐ Y	☑ N	
Foods	☐ Y	☑ N	
Environmental (for example, tape, latex, bee stings, dust, pollen, animals, etc.)	☑ Y	☐ N	*dust, pollen, cats*

Advance directive information

1. Does patient have health care power of attorney? _____ ☐ Y ☑ N
   Name _____ Phone _____
   If yes, request copy from patient/family and place in chart. Date done:_____ Init. _____
2. Does patient have a living will? ☑ Y ☐ N
3. Educational booklet given to patient/family? ☑ Y ☐ N
4. Advise attending physician if there is a living will or power of attorney ☑ Y ☐ N

Organ and tissue donation

1. Has patient signed an organ and/or tissue donor card? ☑ Y ☐ N
   If yes, request information and place in chart. Date done: *1/28/06*
   If no, would patient like to know more about the subject of donation? ☐ Y ☐ N
2. Has patient discussed his wishes with family? ☑ Y ☐ N

Medications

Does patient use any over-the-counter medications?	Aspirin	☐ Y	☑ N
	Laxatives	☑ Y	☐ N
	Vitamins	☑ Y	☐ N
	Weight loss	☐ Y	☑ N

What does the patient usually take for minor pain relief? *Acetaminophen*

Prescribed medication (presently in use)	Reason	Dose	Last time taken
1. *Proventil*	*asthma*	*2 puffs q4hr*	*1/27/06*
2.			
3.			
4.			

Signature *Kate McCauley, RN*   Date *1/28/06*

ESSENTIAL DOCUMENTATION

Record the date and time of your entry. Include your assessment findings, such as wheezing, diminished breath sounds, prolonged expiration, coughing, dyspnea, use of accessory respiratory muscles, tachycardia, tachypnea, anxiety, apprehension, and cyanosis.

Document the name of the doctor you notified, the time of the notification, and the orders given, such as supplemental oxygen, bronchodilators, corticosteroids, pulmonary function tests, chest X-rays, serum theophylline levels, and ABG analysis.

Document your actions and your patient's response to these therapies. Use the appropriate flow sheets to record intake and output, vital signs, I.V. fluids given, positioning, drugs administered, pulse oximetry, and characteristics of cough and breath sounds. Record what you teach the patient, such as details about the disease process and preventing an acute attack, treatments, drugs, signs and symptoms to report, pursed-lip and diaphragmatic breathing, and use of respiratory equipment. Include emotional support given to the patient and family.

| 3/12/05 | 0840 | Pt. c/o difficulty breathing at 0825 while washing. Pt. sitting upright, using accessory muscles for breathing, nasal flaring and circumoral cyanosis noted. Pt. appeared restless and apprehensive and only able to speak 2 or 3 words at a time. P 124, BP 140/86, RR 36, ax temp 97.2° F, pulse ox. on room air 87%. Breath sounds diminished with expiratory wheezes auscultated bilaterally, expiration longer than inspiration. Dr. Cartwright notified of pt.'s respiratory distress and assessment findings at 0830 and came to see pt. and orders given. Humidified O_2 started at 2 L by NC. Albuterol 2.5 mg given via nebulizer. Encouraged slow deep breaths through pursed lips. Within 10 min, P 92, BP 128/84, RR 24, pulse ox. 96%, lungs clear to auscultation bilaterally. Pt. breathing easier without use of accessory muscles. Reinforced use of diaphragmatic and pursed-lip breathing and use of rescue inhaler for acute attacks. ——————— Pat Coleman, RN |

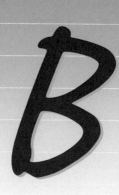

BAD NEWS BY TELEPHONE

It's usually best to relate bad news in person to a patient's family. In reality, however, this may not always be possible. Sometimes you may have the unpleasant task of telephoning a patient's family with news of a patient's deteriorating condition or death. Check the patient's chart for the designated contact person. Don't leave the bad news on the answering machine. Do leave your name and number so that the family member can reach you. Know whether your facility's policy specifies whether a nurse may relate bad news by telephone.

ESSENTIAL DOCUMENTATION

Be sure to chart the name of the family member notified and the date and time of notification. Include the information that was relayed and the family member's response. Include any support given.

4/15/05	0600	Pt. transferred to ICU on portable monitor with
		belongings. Mrs. Peterson, pt.'s wife, notified at 0545 of
		pt.'s irregular heartbeat (SVT) and the need for closer
		monitoring. Mrs. Peterson verbally consented to the
		transfer and stated she's on her way to the hospital to
		be with her husband. When questioned, she said she felt
		calm enough to drive herself to hospital. ————
		———————— Barbara Metcalf, RN

BLADDER IRRIGATION, CONTINUOUS

Continuous bladder irrigation can help prevent urinary tract obstruction by flushing out small blood clots that form after prostate or bladder surgery. It may also be used to treat an irritated, inflamed, or infected bladder lining.

This procedure requires placement of a triple-lumen catheter. One lumen controls balloon inflation, one allows irrigant inflow, and one allows irrigant outflow. The continuous flow of irrigating solution through the bladder also creates a mild tamponade that may help prevent venous hemorrhage. Although the patient typically receives the catheter while he's in the operating room after prostate or bladder surgery, if he isn't a surgical patient he may have it inserted at the bedside by the doctor.

ESSENTIAL DOCUMENTATION

Each time you finish a container of solution, record the date, time, and type and amount of fluid given on the intake and output record. Include any medications added to the solution. Also, record the time and amount of fluid each time you empty the drainage bag. Note the appearance of the drainage and any complaints by the patient. Document any changes in the patient's condition (such as a distended bladder, clots, or bright red outflow), the name of the doctor notified and time of notification, and actions taken. (See *Documenting bladder irrigation*, page 40.)

8/11/05	2300	2000 ml NSS irrigating solution hung at 2250, infusing through intake flow port at 100 gtts/min. Drainage bag emptied for 2500 ml of pink-tinged fluid with few small clots. No c/o discomfort. No bladder distention palpated. See I/O record for totals. — James Black, RN

DOCUMENTING BLADDER IRRIGATION

As this sample shows, you can monitor your patient's fluid balance by using an intake and output record.

Name: *Joseph Klein*

Identification #: *49731*

Admission date: *8/9/05*

INTAKE AND OUTPUT RECORD

	INTAKE						OUTPUT				
	Oral	Tube feeding	Instilled	I.V. and IVPB	TPN	Total	Urine	Emesis Tubes	NG	Other	Total
Date 8/11/05			*NSS Bladder irr.*								
0700–1500	250		800	1000		2050	2000				2000
1500–2300	200		800	1000		2000	2500				2500
2300–0700	100		800	1000		1900	1500				1500
24hr total	550		2400	3000		5950	6000				6000
Date											
24hr total											
Date											
24hr total											
Date											
24hr total											

Key: IVPB = I.V. piggyback   TPN = total parenteral nutrition   NG = nasogastric

Standard measures

Styrofoam cup	240 ml	Water (large)	600 ml	Milk (large)	600 ml	Ice cream,	120 ml
Juice	120 ml	Water pitcher	750 ml	Coffee	240 ml	sherbet, or gelatin	
Water (small)	120 ml	Milk (small)	120 ml	Soup	180 ml		

BLANK SPACES IN CHART OR FLOW SHEET

Blank spaces shouldn't be left in a patient's chart or flow sheet. Follow your facility's policy regarding blank spaces on forms. A blank space may imply that you failed to give complete care or assess the patient fully. Because flow sheets have increased in size, nurses may be required to fill in only those fields or prompts that apply to their patient. It's now common for health care facilities to have a written policy on how to complete such forms correctly. Leaving blank spaces in the nurse's note also allows others to add information to your note.

ESSENTIAL DOCUMENTATION

If information requested on a form doesn't apply to a particular patient, your facility's policy may require you to write "N/A" (not applicable) or draw a line through empty spaces.

When writing your nurse's notes, draw a line through any blank space after your entry, and sign your name on the far right side of the column. If you don't have enough room to sign your name after the last word in the entry, draw a line from the last word to the end of the line. Then drop down to the next line, draw a line from the left margin almost to the right margin, and sign your name on the far right side.

| 3/9/05 | 1500 | 20 yo. male admitted to room 418B by wheelchair. #20 angiocath inserted in ℚ antecubital vein with I.V. of 1000 ml D₅ ½ NSS infusing at 125 ml/hr. O₂ at 2 L/min via NC. Demerol 50 mg given I.M. for abdominal pain in ℚ ventogluteal site. Relief reported. ———————————————— David Dunn, RN |

BLOOD TRANSFUSION

A blood transfusion provides whole blood or a blood component, such as packed cells, plasma, platelets, or cryoprecipitates, to replace losses from surgery, trauma, or disease. No matter which blood product you administer, you must use proper identification and crossmatching procedures to ensure that the correct patient receives the correct blood product for transfusion.

ESSENTIAL DOCUMENTATION

Before administering the blood transfusion, clearly document that you matched the label on the blood bag to the:

- patient's name
- patient's identification number
- patient's blood group or type
- patient's and donor's Rh factor
- crossmatch data
- blood bank identification number
- expiration date of the product.

In addition, document that the blood or blood component and the patient were matched by two licensed health care professionals at the patient's bedside according to facility policy, that both of you signed the slip that comes with the blood, and that both of you verified the information is correct.

When you have determined that all the information is correct and matches, the consent form has been signed, and the patient's vital signs are within acceptable parameters per your facility's policy, you may administer the transfusion. On the transfusion record, document the:

- date and time that the transfusion was started and completed
- name and credentials of the health care professional who verified the information
- type and gauge of the catheter
- total amount of the transfusion
- patient's vital signs before, during, and after the transfusion, according to facility policy
- infusion device used (if any) and its flow rate
- blood-warming unit used (if any)
- amount of normal saline solution used (if any)
- patient's response to the transfusion.

If the patient receives his own blood, document the amount of autologous blood retrieved and reinfused in the intake and output records. Also, monitor and document laboratory data during and after the autotransfusion as well as the patient's pretransfusion and posttransfusion vital signs. Pay particular attention to the patient's coagulation profile, hematocrit, and hemoglobin, arterial blood gas, and calcium levels.

12/16/05	1015	Pt. to be transfused with 1 unit of PRBCs over 4 hr, according to written orders of Dr. Mays. Label on the blood bag checked by me and Nancy Gallager, RN, who verified the following information on the blood slip: 1 unit PRBCs for George Andrews, #123456, pt. and donor O+, Rh+ compatible crossmatch, blood bank #54321, expiration date 12/23/05. ———— Maryann Belinsky, RN
12/16/05	1030	Infusion of 1 unit of PRBCs started at 1025 through 18G catheter in ① forearm at 15 ml/hr using blood transfusion tubing. P 82, BP 132/84, RR 16, oral T 98.2° F. Remained with pt. for 1st 15 min. and increased rate to 60 ml/hr. ———— Maryann Belinsky, RN
12/16/05	1045	No c/o itching, chills, wheezing, or headache. No evidence of vomiting, swelling, laryngeal edema, or fever noted. PRBCs increased to 63 ml/hr. P 84, BP 128/82, RR 17, oral T 97.9° F. ———— Maryann Belinsky, RN
12/16/05	1430	Transfusion of 1 unit PRBCs complete. P 78, BP 130/78, RR 16, oral T 98.0° F. No c/o itching, chills, wheezing, or headache. No evidence of vomiting, swelling, laryngeal edema, or fever noted. ———— Maryann Belinsky, RN

BLOOD TRANSFUSION REACTION

During a blood transfusion, the patient is at risk for developing a transfusion reaction. If he develops a reaction, immediately take the following steps:

- Stop the transfusion.
- Take down the blood tubing.
- Hang new tubing with normal saline solution running to maintain vein patency.
- Notify the doctor and follow facility policy for a blood transfusion reaction.
- Notify the blood bank and laboratory.

ESSENTIAL DOCUMENTATION

Be sure to document the time and date of the reaction, type and amount of infused blood or blood products, time you started the transfusion, and time you stopped it. Also, record clinical signs of the reaction in order of occurrence, the patient's vital signs, urine specimen or blood samples sent to the laboratory for analysis, treatment given, and the patient's response to treatment. Indicate that you sent the blood transfusion equipment (discontinued bag of blood, administration set, attached I.V. solutions, and all related forms and labels) to the blood bank. Some health care facilities require the completion of a transfusion reaction report that must be sent to the blood bank. (See *Transfusion reaction report,* pages 44 and 45.) Docu-
(Text continues on page 46.)

AccuChart

TRANSFUSION REACTION REPORT

If your facility requires a transfusion reaction report, you'll include the following types of information.

TRANSFUSION REACTION REPORT

Nursing report

1. Stop transfusion immediately. Keep I.V. line open with saline infusion.
2. Notify responsible physician.
3. Check all identifying names and numbers on the patient's wristband, unit, and paperwork for discrepancies.
4. Record patient's posttransfusion vital signs.
5. Draw posttransfusion blood samples (clotted and anticoagulated) avoiding mechanical hemolysis.
6. Collect posttransfusion urine specimen from patient.
7. Record information as indicated below.
8. Send discontinued bag of blood, administration set, attached I.V. solutions, and all related forms and labels to the blood bank with this form completed.

Clerical errors
- ☑ None detected
- ☐ Detected

Vital signs

	Pre-TXN	Post-TXN
Temp.	98.4°	97.6°F
B.P.	120/60	160/88
Pulse	88	104

- ☐ Urticaria
- ☐ Fever
- ☑ Chills
- ☐ Chest pain
- ☐ Hypotension
- ☐ Nausea
- ☐ Flushing
- ☐ Dyspnea
- ☐ Headache
- ☐ Perspiration
- ☐ Shock
- ☐ Oozing
- ☐ Back pain
- ☐ Infusion site pain
- ☐ Hemoglobin-uria
- ☐ Oliguria or anuria
- ☐ Cyanosis of lips noted

Reaction occurred

During administration? _Yes_
After administration? _____
How long? _____
Medications added? _No_
Previous I.V. fluids? _NSS at 30 ml/hr_
Blood warmed? _No_

Specimen collection

Blood: Difficulty collecting? _No_
Urine: Voided _Yes — sent to lab_   Catheterized _____

Comments:
Given diphenhydramine 50 mg IM

Signature _Maryann Belinsky, RN_   Date _2/13/05_

BLOOD BANK REPORT

Unit #
_22FM80507_
Component Returned
Yes
Volume Returned
_185 ml_

1. Clerical errors
- ☑ None detected
- ☐ Detected

Comments:

2. Hemolysis

Note: If hemolysis is present in the posttransfusion sample, a posttransfusion urine sample must be tested for free hemoglobin immediately.

	None	Slight	Moderate	Marked
Patient pre-TXN sample	☑	☐	☐	☐
Patient post-TXN sample	☑	☐	☐	☐
Blood Bag	☑	☐	☐	☐
Urine HGB (centrifuged)	☐	☐	☑	☐

TRANSFUSION REACTION REPORT *(continued)*

BLOOD BANK REPORT *(continued)*

3. Direct antiglobulin test

Pretransfusion _____ Posttransfusion _____

If No. 2 and No. 3 are negative, steps 4 through 6 aren't required. Report results to the blood bank physician. Steps 7 and 8 or further testing will be done as ordered by blood bank physician.

4. ABO and Rh Groups

Repeat testing	Cell reaction with							Serum reaction with		ABO/Rh
	Anti-A	Anti-B	Anti-A,B	Anti-D	Cont.	Du	Cont.	CCC	A1 cells	B cells
Pretransfusion										
Posttransfusion										
Unit #										
Unit #										

5. Red cell antibody screen

		Saline/AB				INT
Pretransfusion	Cell	RT	37° C	AHG	CCC	
Date of sample	I					
	II					
By:	Auto					

		Saline/AB				INT
Posttransfusion	Cell	RT	37° C	AHG	CCC	
Date of sample	I					
	II					
By:	Auto					

Specificity of antibody detected:

6. Crossmatch compatibility testing

Use patient pre-TXN and post-TXN serum and the suspected unit red cells obtained from inside the container or from a segment still attached to bag. Observe appearance of blood in bag and administration tubing.

		Albumin			INT
Pretransfusion	RT	37° C	AHG	CCC	
Unit #					
Unit #					

		Albumin			INT
Posttransfusion	RT	37° C	AHG	CCC	
Unit #					
Unit #					

All units on hold for future transfusion must be recrossmatched with the posttransfusion sample.

7. Bacteriologic testing

Pretransfusion _____ Posttransfusion _____

8. Other testing results

Total bilirubin   **Coagulation studies**   **Urine output studies**

Patient pre-TXN _____ mg/dl

Patient 6 hrs. post-TXN _____ mg/dl

Pathologist's conclusions:

Signature _____ Date _____

AVOID BLOCK CHARTING

Be specific about times in your charting, especially the exact time of sudden changes in the patient's condition, significant events, doctor notification, and nursing actions. Don't chart in blocks of time such as 0700 to 1500. This looks vague, implies inattention to the patient, and makes it hard to determine when specific events occurred. If your patient's chart is used as evidence in a lawsuit, the patient's lawyer may use your block charting to show that you didn't provide timely nursing care or that you didn't act fast enough when your patient developed a problem.

These examples show the correct and incorrect ways to chart times.

Correct:

11/2/05	0600	Pt. complained of nausea, then vomited 300 ml light brown emesis around NG tube. NG tube irrigated with 100 ml NSS 80 ml clear fluid return. — Ann Cook, RN
11/2/05	0700	NG tube drained 140 ml light brown fluid over past hr ————————————————— Ann Cook, RN

Incorrect:

11/2/05	1500–2300	Pt. has NG tube in — vomited once — irrigated with NSS 100 ml. No vomiting remainder of shift. ——— ————————————————— Amy Mars, RN

ment your follow-up care. Be sure to time each note and avoid block charting. (See *Avoid block charting.*)

2/13/05	1400	Pt. reports chills. Cyanosis of lips noted at 1350. Transfusion of packed RBCs stopped. Approximately 100 ml of blood infused. Transfusion started 1215, stopped at 1350. Tubing changed. I.V. of 1000 ml NSS infusing at 30 ml/hr rate in ® forearm. Notified Dr. Cahill and blood bank. BP 168/88, P 104, RR 25, rectal T 97.6° F. Blood sample taken from PRBCs. Two red-top tubes of blood drawn from pt. sent to lab. Urine specimen obtained from catheter. Urine specimen sent to lab for U/A. Administered diphenhydramine 50 mg I.M. per order of Dr. Cahill. Two blankets placed on pt. Blood transfusion equipment sent to blood bank. Transfusion reaction report filed. ————— Maryann Belinsky, RN
	1415	Pt. reports he's getting warmer. BP 148/80, P 96, RR 20, T 97.6° F. ———————— Maryann Belinsky, RN
	1430	Pt. no longer complaining of chills. I.V. of 1000 ml NS infusing at 125 ml/hr in ® arm. BP 138/76, P 80, RR 18, T 98.4° F. ————————— Maryann Belinsky, RN

BONE MARROW ASPIRATION AND BIOPSY

A specimen of bone marrow – the major site of blood cell formation – may be obtained by aspiration or needle biopsy. The procedure allows evaluation of overall blood composition by studying blood elements and precursor cells as well as abnormal or malignant cells. Aspiration removes cells through a needle inserted into the marrow cavity of the bone; a biopsy removes a small, solid core of marrow tissue through the needle.

Aspirates aid in diagnosing various disorders and cancers, such as oat cell carcinoma, leukemia, and such lymphomas as Hodgkin's disease. Biopsies are commonly performed simultaneously to stage the disease and monitor response to treatment.

ESSENTIAL DOCUMENTATION

Document patient education regarding what to expect before and after the procedure and that informed consent has been obtained, if necessary. Many facilities have a separate patient education form for documenting what you teach and how the patient responds to the teaching. When assisting the doctor with a bone marrow aspiration or biopsy, document the name of the doctor performing the procedure and the date and time of the procedure. Also, describe the patient's response to the procedure and the location and condition of the aspiration or biopsy site, including bleeding and drainage. Record the patient's vital signs before and after the procedure, and observe the site for bleeding and drainage. Document any pertinent information about the specimen sent to the laboratory.

1/30/06	1000	Explained what to expect before, during, and after bone
		marrow aspiration and answered pt.'s questions. Refer
		to pt. education sheet for specific instructions and pt.
		responses. Informed consent form signed by pt.
		Preprocedure BP 148/86, P 92, RR 24, oral T 98.6° F.
		Assisted Dr. Shelbourne with bone marrow aspiration of
		℞ iliac crest at 0915. No bleeding or drainage at site.
		Pt. denies any discomfort and is resting comfortably in
		bed talking with wife and daughter. Specimen sent to
		lab, as ordered. BP 142/82, P 88, RR 22, oral T 98.8° F.
		Maintaining bed rest. No bruising or bleeding noted at
		site. ———————————— Margaret Little, RN

BRAIN DEATH

Brain death is commonly defined as the irreversible cessation of all brain function, including the brain stem. The Uniform Determination of Death Act (1980) established the standards for diagnosing brain death. The American Academy of Neurology (AAN) used these standards to develop practice guidelines in 1995. Other organizations have also published guidelines for diagnosing brain death. That's why it's important to know your state's laws regarding the definition of brain death as well as your facility's policy. (See *Know your state's laws concerning brain death*.)

The current AAN guidelines recommend that a doctor examine the patient to confirm the presence of the three cardinal signs of brain death:
- coma or unresponsiveness
- absence of brain stem function
- apnea.

To make this determination, the doctor should test the patient for responsiveness or movement, brain stem reflexes (pupillary, corneal, gag/cough, oculocephalic, and oculovestibular), and apnea. He should aslo evaluate laboratory and diagnostic test results to eliminate other causes of coma. Although standards may vary by state or facility, the AAN recommends that the doctor perform the examination twice, at least 6 hours apart.

ESSENTIAL DOCUMENTATION

Your nurse's note for a patient undergoing testing for brain death should include:
- family teaching and emotional support given
- date and time of the examination
- the name of the person performing the test
- the patient's response and any action taken (If you notified anyone about the test and results, include the date and time of notification, the name of the person notified, the person's response, and any action taken.)

KNOW YOUR STATE'S LAWS CONCERNING BRAIN DEATH

In states without laws defining death or without judicial precedents, the common law definition of death (cessation of circulation and respiration) is still used. In these states, doctors are understandably reluctant to discontinue artificial life support for brain-dead patients. If you're likely to be involved with patients on life-support equipment, protect yourself by finding out how your state defines death.

- time of brain and cardiopulmonary death (Include any evidence such as ECG strips.)

In addition, individuals performing the tests, such as a respiratory therapist, will need to complete their documentation in appropriate sections of the chart.

6/1/05	0800	Dr. Malone in to speak with pt.'s son, Mark Newton, who has health care POA, about pt.'s condition. Pt verbalized understanding about probable brain death due to subarachnoid hemorrhage. Son agreed to tests to determine brain death. Son was teary and spent a few minutes verbalizing about his father's good qualities. When offered, stated he didn't want a visit by clergy or social worker. —————————————— Dawn Silfies, RN
	0815	Dr. Malone performed clinical exam. See Physical Progress Notes for full report. Son present for exam. Dr. Malone explained to son pt.'s lack of response and absence of reflexes. Son understands that another dr. not involved with his father's care will repeat the exam in 6 hours. ————————————— Dawn Silfies, RN
	0830	ABG results obtained by Michael Burke, RPT, with pt. on ventilator. Results pH 7.40, PO₂ 100, Pco₂ 40. Pt. taken off ventilator by respiratory therapist and placed on 100% O₂ via T-piece. Dr. Malone in attendance. Cardiac monitor showing NSR at a rate of 70, O₂ sat. via continuous pulse oximetry 99%. Within 1 minute of testing, heart rate 150 with PVCs, and O₂ sat. dropped to 91%. Pt. without spontaneous respirations. ABGs drawn by respiratory therapist showed pH 7.32, PO₂ 60, Pco₂ 65. Pt. placed back on ventilator. Son verbalized understanding of the results showing apnea. Son states he will stay with his dad until exam at 1430 with Dr. Porter. Dr. Malone will meet with son at 1500 to discuss results and plan. ————————— Dawn Silfies, RN

BURNS, ASSESSING RISK FOR

Burns are a common cause of injury to patients. Patients are burned by spilled hot food or liquids, hot baths, and electrical equipment. Always assess the risk of burns, and take appropriate precautions. For example, caution patients with hand tremors not to handle hot foods or liquids by themselves, or instruct them to wait for the food or liquid to cool. Teach patients with decreased sensation in their feet or hands to test bath water with an unaffected extremity or to use a bath thermometer. Explain to patients taking medication causing drowsiness that they may be more prone to burns and need to be cautious.

ESSENTIAL DOCUMENTATION

Document your patient teaching regarding burn prevention and nursing measures taken to prevent burns. If a patient does burn himself, document the date and time of the burn, how the burn occurred, your assessment findings, the name of the doctor notified and the time of notification, treatments given, and patient response. You'll also need to file an incident report.

9/8/05	1100	Pt. dropped hot cup of tea on ® thigh. 4 cm X 3 cm
		area on inner ® thigh slightly pink, sensitive to touch, no
		edema or blisters. Dr. Adler notified. Cold compresses
		ordered and applied. Pt. tolerated cold compress well.
		Tylenol Extra-Strength 500 mg X 1 given with relief. Pt.
		instructed to test temp. of hot beverages by sampling
		them using spoon. Once beverage is no longer hot, pt.
		may pick up cup. Also instructed to call for assistance if
		he's unsure of temp. of beverage or feels unable to hold
		cup. ———————————— Colleen Cameron, RN

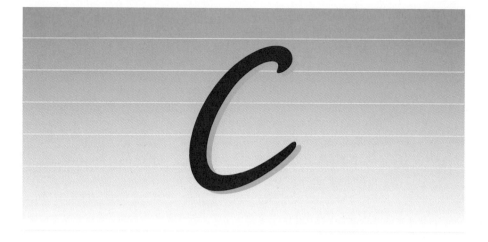

CARDIAC MONITORING

Because it allows continuous observation of the heart's electrical activity, cardiac monitoring is useful not only for assessing cardiac rhythm, but also for gauging a patient's response to drug therapy and for preventing complications associated with diagnostic and therapeutic procedures. Like other forms of electrocardiography, cardiac monitoring uses electrodes placed on the patient's chest to transmit electrical signals that are converted into a tracing of cardiac rhythm on an oscilloscope. Cardiac monitoring may be hardwire monitoring, in which the patient is connected to a monitor at bedside, or telemetry, in which a small transmitter connected to the patient sends an electrical signal to a monitor screen for display.

ESSENTIAL DOCUMENTATION

In your note, document the date and time that monitoring began and the monitoring leads used. Attach all rhythm strip readings to the record. Be sure to label the rhythm strip with the patient's name, his room number, and the date and time. Measure and document the PR interval, QRS duration, and QT interval along with an interpretation of the rhythm. Also, document any changes in the patient's condition, and place a rhythm strip in the chart.

If cardiac monitoring will continue after the patient's discharge, document which caregivers can interpret dangerous rhythms and can perform cardiopulmonary resuscitation. Also, teach troubleshooting techniques to use if the monitor malfunctions, and document your teaching efforts or referrals (for example, to equipment suppliers).

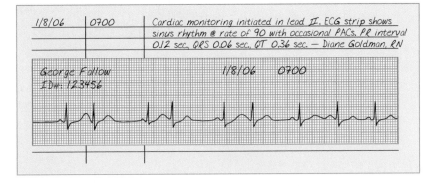

1/8/06	0700	Cardiac monitoring initiated in lead II. ECG strip shows
		sinus rhythm @ rate of 90 with occasional PACs. PR interval
		0.12 sec., QRS 0.06 sec., QT 0.36 sec. — Diane Goldman, RN

George Fallow
ID# 123456   1/8/06   0700

CARDIAC TAMPONADE

In cardiac tamponade, a rapid, unchecked rise in intrapericardial pressure impairs diastolic filling of the heart. The rise in pressure usually results from blood or fluid accumulation in the pericardial sac. If fluid accumulates rapidly, the patient requires emergency lifesaving measures.

Cardiac tamponade may be idiopathic (Dressler's syndrome) or may result from effusion, hemorrhage from trauma or nontraumatic causes, pericarditis, acute myocardial infarction, chronic renal failure during dialysis, drug reaction, or connective tissue disorders.

If you suspect cardiac tamponade in your patient, notify the doctor immediately and prepare for pericardiocentesis (needle aspiration of the pericardial cavity), emergency surgery (usually a pericardial window), or both. Anticipate I.V. fluids, inotropic drugs, and blood products to maintain blood pressure until treatment is performed.

ESSENTIAL DOCUMENTATION

Note the date and time that you detect signs of tamponade. Include your assessment findings, such as neck vein distention, decreased arterial blood pressure, pulsus paradoxus, narrow pulse pressure, muffled heart sounds, acute pain, dyspnea, diaphoresis, anxiety, restlessness, pallor or cyanosis, rapid and weak pulses, and hepatomegaly. Record the name of the doctor notified and the time of notification. Make a note of diagnostic tests ordered by the doctor, such as an ECG or chest X-ray, and the findings. Document treatments and procedures and the patient's response. Note any patient teaching provided. Frequency of vital signs and titration of drugs and patient responses may be documented on the appropriate flow sheets.

6/5/05	1320	BP at 1300 90/40 via cuff on ® arm. Last BP at 1245 was
		120/60. Drop of 17 mm Hg in systolic BP noted during
		inspiration. P 132 and regular, RR 34, oral T 97.2° F. See
		frequent vital sign sheet for q15min VS. Neck veins
		distended with pt. in semi-Fowler's at 45-degrees, heart
		sounds muffled, peripheral pulses weak. Pt. anxious and
		dyspneic, skin pale and diaphoretic. Pt. c/o chest soreness
		from MVA and hitting steering wheel. Slight ecchymosis
		visible across chest. Pt. awake, alert, and oriented to time,
		place, and person. Dr. Hoffmann notified at 1305. Stat
		portable CXR shows slightly widened mediastinum and
		enlargement of the cardiac silhouette. ECG shows sinus
		tachycardia with rate of 130. 200-ml bolus of NSS given.
		Dopamine 400 mg in 250 D₅W started via distal port of ®
		subclavian TLC at 4 mcg/kg. Urine output is 25 ml for last
		hr. Awaiting Dr. Brown's arrival for pericardiocentesis.
		Explained the procedure to pt. and wife and answered
		their questions. ———————————— Cindy Rogers, RN

CARDIOPULMONARY ARREST AND RESUSCITATION

Guidelines established by the American Heart Association direct you to keep a written, chronological account of a patient's condition throughout cardiopulmonary resuscitation (CPR). If you're the designated recorder, document therapeutic interventions and the patient's responses as they occur. Don't rely on your memory later. Writing "recorder" after your name indicates that you documented the event but didn't participate in the code.

The form used to chart a code is the code record. It incorporates detailed information about your observations and interventions as well as drugs given to the patient. Remember, the code response should follow Advanced Cardiac Life Support guidelines.

Some facilities use a resuscitation critique form to identify actual or potential problems with the resuscitation process. This form tracks personnel responses and response times as well as the availability of appropriate drugs and functioning equipment.

ESSENTIAL DOCUMENTATION

The code record is a precise, quick, and chronological recording of the events of the code. (See *The code record,* page 54.) Document the date and time the code was called. You'll also need to record the patient's name, location of the code, person who discovered the patient, the patient's condi-

ACCUCHART

THE CODE RECORD

Here's an example of the completed resuscitation record for inclusion in your patient's chart.

CODE RECORD

Pg. *1* of *1*

Arrest Date: *11/9/05*
Arrest Time: *0631*
Rm/Location: *431–2*
Discovered by:
C. Brown
☑ RN ☐ MD
☐ Other

Methods of alert:
☐ Witnessed, monitored: rhythm

☐ Witnessed, unmonitored
☑ Unwitnessed, unmonitored
☐ Unwitnessed, monitored; rhythm

Diagnosis: *Post anterior wall MI*

Condition when needed:
☑ Unresponsive
☐ Apneic
☐ Pulseless
☐ Hemorrhage
☐ Seizure

Ventilation management:
Time: *0635*
Method:
oral ET tube
Precordial thump:

CPR initiated at:
0631

Previous airway:
☐ ET tube
☐ Trach
☑ Natural

Addressograph

CPR PROGRESS NOTES

	VITAL SIGNS						I.V. PUSH					INFUSIONS				ACTIONS/PATIENT RESPONSE
Time	Pulse CPR	Resp. rate Spont; bag	Blood pressure	Rhythm	Defib (Joules)	Atropine	Epinephrine	Lidocaine	NA bicarb	Other	Lidocaine	Procaine	Isuprel	Dopamine		Responses to therapy, procedures, labs drawn/results
0631	CPR	Bag	0	V fib	200											No change.
0632		Bag	0	V fib	300											ABGs drawn. Ⓡ fem pressure applied.
0633	CPR	Bag	0	Asystole	360		1 mg									No change
0635	40	Bag	60 palp	SB PVCs				75			✓					Oral intubation by Dr. Hart
0645	60	Bag	80/40	SB PVCs							✓					CCU ready for patient

ABGs & Lab Data

Time Spec Sent	pH	PCO	Po₂	HCO₃⁻	Sat%	Fio₂	Other
0633	7.1	76	43	14	80%		

Resuscitation outcome
☑ Successful ☑ Transferred to *CCU* at *0648*
☐ Unsuccessful — Expired at _____
Pronounced by: _____ MD
Family notified by: *S. Quinn, RN*
Time: *0645*
Attending notified by: *S. Quinn, RN* Time *0645*
Code Recorder *S. Quinn, RN*
Code Team Nurse *B. Mullen, RN*
Anesthesia Rep. *J. Hanna, RN*
Other Personnel *Dr. Hart*
B. Russo, RT

tion, and whether the arrest was witnessed or unwitnessed. Record the name of the doctor notified, the time of notification, and list other members who participated in the code. Record the exact time for each code intervention, and include vital signs, heart rhythm, laboratory results (such as arterial blood gas or electrolyte levels), type of treatment (such as CPR, defibrillation, or cardioversion), drugs (name, dosage, and route), procedures (such as intubation, temporary or transvenous pacemaker, and central line insertion), and patient response. Record the time that the family was notified. At the end of the code, indicate the patient's status and the time that the code ended. Some facilities require that the doctor leading the code and the nurse recording the code review the code sheet and sign it.

In your nurse's note, record the events leading up to the code, your assessment findings prompting you to call a code, who initiated CPR, and other interventions performed before the code team arrived. Include the patient's response to interventions. Indicate in your note that a code sheet was used to document the events of the code.

11/9/05	0650	Summoned to pt.'s room at 0630 by a shout from roommate. Found pt. unresponsive in bed without respirations or pulse. Roommate stated, "He was talking to me, then all of a sudden he started gasping and holding his chest." Code called at 0630. Initiated CPR with Ann Barrow, RN. Code team arrived at 0632 and continued resuscitative efforts. (See code record.) ———————————————— Connie Brown, RN

CARDIOVERSION, SYNCHRONIZED

Used to treat tachyarrhythmias, cardioversion delivers an electric charge to the myocardium at the peak of the R wave. This causes immediate depolarization, interrupting reentry circuits and allowing the sinoatrial node to resume control. Synchronizing the electric charge with the R wave ensures that the current won't be delivered on the vulnerable T wave and thus disrupt repolarization.

Indications for cardioversion include stable paroxysmal atrial tachycardia, unstable paroxysmal supraventricular tachycardia, atrial fibrillation, atrial flutter, and ventricular tachycardia. Cardioversion may be an elective or urgent procedure, depending on how well the patient tolerates the arrhythmia.

ESSENTIAL DOCUMENTATION

Document the date and time of the cardioversion. Record the signing of a consent form and any patient teaching. Include any preprocedure activities, such as withholding food and fluids, withholding drugs, removing dentures, administering a sedative, and obtaining a 12-lead ECG. Document vital signs, and obtain a rhythm strip before starting. Note that the cardioverter was on the synchronized setting, how many times the patient was cardioverted, and the voltage used each time. After the procedure, obtain vital signs, place a rhythm strip in the chart, and record that a 12-lead ECG was obtained. Assess and document the patient's level of consciousness, airway patency, respiratory rate and depth, and use of supplemental oxygen until he's awake. Indicate the specific time of each assessment and avoid block charting.

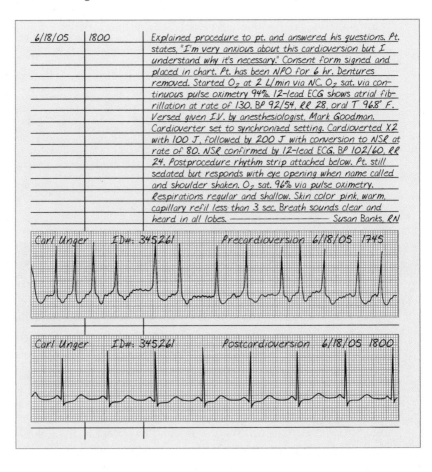

6/18/05	1800	Explained procedure to pt. and answered his questions. Pt.
		states, "I'm very anxious about this cardioversion but I
		understand why it's necessary." Consent form signed and
		placed in chart. Pt. has been NPO for 6 hr. Dentures
		removed. Started O₂ at 2 L/min via NC. O₂ sat. via con-
		tinuous pulse oximetry 94%. 12-lead ECG shows atrial fib-
		rillation at rate of 130. BP 92/54, RR 28, oral T 96.8° F.
		Versed given I.V. by anesthesiologist, Mark Goodman.
		Cardioverter set to synchronized setting. Cardioverted X2
		with 100 J, followed by 200 J with conversion to NSR at
		rate of 80. NSR confirmed by 12-lead ECG. BP 102/60, RR
		24. Postprocedure rhythm strip attached below. Pt. still
		sedated but responds with eye opening when name called
		and shoulder shaken. O₂ sat. 96% via pulse oximetry.
		Respirations regular and shallow. Skin color pink, warm,
		capillary refill less than 3 sec. Breath sounds clear and
		heard in all lobes. ———————— Susan Banks, RN

Carl Unger   ID#: 345261   Precardioversion 6/18/05 1745

Carl Unger   ID#: 345261   Postcardioversion 6/18/05 1800

CARE GIVEN BY SOMEONE ELSE

Unless you document otherwise, anyone reading your notes assumes that they're a firsthand account of care provided. In some settings, nursing assistants and technicians aren't allowed to make formal charting entries. If this is the case in your facility, determine what care was provided, assess the patient and the task performed (for example, a dressing change), and document your findings.

If your facility allows unlicensed personnel to chart, you may have to countersign their notes. If your facility's policy states that the unlicensed person must provide care in your presence, don't countersign unless you actually witness her actions. If the policy says you don't have to be there, your countersignature indicates the note describes care that the other person had the authority and competence to perform and that you verified the procedure was performed. Unless your facility authorizes or requires you to witness someone else's notes, your signature will make you responsible for anything put in the notes above it. So if another nurse asks you to document her care or sign her notes, tell her you refuse.

ESSENTIAL DOCUMENTATION

If nursing assistants and technicians aren't allowed to chart, be sure to record the full names – not just initials – and titles of unlicensed personnel who provided care, and describe the care performed and your assessment of the patient.

| 10/23/05 | 0600 | Morning care provided by Kevin Lawson, NA, who stated that pt. moaned when being turned. When I questioned pt., she stated that her abdominal incision hurt. Rated pain as 6 on a scale of 0 to 10, w/10 being the worst pain imaginable. Incision dry and intact. No redness or drainage noted. P 92, BP 150/88, RR 18, oral T 98.7° F. Medicated with Tylenol 650 mg P.O. at 0550. ——— Camille Dunn, RN |

CAREGIVER STRAIN

Illness in a family member commonly takes a toll on other family members and caregivers. In fact, family members under great stress from trying to carry out their own roles while also caring for a sick person are at risk for burnout. If the patient has a long-term illness such as Alzheimer's disease, the caregiver could be facing years of hard work. Signs of stress in a caregiver include muscular aches, headache, insomnia, illness, unexplained pain or GI complaints, fatigue, weight loss, grinding teeth, inability to concentrate, mood swings, use of tranquilizers or alcohol, decreased socialization, depression, forgetfulness, feelings of despair, and thoughts of suicide.

Refer caregivers at risk for or showing signs of strain to social services. Educate caregivers about signs and symptoms of stress to report to their doctor or nurse. Help them identify support systems and tell them about community services that are available.

ESSENTIAL DOCUMENTATION

Record the date and time of your entry. Identify the individual at risk for or experiencing caregiver strain. Describe subjective and objective signs of caregiver strain. Use the caregiver's own words in quotes, when possible. Include education and support given and the caregiver's response. Identify referrals made to services, such as social services, chaplain, support groups, Meals on Wheels, and respite care.

Family education may also be documented on a patient education flow sheet, depending on facility policy. Appropriate notes should also be recorded on discharge planning forms.

6/2/05	1830	While visiting her father, Sandy Peterson, stated, "I'm
		very tired and worried about my father. I've been
		caring for him alone since my sister moved out of
		state. This is my father's second stroke, and he isn't
		responding as well as I'd hoped. I don't know if I'll be
		able to continue to care for him at home." Daughter
		states she's having problems sleeping and feels she's
		alone. She also reports weight loss, headaches, and
		forgetfulness. Explained caregiver strain to her, includ-
		ing s/s to report to her doctor. She verbalized under-
		standing and said she recognized s/s in herself. Stated
		shell make an appointment to see her doctor. Gave her
		pamphlet on Stroke Support Group for Families and
		phone numbers for information on respite care and
		Adult Day Programs. Eileen Murphy, MSW, in social
		services contacted and will make appointment to see
		daughter. ———————————————— Mary Albright, RN

CARE PLAN, STANDARDIZED

The standardized care plan is written to address patient outcomes, nursing actions, and broad interventions that are common to patients with a particular need or problem and are part of the patient's medical record. The standardized care plan is used to save documentation time and improve the quality of care. The nurse may use a standardized care plan as an initial tool for planning care for patients. However, it must be developed and personalized based on the unique needs of the patient. Standardized care plans may be written with general outcomes and interventions or with spaces left blank so that individualized patient outcomes and interventions can be incorporated. Such care plans are commonly published in nursing care plan textbooks.

ESSENTIAL DOCUMENTATION

The standardized care plan should include:

■ related factors and signs and symptoms for a nursing diagnosis. For instance, the form will provide a root diagnosis such as "Pain R/T..." You might fill in "inflammation as exhibited by grimacing, expressions of pain."

■ time limits for the outcomes. To a root outcome statement of "Patient will perform postural drainage without assistance," you might add "for 15

AccuChart

USING A STANDARDIZED CARE PLAN

The standardized care plan below is for a patient with a nursing diagnosis of *Decreased cardiac output*. To customize it to your patient, you would complete the diagnosis — including related factors and signs and symptoms — and fill in the expected outcomes. You would also modify, add, or delete interventions as necessary.

Date _1/8/06_

Target date _1/9/06_

Nursing diagnosis
Decreased cardiac output _R/T reduced stroke volume secondary to fluid volume overload_

Expected outcomes
Adequate cardiac output (AEB) _> 4 L/min_
Heart rate: _Apical rate < 90_
BP: _140/80 mm Hg_
Pedal pulse: _palpable and regular_
Radial pulse: _palpable and regular_
Cardiac rhythm: _normal sinus rhythm_
Cardiac index: _2.2 to 4 L/min/m²_
Pulmonary artery wedge pressure (PAWP): _10 mm Hg_
Pulmonary artery pressure (PAP): _20/12 mm Hg_
$S\bar{v}o_2$: _Between 60% and 80%_
Urine output in ml/hr: _> 30 ml/hr_

Date _1/8/06_

Interventions
- Monitor ECG for rate and rhythm; note ectopic beats. If arrhythmias occur, note patient's response. Document and report findings and follow appropriate arrhythmia protocol.
- Monitor $S\bar{v}o_2$, T, R, and central pressures continuously.
- Monitor other hemodynamic pressures q _1_ hr and p.r.n.
- Auscultate for heart sounds and palpate peripheral pulses q _2_ hr and p.r.n.
- Monitor I & O q _1_ hr. Notify doctor if output < 30 ml/hr × 2 hr.
- Administer medications and fluids as ordered, noting effectiveness and adverse reactions. Titrate vasoactive drugs p.r.n. Follow appropriate vasoactive drug protocol to wean pt. as tolerated.
- Monitor O_2 therapy or other ventilatory assistance.
- Decrease patient's activity to reduce O_2 demands. Increase as tolerated.
- Assess and document LOC. Assess for changes q _1_ hr and p.r.n.
- Additional interventions:
  Inspect for pedal and sacral edema q2hr.

minutes immediately upon awakening in the morning by 2/8/05." The expected outcome should also be realistic, achievable, measurable, observable, behavioral, patient centered, and mutually agreed upon.

■ frequency of interventions. You can complete an intervention such as "Perform passive range-of-motion exercises" with "twice per day: 1 × each in the morning and evening."

■ specific instructions for interventions. For a standard intervention such as "Elevate patient's head of bed," you might specify "Before sleep, elevate the patient's head on three pillows."

Refer to *Using a standardized care plan* for sample documentation.

CARE PLAN, TRADITIONAL

The nursing care plan serves as a written guide to facilitate continuity of care for individual patients. The care plan provides an avenue for communication among health care providers who interact to deliver comprehensive care.

The traditional care plan is initiated when the patient is admitted and continues throughout the hospitalization. The patient's problem, expected outcomes, specific interventions, and evaluations, along with the date that the problem was resolved, are typical components of the traditional care plan. The traditional care plan is written from scratch and is rarely used today because of the time required to write one for each patient. It is, however, specific to the patient so that all health care workers understand the precise patient problem, expected outcomes, and individualized interventions.

ESSENTIAL DOCUMENTATION

The traditional care plan includes dates for problem identification and resolution, the problem (written as a nursing diagnosis), the expected patient outcomes, individualized nursing interventions, and evaluation of the expected outcome. (See *Using a traditional care plan,* page 62.)

AccuChart

USING A TRADITIONAL CARE PLAN

Here's an example of a traditional care plan. It shows how these forms are typically organized. Remember that a traditional care plan is written from scratch for each patient.

DATE	NURSING DIAGNOSIS	EXPECTED OUTCOMES	INTERVENTIONS	REVISION (INITIALS AND DATE)	RESOLUTION (INITIALS AND DATE)
1/8/06	Decreased cardiac output R/T reduced stroke volume secondary to fluid volume overload	Lungs clear on auscultation by 1/10/06 BP will return to baseline by 1/10/06	Monitor for signs and symptoms of hypoxemia, such as dyspnea, confusion, arrhythmias, restlessness, and cyanosis. Ensure adequate oxygenation by placing patient in semi-Fowler's position and administering supplemental O_2 as ordered. Monitor breath sounds q4hr. Administer cardiac medications as ordered and document pt.'s response, drugs' effectiveness, and adverse reactions. Monitor and document heart rate and rhythm, heart sounds, and BP. Note the presence or absence of peripheral pulses.		
			KK		

REVIEW DATES		
Date	Signature	Initials
1/8/06	Karen Kramer, RN	KK

CAST CARE

A cast is a hard mold that encloses a body part, usually an extremity, to provide immobilization without discomfort. It can be used to treat injuries, correct orthopedic conditions, or promote healing after general or plastic surgery, amputation, or neurovascular repair. Care of the cast involves assessment of the limb for neurovascular function, prevention of complications, and patient and family education. Complications include compartment syndrome, palsy, paresthesia, ischemia, ischemic myosis, pressure necrosis, and misalignment or nonunion of fractured bones.

ESSENTIAL DOCUMENTATION

Record the date and time of, and the reason for, cast application and skin condition of the extremity before the cast was applied. Document diagnostic tests performed and the results. Note any contusions, redness, or open wounds. Assess and document the results of neurovascular checks, before and after application, bilaterally. Include the location of special devices, such as felt pads or plaster splints. Document patient education and whether written instructions were given. Patient education may be documented in emergency department (ED) notes, nurse's notes, patient education forms, or discharge sections of the chart.

| 6/5/05 | 1400 | X-ray shows simple Ⓛ radial fracture. Fiberglass cast applied to Ⓛ forearm by Dr. Brown at 1330. Before cast application, 5 cm X 10 cm area of bruising at fracture site, no open wounds noted. Radial pulses strong, capillary refill less than 3 sec, hands warm, no finger edema bilaterally. C/o pain at fracture site. No numbness or tingling, able to move fingers and feel light touch in either hand. After cast application, Ⓛ forearm elevated on 2 pillows. Rough edges of cast petaled. Neurovascular status remains unchanged. Pt. and family told to keep Ⓛ forearm elevated on pillows. Instructed them to call the doctor if pt. is unable to move fingers, if numbness or tingling develops in fingers of Ⓛ hand, or if pain increases despite taking pain medication as ordered. Explained s/s of infection to report. Told them not to insert anything into cast. Written discharge instructions for cast care given to pt. and family. Answered their questions and gave phone # of ED and doctor's office to call with any problems or questions. ——Joyce Chow, RN |

CENTRAL VENOUS CATHETER INSERTION

A central venous (CV) line is a sterile catheter that's inserted through a major vein, such as the subclavian vein or sometimes the jugular vein. CV therapy offers several benefits. It allows CV pressure monitoring, which indicates blood volume or pump efficiency. It permits aspiration of blood samples for diagnostic tests. It also allows administration of I.V. fluids (in large amounts, if necessary) in emergencies or when decreased peripheral circulation causes peripheral veins to collapse. CV lines help when prolonged I.V. therapy reduces the number of accessible peripheral veins, when solutions must be diluted (for large volumes or for irritating or hypertonic fluids such as total parenteral nutrition solutions), and when long-term access is needed to the patient's venous system. A peripherally inserted central catheter (PICC) is inserted in a peripheral vein, such as the basilic vein, and used for infusion and blood sampling only.

ESSENTIAL DOCUMENTATION

When you assist the doctor who inserts a CV line, document the time and date of insertion; type, length, and location of the catheter; solution infused; the doctor's name; and the patient's response to the procedure. If the ports aren't being used, document that they have needle-free injection caps and include any orders related to maintaining patency. You'll also need to document the time of the X-ray performed to confirm placement, the location of the catheter tip, and your notification of the doctor. Note whether the catheter is sutured in place and the type of dressing applied. For a PICC, record the length of the external catheter.

2/24/05	1100	Procedure explained to pt. and consent obtained by Dr.
		Chavez. Pt. in Trendelenburg's position and 20.3 cm
		TLC placed by Dr. Chavez on first attempt in ® sub-
		clavian vein. Cath sutured in place with 3-0 silk, and
		sterile dressing applied per protocol. Needle-free
		injection caps placed on all lines. Lines flushed with
		100 units heparin. Portable CXR obtained to confirm
		line placement. Results pending. P 110, BP 90/58, RR 24,
		oral T 97.9° F. Pt. sitting in semi-Fowler's position and
		breathing easily, lungs clear bilaterally. — Louise Flynn, RN
	2350	Received telephone report from Dr. Turner in radiology confirming
		proper placement of CV line in superior vena cava. Dr. Chavez
		notified by phone of report. ———————— Joyce Williams, RN

CENTRAL VENOUS CATHETER OCCLUSION

A central venous (CV) catheter may become occluded because of kinks in the tubing, closed clamps, the presence of a blood clot or fibrin sheath, or crystalline adherence. Signs of occlusion include the inability to draw blood, infuse a solution, or flush the catheter. If you suspect CV catheter occlusion, check the tubing for kinks. You may need to remove the dressing to check for kinks under it. Check the infusion pump system, and ensure that all clamps are open. Ask the patient to cough or change position. Attempt to withdraw blood or gently flush with normal saline solution. Don't force the flush through the catheter because this may dislodge a clot. For a multilumen catheter, label the occluded lumen "Occluded: Do not use." Depending on the catheter, a thrombolytic may be used to lyse a clot or dissolve a fibrin sheath. A new CV line may be inserted.

ESSENTIAL DOCUMENTATION

Document the date and time of the occlusion. Record evidence of catheter occlusion. Describe your actions and the results. Include the name of the doctor notified, the time of notification, and any orders given. Depending on your facility's policy, you may also need to document the occlusion on the I.V. therapy flow sheet.

7/4/05	1220	Unable to aspirate blood from blue distal port of TLC.
		Infusion pump alarm indicates occlusion. Unable to
		flush line with NSS. All clamps checked and are open.
		No kinks noted in tubing. Dsg removed, no kinks noted
		under dsg. Site re-dressed according to protocol. Pt.
		changed from supine to ℝ and Ⓛ lateral position and
		asked to cough; still unable to obtain blood return or
		flush with NSS. Blue distal port labeled "occluded." Dr.
		Brown notified of the occlusion at 1210. ————————
		———————————————————————— Ruth Clark, RN

CENTRAL VENOUS CATHETER REMOVAL

When a central venous (CV) line is no longer necessary, it's removed by the doctor or by a specially trained nurse. Be sure to verify your facility's policy and protocols related to CV line removal by a registered nurse.

ESSENTIAL DOCUMENTATION

After assisting with a CV line's removal or performing the CV line removal yourself, record the name of the person discontinuing the line, the time and date of the removal, the length of time that pressure was held to the site, and the type of dressing applied. Note the length of the catheter and the condition of the insertion site. Also, document collecting any catheter specimens for culture or other analysis.

2/24/05	1100	20.3 cm CV catheter removed by Dr. Romero at 1045 and pressure held for 5 min. Catheter tip present, sent to laboratory for culture. Povidone-iodine applied to insertion site and covered with gauze pad and transparent semipermeable dressing. No drainage, redness, or swelling noted at insertion site. ————— Louise Flynn, RN

CENTRAL VENOUS CATHETER SITE CARE

Central venous catheter site care and frequency of care will vary according to the type of catheter and the facility's policy. Site care is performed using aseptic technique. After the catheter is inserted, use normal saline solution to remove dried blood from the insertion site.

The insertion site should be visually inspected and palpated daily through an intact dressing. Chlorhexidine is replacing povidone-iodine and alcohol as the antiseptic of choice because of its increased efficacy. Don't apply ointment to the insertion site.

When the dressing is removed, inspect the site for signs and symptoms of infection, such as discharge, inflammation, and tenderness. Frequency of site care varies from daily to every 48 hours for gauze dressings to every 3 to 7 days for transparent dressings. Dressings should always be changed if they become soiled or lose integrity.

ESSENTIAL DOCUMENTATION

After you've completed the dressing change, label the dressing with the time, date, and your initials. In your documentation, record the date and time of site care. Depending on facility policy, this documentation may be in the nurse's notes or I.V. therapy flow sheet. Note the marking indicating catheter length, appearance of the insertion site, method of cleaning site, and type of dressing applied. Describe any drainage on the dressing. If complications are noted, record the name of the doctor notified, the time of notification, and any orders given.

9/25/05	1220	® subclavian TLC dressing removed. Suture intact, insertion site without redness or drainage, catheter marking at 12 cm. Pt. denies tenderness. Using sterile technique, area and insertion site cleaned with chlorhexidine. Catheter secured with tape and covered with semipermeable membrane dressing. — Nick Cerone, RN

CENTRAL VENOUS PRESSURE MONITORING

To monitor central venous pressure (CVP), the doctor inserts a catheter through a vein and advances it until the tip lies in or near the right atrium and end-diastolic pressure is seen on the monitor. When connected to a monitoring device, the catheter measures CVP, which is an index of right ventricular function. CVP monitoring helps to assess cardiac function, evaluate venous return to the heart, and indirectly gauge how well the heart is pumping. CVP monitoring may be done intermittently (with a water manometer) or continuously (with a water manometer or pressure monitoring system) with readings recorded in centimeters of water or millimeters of mercury.

ESSENTIAL DOCUMENTATION

Record CVP readings on a flow sheet or in your note, according to your facility's policy. I.V. fluids may be documented on the I.V. flow sheet as well. When writing your note, record the date and time of assessment. Record the CVP reading, the patient's position, and whether the transducer was at the zero reference point. Describe the appearance of the waveform and your evaluation. Place a printout of recordings, if available, in the patient's chart. Include any relevant assessments of the patient. Document the name of the doctor notified, the time of notification, and whether any actions were taken.

10/5/05	0500	® subclavian CVP attached to monitor with pressure bag
		setup of 500 ml NSS with 1000 units of heparin added.
		Line balanced and calibrated as per protocol. Normal
		CVP waveform on monitor shows reading of 4 cm H₂O.
		Urine output 25 ml in past hr. Mucous membranes dry,
		Skin tents when pinched. P 110, BP 110/72, RR 18, oral T
		99.0° F. Dr. Brown notified of dropping CVP reading and
		physical assessment findings. Fluid challenge of 500 ml
		NSS over 1 hr via CVP line started. — Joanne Nunez, RN

CHEST PAIN

When your patient complains of chest pain, you'll need to act quickly to determine its cause. That's because chest pain may be caused by a disorder as benign as epigastric distress (indigestion) or as serious and life-threatening as acute myocardial infarction.

Essential documentation

Record the date and time of the onset of chest pain. Question your patient about his pain, and record the responses using the patient's own words, when appropriate. Include the following:

- What the patient was doing when the pain started
- How long the pain lasted, if it had ever occurred before, and whether the onset was sudden or gradual
- Whether the pain radiates
- Factors that improve or aggravate the pain
- The exact location of the pain (Ask him to point to the pain and record his response. For example, he may move his hand vaguely around his abdomen or may point with one finger to his left chest.)

■ Severity of the pain. (Ask the patient to rank the pain on a 0 to 10 scale, with 0 indicating no pain and 10 indicating the worst pain imaginable.)

Record the patient's vital signs and a quick assessment of his body systems. Document the time and name of any individuals notified, such as the doctor, nursing supervisor, or admission's department (if the patient is transferred). Record your actions and the patient's responses. Include any patient education and emotional support you provided.

| 8/9/05 | 0410 | Pt. c/o sudden onset of a sharp chest pain while sleeping. Points to center of chest, over sternum. States, "It feels like an elephant is sitting on my chest." Pain radiates to the neck and shoulders. Rates pain as 7 on a scale of 0 to 10, w/ 10 being the worst pain imaginable. P 112, BP 90/62, RR 26. Lungs have fine crackles in the bases on auscultation. Dr. Romano notified and orders received. Morphine 2 mg I.V. given. O₂ at 4 L/min started by NC. Continuous pulse oximetry started with O₂ sat. 94%. 12-lead ECG and MI profile obtained. All procedures explained to pt. Reassured pt. that he's being closely monitored. ———————— Martha Wolcott, RN |
| | 0415 | Dr. Romano here to see patient. Pt. states pain is now a 5 on a scale of 0 to 10. Morphine 2 mg I.V. repeated. ECG interpreted by Dr. Romano to show acute ischemia. Pt. prepared for transport to CCU. —— Martha Wolcott, RN |

CHEST PHYSIOTHERAPY

Chest physiotherapy includes postural drainage, chest percussion and vibration, and coughing and deep-breathing exercises. Together, these techniques move and eliminate secretions, reexpand lung tissue, and promote efficient use of respiratory muscles. Of critical importance to the bedridden patient, chest physiotherapy helps prevent or treat atelectasis and may help prevent pneumonia.

ESSENTIAL DOCUMENTATION

Whenever you perform chest physiotherapy, document the date and time of your interventions; the patient's position for secretion drainage and the length of time the patient remains in each position; the chest segments percussed or vibrated; and the characteristics of the secretion expelled, including color, amount, odor, viscosity, and the presence of blood. Also, record indications of complications, the nursing actions taken, and the patient's tolerance of the treatment.

12/20/05	1415	Pt. placed on Ⓛ side with foot of bed elevated. Chest PT
		and postural drainage performed for 10 min. from
		lower to middle then upper lobes, as ordered. Pt. had
		productive cough and expelled large amt. of thick, yellow,
		odorless sputum. Lungs clear after chest PT. After chest
		PT, pt. stated he was tired and asked to lie down.
		————————————— Jane Goddard, RN

CHEST TUBE CARE

Inserted into the pleural space, the chest tube allows blood, fluid, pus, or air to drain and allows the lung to reinflate. Chest drainage uses gravity or suction to restore negative pressure and remove material that collects in the pleural cavity. An underwater seal in the drainage system allows air and fluid to escape from the pleural cavity but doesn't allow air to reenter.

Caring for the patient with a chest tube involves maintaining suction, monitoring for and preventing air leaks, monitoring drainage, promoting pulmonary hygiene, promoting patient comfort, performing dressing changes and site care, and preventing, detecting, and treating complications.

ESSENTIAL DOCUMENTATION

Record the date and time of your entry. Identify the chest tube location; type and amount of suction; type, amount, and consistency of drainage; and presence or absence of bubbling or fluctuation in the water-seal chamber. If site care was performed, record the appearance of the site and the type of dressing applied. Document the patient's respiratory status and any pulmonary hygiene performed. Note the patient's level of pain, any comfort measures performed, and the results. Include interventions to prevent complications. If any complications occurred, record your interventions and the results. Note the name of the doctor notified of problems and the time of notification.

| 5/31/05 | 1350 | Received pt. from recovery room at 1325. ℞ midaxillary CT with 20 cm of H_2O in Pleur-evac suction control chamber. Collection chamber has 100 ml of serosanguineous fluid. No clots noted. Level of drainage dated and timed. Water level fluctuating with respirations in water-seal chamber. All CT connections taped, and 2 rubber-tipped clamps placed at bedside. Dried blood on CT dsg. Dsg removed, one suture noted. Dried blood cleaned from skin with NSS and gauze. Antimicrobial ointment applied to insertion site and re-dressed using sterile 4" X 4" petroleum jelly gauze around site and secured with tape. No crepitus noted. Breath sounds clear with diminished breath sounds in ℞ lower lobe. P 98, BP 132/82, RR 28 shallow and labored, oral T 99.1° F. Skin pale, warm, and dry, mucous membranes pink. O_2 sat. 97% on 50% face mask. Pt. c/o aching pain at CT site and refused to take deep breaths and cough due to pain. Morphine sulfate 2 mg I.V. given at 1335. Pt. able to C&DB within 15 min after administration. ——————————— Mary Ann Pfister, RN |
| | | |

CHEST TUBE INSERTION

Insertion of a chest tube permits drainage of air or fluid from the pleural space. Usually performed by a doctor with a nurse assisting, this procedure requires sterile technique. Insertion sites vary, depending on the patient's condition. For pneumothorax, the second intercostal space is the usual site because air rises to the top of the intrapleural space. For hemothorax or pleural effusion, the sixth to the eighth intercostal spaces are common sites because fluid settles to the lower levels of the intrapleural space. For removal of air and fluid, a chest tube is inserted into a high site as well as a low site.

Following insertion, one or more chest tubes are connected to a thoracic drainage system that removes air, fluid, or both from the pleural space and prevents backflow into that space, thus promoting lung reexpansion. Inserting a chest tube requires close observation of the patient and verification of proper placement.

ESSENTIAL DOCUMENTATION

Document the date and time of chest tube insertion. Include the name of the doctor performing the procedure. Identify the insertion site and the type of drainage system and suction used. Record the presence of drainage and bubbling. Drainage should also be included on the patient's intake and output record. Record the type, amount, and consistency of drainage. Document the patient's vital signs, auscultation findings, any complications, and nursing actions taken. Record any patient education performed. This may also need to be recorded on a patient teaching record, depending on your facility's policy.

| 9/30/05 | 1100 | Pt. consented to insertion of chest tube after discussing risks and complications with Dr. Brown. Informed consent signed. Preinsertion P 98, RR 32, BP 118/72, oral T 97.9° F. Assisted Dr. Brown with sterile insertion of #22 CT into pt.'s Ⓛ lower midaxillary area. Tube secured with one suture. CT connected to Pleur-evac with 20 cm of suction, which immediately drained 100 ml of serosanguineous drainage. No air leaks evident with the system. Postinsertion P 80, RR 24, BP 120/72. Respirations shallow, unlabored. Slightly decreased breath sounds in Ⓛ post. lower lobe, otherwise breath sounds clear bilaterally. O₂ sat. 99% after CT insertion. Equal lung excursion noted. No crepitus palpated. Petroleum jelly gauze applied to CT insertion site and occlusive dressing applied. Tubing secured to pt. to prevent dislodgment. Pt. reports only minimal discomfort at insertion site. Upright portable CXR obtained, and Dr. Brown notified. C&DB exercises and use of incentive spirometer reviewed with pt.; pt. verbalized understanding and was able to inspire 900 ml of volume. —————— Carol Slane, RN |

CHEST TUBE REMOVAL

After the patient's lung has reexpanded, you may assist the doctor in removing the chest tube. In many facilities, other health care professionals such as advanced practice nurses (clinical nurse specialists or nurse practitioners) are trained to perform chest tube removal.

ESSENTIAL DOCUMENTATION

Document the date and time of chest tube removal and the name of the person who performed the procedure. Record the patient's vital signs and the findings of your respiratory assessment before and after chest tube removal. Note whether an analgesic was administered before the removal and how long after administration the chest tube was removed. Describe the patient's tolerance of the procedure. Record the amount of drainage in the collection bottle and the appearance of the wound at the chest tube site. Describe the type of dressing applied. Include any patient education performed.

| 10/9/05 | 1300 | Explained to pt. that CT was being removed because (L) lung is now reexpanded. Explained how to perform Valsalva's maneuver when tube is removed. Pt. was able to give return demonstration. Administered Percocet 2 tabs P.O. 30 min before removal. Preprocedure P 88, BP 120/80, RR 18, oral T 97.8° F. Respirations regular, deep, unlabored. No use of accessory muscles. Full respiratory excursion bilaterally. Breath sounds clear bilaterally. No drainage in collection chamber since 0800. #20 CT removed without difficulty by Dr. Smith. CT wound clean. No drainage or redness noted. Petroleum jelly gauze dressing placed over insertion site, covered with 4" X 4" gauze dressing, and secured with 2" tape. Postprocedure breath sounds remain clear, full respiratory excursion bilaterally, breathing comfortably in semi-Fowler's position, no subcutaneous crepitus noted. P 86, BP 132/84, RR 20. Pt. without complaints of pain or shortness of breath. Reminded him of importance of continuing to use incentive spirometer q1hr. CXR performed at 1255. Results not yet available. ———————————————————— Marcy Wells, RN |

CHEST TUBE REMOVAL BY PATIENT

The accidental or intentional removal of a chest tube by the patient can introduce air into the pleural space, leading to the potentially life-threatening complication of pneumothorax. As a precaution, sterile petroleum jelly gauze should be kept at the patient's bedside at all times. Moreover, inappropriate removal of a chest tube can damage the surrounding tissue.

If your patient removes his chest tube, immediately cover the site with sterile petroleum jelly gauze and tape it in place. Stay with the patient and assess his vital signs, respiratory status, and observe for signs and symptoms of pneumothorax. Call for help and instruct a coworker to notify the doctor and gather the equipment needed for reinsertion of the chest tube. If the patient isn't in respiratory distress, the doctor may order a chest X-ray to determine if the chest tube needs to be reinserted.

ESSENTIAL DOCUMENTATION

Record the date and time of your entry. Describe how you discovered that the patient removed his chest tube. Use the patient's own words, if appropriate, to describe what happened. Record your immediate actions and the patient's response. Document vital signs and your cardiopulmonary assessment, in particular noting whether the patient has any signs or symptoms of pneumothorax, such as hypotension, distended neck veins, absent breath sounds, tracheal shift, hypoxemia, weak and rapid pulse, dyspnea, tachypnea, diaphoresis, or chest pain. Note the name of the doctor notified, the time of notification, and any orders given, such as preparing for chest tube reinsertion, administering supplemental oxygen, or obtaining a chest X-ray. Document any support or education given. If the patient requires reinsertion of a chest tube, follow the documentation guidelines for chest tube insertion. (See "Chest tube insertion," page 71.)

4/15/05	0815	Upon entering room at 0740 to give pt. his 0800
		meds, noted chest tube lying on floor. Pt. stated, "This
		tube was hurting me so I was rubbing it. Next thing I
		know it was lying on the floor." Immediately covered
		site with petroleum jelly gauze taped in place over Ⓛ
		chest wound. No external trauma to insertion site, no
		drainage or bleeding noted. Pt. didn't appear to be in
		acute distress. Pt. in bed in semi-Fowler's position,
		breathing comfortably at rate of 22, P 94, BP 110/74.
		Breath sounds clear bilaterally with Ⓛ lower lobe sounds
		slightly diminished. Neck veins not distended, no
		dyspnea noted, trachea in midline, skin warm and dry,
		no c/o chest pain. Stayed with pt. while Brian Mott, LPN,
		notified Dr. Finnegan at 0745. Dr. came to see pt. at
		0750. CXR done, showing Ⓛ lung mostly inflated.
		Decision made by Dr. Finnegan not to reinsert chest
		tube at this time. Pt.'s cardiopulmonary status to be
		assessed q15min for 1st hr, then q1hr for next 4 hr,
		then q4hr thereafter. Reviewed C&DB exercises with pt.
		and reminded him to do them every hr. ————————
		———————————————— Sarah Clarke, RN

CLINICAL PATHWAY

A clinical pathway, also known as a *critical pathway,* integrates the principles of case management into nursing documentation. It outlines the standard of care for a specific diagnosis-related group. It incorporates multidisciplinary diagnoses and interventions, such as nursing-related problems, combined nursing and medical interventions, and key events that must occur for the patient to be discharged by a target date.

A clinical pathway is usually organized by categories according to the patient's diagnosis, which dictates his expected length of stay, daily care guidelines, and expected outcomes. These categories, specified for each day, include consultations, diagnostic tests, treatments, drugs, procedures, activities, diet, patient teaching, discharge planning, and anticipated outcomes. Other events or interventions may be added, and the pathway's categories may be presented in various formats and combinations.

Within the managed care system, clinical pathways set the standard for tracking patient progress. They provide the nursing staff with necessary written criteria to guide and monitor patient care. In some health care facilities, the nursing diagnosis forms the clinical pathway's basis for patient care.

ESSENTIAL DOCUMENTATION

Record whether your patient's progress follows what is outlined in the clinical pathway by choosing either "variance," if the patient's progress deviates from the standard, or "no variance," if the patient's progress is following the standard. This is recorded for each shift and signed by the nurse. (See *Following a clinical pathway,* pages 76 and 77.)

(Text continues on page 78.)

ACCUCHART

FOLLOWING A CLINICAL PATHWAY

At any point in a treatment course, a glance at the clinical pathway allows you to compare the patient's progress and your performance as a caregiver with care standards. Below is a sample pathway.

CLINICAL PATHWAY: COLON RESECTION WITHOUT COLOSTOMY

	Patient visit	Presurgery Day 1	O.R. Day	Postop Day 1
Assessments	History and physical with breast, rectal, and pelvic exam Nursing assessment	Nursing admission assessment	Nursing admission assessment on TBA patients in holding area Review of systems assessment*	Review of systems assessment*
Consults	Social services consult Physical therapy consult	Notify referring physician of impending admission	Type and screen for patients in holding area with Hgb < 10	
Labs and diagnostics	Complete blood count (CBC) Coagulation profile ECG Chest X-ray (CXR) Chem profile CT ABD w/wo contrast CT pelvis Urinalysis Barium enema & flex sigmoidoscopy/colonoscopy Biopsy report	Type and screen for patients with hemoglobin (Hgb) < 10		CBC
Interventions	Many or all of the above labs/diagnostics will have already been done. Check all results and fax to the surgeon's office.	Admit by 8 a.m. Check for bowel prep orders Bowel prep* Antiembolism stockings Incentive spirometry Ankle exercises* I.V. access* Routine vital signs (VS)* Pneumatic inflation boots	Shave and prep in O.R. Nasogastric (NG) tube maint.* Intake and output (I/O) VS per routine* Catheter care* Incentive spirometry* Ankle exercises* I.V. site care* Head of bed (HOB) 30°* Safety measures* Wound care* Mouth care*	NG tube maintenance* I/O* VS per routine* Catheter care* Incentive spirometry* Ankle exercises* I.V. site care* HOB 30°* Safety measures* Wound care* Mouth care* Antiembolism stockings
I.V.s		I.V. fluids, $D_5\frac{1}{2}$ NSS	I.V. fluids, D_5LR	I.V. fluids, D_5LR
Medication	Prescribe GoLYTELY/NuLYTELY 10a — 2p Neomycin @ 2p, 3p, and 10p Erythromycin @2p, 3p, and 10p	GoLYTELY/NuLYTELY 10a — 2p Erythromycin @ 2p, 3p, and 10p Neomycin @ 2p, 3p and 10p	Preop antibiotics (ABX) in holding area Postop AB × 2 doses PCA (basal rate 0.5 mg) SubQ heparin	PCA (basal rate 0.5 mg) SubQ heparin
Diet/GI	Clears presurgery day NPO after midnight	Clears presurgery day NPO after midnight	NPO/NG tube	NPO/NG tube
Activity	Preop teaching	Reinforce preop teaching	4 hours after surgery, ambulate with abdominal binder* Discontinue pneumatic inflation boots after patient ambulates	Ambulate t.i.d. with abdominal binder* May shower Physical therapy b.i.d.

KEY:
* = NSG activities
V = Variance
N = No variance

Signatures:

	1. 2. 3.	1. 2. 3.	1. 2. 3.	1. 2. 3.
	V V V N N N	V V V N N N	V V V N N N	V V V N N N
	1. M. Connel, RN 2. ___ 3. ___	1. M. Connel, RN 2. C. Roy, RN 3. J. Kane, RN	1. L. Singer, RN 2. J. Smith, RN 3. P. Joseph, RN	1. L. Singer, RN 2. J. Smith, RN 3. P. Joseph, RN

FOLLOWING A CLINICAL PATHWAY
(continued)

CLINICAL PATHWAY: COLON RESECTION WITHOUT COLOSTOMY

	Postop Day 2	Postop Day 3	Postop Day 4	Postop Day 5
Assessments	Review of systems assessment*	Review of systems assessment*	Review of systems assessment*	Review of systems assessment*
Consults		Dietary consult		Oncology consult if indicated (or to be done as outpatient)
Labs and diagnostics	Electrolyte 7 (EL-7) CXR	CBC EL-7	Pathology results on chart	CBC EL-7
Interventions	Discontinue NG tube if possible* (per guidelines) I/O* VS per routine* Discontinue catheter* Ambulating* Incentive spirometry* Ankle exercises* I.V. site care* HOB 30°* Safety measures* Wound care* Mouth care* Antiembolism stockings	I/O* VS per routine* Incentive spirometry* Ankle exercises* I.V. site care* Safety measures* Wound care* Antiembolism stockings	I/O* VS per routine* Incentive spirometry* Ankle exercises* I.V. site care* Safety measures* Wound care* Antiembolism stockings	Consider staple removal Replace with Steri-Strips Assess that patient has met discharge criteria*
I.V.s	I.V. fluids $D_5\frac{1}{2}$ NSS+ MVI	I.V.-Heplock	Heplock	Discontinue Heplock
Medication	PCA (5 mg basal rate)	Discontinue PCA P.O. analgesia Resume routine home meds	P.O. analgesia	P.O. analgesia
Diet/GI	Discontinue NG tube per guidelines: (Clamp tube at 8 a.m. if no N/V and residual < 200 ml, Discontinue tube @ 12 noon)* (Check with doctor first)	Clears if pt. has BM/flatus Advance to postop diet if tolerating clears (at least one tray of clears)*	House	House
Activity	Ambulate q.i.d. with abdominal binder* May shower Physical therapy b.i.d.	Ambulate at least q.i.d. with abdominal binder* May shower Physical therapy b.i.d.	Ambulate at least q.i.d. with abdominal binder* May shower Physical therapy b.i.d.	
Teaching	Reinforce preop teaching* Patient and family education p.r.n.* re: family screening	Reinforce preop teaching* Patient and family education p.r.n.* re: family screening Begin discharge teaching	Reinforce preop teaching* Patient and family education p.r.n.* Discharge teaching re: reportable s/s, F/U and wound care*	Review all discharge instructions and Rx ncluding* follow-up appointments: with surgeon within 3 weeks, with oncologist within 1 month if indicated

KEY:
* = NSG activities
V = Variance
N = No variance

Signatures:

1. 2. 3.	1. 2. 3.	1. 2. 3.	1. 2. 3.
V V V	V V V	V V V	V V V
Ⓝ Ⓝ Ⓝ	Ⓝ Ⓝ Ⓝ	Ⓝ Ⓝ Ⓝ	Ⓝ N N
1. *A. McCarthy, RN*	1. *A. McCarthy, RN*	1. *L. Singer, RN*	1. *L. Singer, RN*
2. *R. Mayer, RN*	2. *R. Mayer, RN*	2. *J. Smith, RN*	2. _____
3. *P. Drake, RN*	3. *P. Drake, RN*	3. *P. Joseph, RN*	3. _____

COLD APPLICATION

The application of cold constricts blood vessels; inhibits local circulation, suppuration, and tissue metabolism; relieves vascular congestion; slows bacterial activity in infections; reduces body temperature; and may act as a temporary anesthetic during brief, painful procedures. Because treatment with cold also relieves inflammation, reduces edema, and slows bleeding, it may provide effective initial treatment after eye injuries, strains, sprains, bruises, muscle spasms, and burns. However, cold doesn't reduce existing edema because it inhibits reabsorption of excess fluid.

ESSENTIAL DOCUMENTATION

Record the time, date, and duration of cold application; the site of application; and the type of device used, such as an ice bag or collar, K pad, cold compress, or chemical cold pack. Indicate the temperature or temperature setting of the device. Before and after the procedure, record the patient's vital signs and the appearance of his skin. Document any signs of complications, interventions, and the patient's response. Describe the patient's tolerance of treatment.

11/14/05	1300	Before cold application, oral T 98.6° F, BP 110/70, P 80,
		RR 18. ® groin site warm and dry, without redness,
		edema, or ecchymosis. Ice bag covered with towel applied
		to ® groin for 20 min. Postprocedure T 98.6° F,
		BP 120/70, P 82, RR 20. ® groin site cool and dry,
		without redness, edema, graying, mottling, blisters, or
		ecchymosis. No c/o burning or numbness. Pt. is resting
		comfortably. ———————— Greg Pearson, RN

COMMUNICABLE DISEASE, REPORTING

The Centers for Disease Control and Prevention, the Occupational Safety and Health Administration, the Joint Commission on Accreditation of Healthcare Organizations, and the American Hospital Association all require health care facilities to document and report certain diseases acquired in the community or in hospitals and other health care facilities. (See *Reporting communicable diseases.*)

REPORTING COMMUNICABLE DISEASES

According to the Centers for Disease Control and Prevention (2005), certain diseases must be reported to local health authorities. Because regulations vary among communities and states and because different agencies focus on different data, the list of reportable diseases that appears below isn't conclusive and may change periodically.

- Acquired immunodeficiency syndrome (AIDS)
- Anthrax
- Arboviral neuroinvasive and nonneuroinvasive diseases
    - California serogroup virus disease
    - Eastern equine encephalitis virus disease
    - Powassan virus disease
    - St. Louis encephalitis virus disease
    - West Nile virus disease
    - Western equine encephalitis virus disease
- Botulism (foodborne, infant, other)
- Brucellosis
- Chancroid
- Cholera
- Coccidioidomycosis
- Cryptosporidiosis
- Cyclosporiasis
- Diphtheria
- Ehrlichiosis (human granulocytic, human monocytic, human, other or unspecifed)
- Enterohemorrhagic *Escherichia coli* (O157:H7; shiga toxin positive, serogroup non-O157; shiga toxin+ [not serogrouped])
- Giardiasis
- Gonorrhea
- *Haemophilus influenzae*, invasive disease
- Hansen disease (leprosy)
- Hantavirus pulmonary syndrome
- Hemolytic uremic syndrome, postdiarrheal
- Hepatitis, viral, acute (A, B, B perinatal, C)
- Hepatitis, viral, chronic (B, C past or present)
- Human immunodeficiency virus (HIV) infection
- Influenza-associated pediatric mortality
- Legionellosis
- Listeriosis
- Lyme disease
- Malaria
- Measles
- Meningococcal disease
- Mumps
- Pertussis
- Plague
- Poliomyelitis, paralytic
- Psittacosis
- Q Fever
- Rabies
- Rocky Mountain spotted fever
- Rubella or rubella congenital syndrome
- Salmonellosis
- Severe acute respiratory syndrome-associated coronavirus (SARS-CoV) disease
- Shigellosis
- Smallpox
- Streptococcal disease, invasive, group A
- Streptococcal toxic shock syndrome
- *Streptococcus pneumoniae*, drug resistant, invasive disease
- Syphilis (primary, secondary, latent, neurosyphilis, congenital)
- Tetanus
- Toxic shock syndrome
- Trichinellosis (trichinosis)
- Tuberculosis
- Tularemia
- Typhoid fever
- Vancomycin — intermediate *Staphylococcus aureus* (VISA)
- Vancomycin — resistant *Staphylococcus aureus* (VRSA)
- Varicella (morbidity)
- Varicella (deaths only)
- Yellow fever

Generally, the health care facility's infection control department reports diseases to the appropriate local authorities. These authorities notify the state health department, which in turn reports the diseases to the appropriate federal agency or national organization.

ESSENTIAL DOCUMENTATION

Document the date, time, person or department notified (according to your facility's policy and procedure manual), and what you reported.

8/1/05	1400	Notified Ms. Smith, Infectious Disease Coordinator of
		West Brook Memorial Hospital, that the diagnosis of
		West Nile encephalitis has been identified as per Dr.
		John Jones, Infectious Disease. — Tammy Hartwell, RN

CONFUSION

An umbrella term for puzzling or inappropriate behavior or responses, confusion reflects the inability to think quickly and coherently. Depending on its cause, confusion may arise suddenly or gradually and may be temporary or irreversible. Aggravated by stress and sensory deprivation, confusion commonly occurs in elderly hospitalized patients, in whom it may be mistaken for senility.

When severe confusion arises suddenly and the patient also has hallucinations and psychomotor hyperactivity, his condition is classified as delirium. Long-term, progressive confusion with deterioration of all cognitive functions is classified as dementia.

Confusion may result from metabolic, neurologic, cardiopulmonary, cerebrovascular, or nutritional disorders or can result from infection, toxins, drugs, or alcohol.

ESSENTIAL DOCUMENTATION

When your patient is confused, document how you became aware of his confusion. Record the results of your neurologic and cardiopulmonary assessments. Record possible contributing factors, such as abnormal laboratory values, drugs, poor nutrition, poor sleep patterns, infection, surgery, pain, sensory overload or deprivation, and the use of alcohol and nonprescription drugs. Record the time and name of the doctor notified. Note any new orders such as blood work to assess laboratory values or drug changes. Describe your interventions to reduce confusion and to keep your patient safe, and include the patient's response. Document patient teaching and emotional support given.

6/22/05	1300	Upon entering pt.'s room, noted pt. putting on his pajamas.
		When asked what he was doing pt. stated, "It's my bedtime.
		I'm going to sleep." Told pt. it was 1230, lunchtime, and I
		had his lunch for him. Pt. put his pj's back and sat down on
		his bed. Pt. alert, oriented to person, but not place and
		time. Knows the year he was born but stated he was at
		home and that it was fall of 1955. Speech clear but
		fragmented. Unable to repeat back 5 numbers. Moving all
		extremities, hand grasps firm bilaterally. Gait steady with
		walker. P 102, BP 96/62, RR 18, oral T 101.8° F. Lungs clear,
		no use of accessory muscles, skin pink. S₁ and S₂ heart
		sounds, no edema noted, radial and dorsalis pedis pulses
		strong, capillary refill less than 3 sec, skin hot and dry. Pt.
		needed to urinate X2 during assessment. Urinated 100 ml
		each time, urine cloudy, foul odor. No c/o burning on
		urination. Dr. Blake notified at 1245. Urine culture sent to
		lab for C/S. Tylenol 650 mg P.O. given for fever. To be
		given q4hr P.O. p.r.n. for T greater than 101° F. CBC
		w/diff., BUN, creatinine, and electrolytes to be drawn in
		a.m. Pt. reoriented to time and place. Encouraged pt. to
		drink. Brought him ginger ale as he requested. Will check on
		pt. q15min. Family in to visit. Discussed possible UTI as
		cause of confusion. They will assist pt. to bathroom and
		will alert nurse when they leave. — Matilda Jennings, RN

CONTINUOUS RENAL REPLACEMENT THERAPY

Continuous renal replacement therapy (CRRT) is a procedure that filters fluid, solutes, and electrolytes from the patient's blood and infuses a replacement solution. CRRT is used to treat patients with fluid overload who don't require dialysis. Commonly used to treat patients in acute renal failure, CRRT is also used for treating fluid overload that doesn't respond to diuretics and for some electrolyte and acid-base disturbances.

CRRT carries a much lower risk of hypotension than conventional hemodialysis because it withdraws fluid more slowly, at about 200 ml/hour. This procedure can be performed in hypotensive patients who require fluid removal, who can't undergo peritoneal dialysis, or whose requirements for parenteral nutrition would make fluid volume control problematic.

CRRT reduces the risk of other complications and makes maintaining a stable fluid volume and regulating fluid and electrolyte balance easier. CRRT methods vary in complexity and include slow continuous ultra fil-tration (SCUF), continuous arteriovenous hemofiltration (CAVH), and-continuous venovenous hemofiltration (CVVH).

ESSENTIAL DOCUMENTATION

When your patient undergoes CRRT, record the time that the treatment began and the time it ended, and record fluid balance information. Document baseline and hourly vital signs and weight. Record laboratory studies, such as electrolytes, coagulation factors, complete blood count, and blood urea nitrogen and creatinine levels. Weight, vital signs, and laboratory studies may be documented on a specialized flow sheet. Describe the appearance of the ultrafiltrate. Document your inspection of the insertion sites as well as any site care and dressing changes. Make sure you mark the dressing with the date and time of the dressing change. Record your assessment of circulation in the affected leg. Document any drugs given during the procedure. Note any complications, your interventions, and the patient's response. Include the patient's tolerance of the procedure.

| 7/27/05 | 0815 | CAVH started at 0800. See CAVH flow sheet for labs, and hourly VS and I/O. Baseline weight 132.4 lb, P 92, BP 132/74, RR 20, oral T 98.2° F. Ultrafiltrate clear yellow. ⓛ femoral access sites without hematoma, redness, swelling, or warmth. ⓛ foot warm, dorsalis pedis and posterior tibial pulses strong, capillary refill less than 3 sec. Insertion sites cleaned according to protocol and covered with occlusive dressing. Pt. states he's tired and would like to sleep. — Tom Costanza, RN |

CORRECTION TO DOCUMENTATION

When you make a mistake on a chart, correct it promptly. Never erase, cover, completely scratch out, or otherwise obscure an erroneous entry because this may imply a cover-up. If the chart ends up in court, the plaintiff's attorney will be looking for anything that may cast doubt on the chart's accuracy. Erasures or the use of correction fluid or heavy black ink to obliterate an error are red flags.

ESSENTIAL DOCUMENTATION

When you make a mistake documenting on the medical record, correct it by drawing a single line through it and writing the words "mistaken entry" above or beside it. Follow these words with your initials and the date. If appropriate, briefly explain the necessity for the correction. Make sure the mistaken entry is still readable. This indicates that you're only trying to correct a mistake, not cover it up.

1/19/06	0900	*Mistaken entry. J. M. 1/19/06*
		~~*Pt. walked to bathroom. States he experienced no*~~
		~~*difficulty urinating.*~~ —————— *John Mora, RN*

COUNTERSIGNATURE OF COLLEAGUE'S NOTES

Countersigning, or signing off on someone else's entry, requires good judgment. Although countersigning doesn't imply that you performed the procedure, it does imply that you reviewed the entry and approved the care given.

To act correctly and to protect yourself, review your facility's policy on countersigning and proceed accordingly. If your facility interprets countersigning to mean that the licensed practical nurse (LPN), graduate nurse, or nurse's aide performed the nursing actions in the countersigning registered nurse's presence, don't countersign unless you were there when the actions occurred.

On the other hand, if your facility acknowledges that you don't necessarily have time to witness your coworkers' actions, your countersignature implies that the LPN or nurse's aide had the authority and competence to perform the care described. In countersigning, you verify that all required patient care procedures were carried out.

If policy does require you to countersign a subordinate's entries, be careful. Review each entry, and make sure it clearly identifies who did the procedure. If you sign off without reviewing an entry, or if you overlook a problem that the entry raises, you could share liability for any patient injury that results.

ESSENTIAL DOCUMENTATION

When countersigning the notes of a colleague, specifically document that you reviewed the notes and consulted with the technician or assistant on certain aspects of care. Of course, you must document any follow-up care you provide.

10/10/05	1300	Removed dressing from ① ankle ulcer. Ulcer approx.
		4 cm wide X 4 cm long X 1 cm deep, even edges, wound
		bed pink, no drainage, surrounding skin pink and intact.
		Irrigated wound with NSS. Skin surrounding wound
		dried. Hydrocolloid dressing applied.— Mary Lewis, LPN
10/10/05	1345	Note reviewed. Discussed wound with Mary Lewis. Wound size has
		decreased from 5 cm wide X 6 cm long X 2 cm on 10/3/05. Dr.
		Spellman notified and orders given to continue current wound care.
		————————————————————— Tammy Durkin, RN

CRITICAL TEST VALUES, REPORTING

According to the Joint Commission on Accreditation of Healthcare Organizations' 2005 National Patient Safety Goals, critical test results must be reported to a responsible licensed caregiver in a timely manner so that immediate action may be taken. Critical test results include diagnostic tests, such as imaging studies, ECGs, laboratory tests, and other diagnostic studies. These critical test results may be reported verbally (including by telephone), and by fax, e-mail, or other technologies. If the results aren't reported verbally, the person sending the results should confirm that they have been received. Critical test values may be reported to another individual (such as a nurse, unit secretary, or doctor's office staff) who will then report the values to the doctor or licensed caregiver.

ESSENTIAL DOCUMENTATION

Record the date and time you received the critical test result, the person who gave the results to you, the name of the test, and the critical value. Document the name of the doctor or licensed health care provider you notified, the time of the notification, the means of communication used, and any orders given. If the message wasn't relayed verbally, include confirmation that the critical test result was received by the doctor. Note any instructions or information given to the patient. If the message was given to a nurse, unit secretary, or office staff personnel, include that individual's name.

6/4/05	1000	Nanette Lange called from pharmacy at 0945 to report critical PT value of 52 seconds. Results reported by telephone to Dr. Potter at 0948, orders given to hold warfarin, obtain PT level in a.m., and call Dr. Potter with results. Pt. informed about elevated PT and the need to hold warfarin until PT levels drop to therapeutic range. Pt. instructed to report any bleeding to nurse. ———————————— Karen Lane, RN

CRITICISM OF CARE IN THE MEDICAL RECORD

Criticism of a colleague's care in the medical record is inappropriate and reflects badly on all members of the health care team. In a court of law, accusations in the medical record can be used to show that the patient received incompetent care.

Report any criticism of your care by another nurse in the medical record to the nursing supervisor. Don't respond to the criticism in the medical record. Moreover, don't alter the medical record in any way because this is considered tampering. Rather, speak privately with the nurse who criticized you and try to work out your differences. Suggest that she fill out an incident report or variance report, and offer to help her write it. If you have questions about the care given by another nurse, talk with her, speak with your supervisor, and file an incident report or variance report.

ESSENTIAL DOCUMENTATION

If you have a problem with the care given by another nurse, objectively record your findings on an incident report or variance report. (See "Incident report," page 219.) Note the date and time you became aware of the problem. Without blaming a colleague, describe what you assessed or witnessed and your interventions. Record the name of the nursing supervisor and doctor who you notified and the time that you notified them.

ACCUCHART

DOCUMENTING INAPPROPRIATE CARE ON AN INCIDENT REPORT

When you witness a reportable event, you must fill out an incident report. Forms vary, but most include the following information.

INCIDENT REPORT

		Name _Greta Manning_
DATE OF INCIDENT	**TIME OF INCIDENT**	Address _7 Worth Way, Boston, MA_
_11-14-05_	_1500_	Phone _(617) 555-1122_

EXACT LOCATION OF INCIDENT (Bldg, Floor, Room No, Area)
4-Main, Rm. 447

Addressograph if patient _____

TYPE OF INCIDENT
(CHECK ONE ONLY) ☑ PATIENT ☐ EMPLOYEE ☐ VISITOR ☐ VOLUNTEER ☐ OTHER (specify)

DESCRIPTION OF THE INCIDENT (WHO, WHAT, WHEN, WHERE, HOW, WHY)
(Use back of form if necessary) _When making rounds at beginning of shift, pt. c/o pain at I.V. site on ℞ forearm. Dressing removed. Skin around I.V. red, warm & tender. Pt. states "I told the day nurse at lunch time. But she didn't do anything." I.V. line removed._

Patient fall incidents	**FLOOR CONDITIONS** ☐ OTHER _____ ☐ CLEAN & SMOOTH ☐ SLIPPERY (WET)	**FRAME OF BED** ☐ LOW ☐ HIGH	**NIGHT LIGHT** ☐ YES ☐ NO
	WERE BED RAILS PRESENT? ☐ NO ☐ 1 UP ☐ 2 UP ☐ 3 UP ☐ 4 UP	**OTHER RESTRAINTS** (TYPE AND EXTENT)	
	AMBULATION PRIVILEGE ☐ UNLIMITED ☐ LIMITED WITH ASSISTANCE ☐ COMPLETE BEDREST ☐ OTHER		
	WERE OPIOIDS, ANALGESICS, HYPNOTICS, SEDATIVES, DIURETICS, ANTIHYPERTENSIVES, OR ANTICONVULSANTS GIVEN DURING LAST 4 HOURS? ☐ YES ☐ NO DRUG	AMOUNT	TIME

Patient incidents	**PHYSICIAN NOTIFIED** Name of Physician _J. Reynolds, MD_	DATE _11-14-05_	TIME _1515_	COMPLETE IF APPLICABLE
Employee incidents	**DEPARTMENT**	**JOB TITLE**	**SOCIAL SECURITY #**	
	MARITAL STATUS			

All incidents	**NOTIFIED** DATE TIME	**LOCATION WHERE TREATMENT WAS RENDERED**
	NAME, ADDRESS AND TELEPHONE NUMBERS OF WITNESS(ES) OR PERSONS FAMILIAR WITH INCIDENT - WITNESS OR NOT	

SIGNATURE OF PERSON PREPARING REPORT	**TITLE**	**DATE OF REPORT**
Connie Smith	_RN_	_11-14-05_

PHYSICIAN'S REPORT — To be completed for all cases involving injury or illness   (Don't use abbreviations.) (Use back of form if necessary.)

DIAGNOSIS AND TREATMENT
Patient with phlebitis at I.V. site on right forearm. Elevate arm, warm soaks for 20 minutes 3 times a day, Tylenol 650 orally every 4 hours for discomfort. ——— J. Reynolds, MD

DISPOSITION

PERSON NOTIFIED OTHER THAN HOSPITAL PERSONNEL	**DATE**	**TIME**
NAME AND ADDRESS _R. Manning (daughter), address same as pt._	_11-14-05_	_1520_
PHYSICIAN'S SIGNATURE	**DATE**	
J. Reynolds, MD	_11-14-05_	

Include the name, address, and telephone number of witnesses, if appropriate. See the sample incident report for documenting problems with the care given by another nurse. (See *Documenting inappropriate care on an incident report.*)

CULTURAL NEEDS IDENTIFICATION

To provide culturally competent care to your patient, you must remember that your patient's cultural behaviors and beliefs may be different than your own. For example, most people in the United States make eye contact when talking with others. However, people in a number of cultures – including Native Americans, Asians, and people from Arab-speaking countries – may find eye contact disrespectful or aggressive. Identifying your patient's cultural needs is the first step in developing a culturally sensitive care plan.

ESSENTIAL DOCUMENTATION

Record the date and time of your assessment. Depending on your facility's policy, cultural assessment may be part of the admission history form or there may be a separate, more in-depth cultural assessment tool. (See *Identifying your patient's cultural needs,* pages 88 to 90.)

Assess the patient's communication style. Find out if he can speak and read English, his ability to read lips, his native language, and whether an interpreter is required. Observe his nonverbal communication style for eye contact, expressiveness, and ability to understand common signs. Determine social orientation, including culture, race, ethnicity, family role function, work, and religion. Document the patient's spatial comfort level, particularly in light of his conversation, proximity to others, body movement, and space perception. Note his skin color and body structure. Ask about food preferences, family health history, religious and cultural health practices, and definitions of health and illness. Determine the patient's time orientation (past, present, or future).

AccuChart

IDENTIFYING YOUR PATIENT'S CULTURAL NEEDS

A transcultural assessment tool can help promote cultural sensitivity in any nursing setting. Consult your facility's policy on the use of such forms, or incorporate the information included in this sample form when developing your client's care plan.

Date _3/12/05_ Time _1015_ Pt name _Claudette Valiente_ Age _34_ ☐ M ☑ F
Medical dx: _36 weeks pregnant, states "high sugar in my blood"_

Communication (language, voice quality, pronunciation, use of silence and nonverbals)
Subjective data
Can you speak English? ☑ Yes ☐ No _____
Can you read English? ☑ Yes ☐ No _with difficulty_
Are you able to read lips? ☐ Yes ☑ No _____
Native language? _Creole_
Do you speak or read any other language? _No_
How do you want to be addressed? ☐ Mr. ☐ Mrs. ☐ Ms. ☑ First name ☐ Nick Name _____

Objective data
How would you characterize the nonverbal communication style? _Very open_
Eye contact: ☐ Direct ☑ Peripheral gaze or no eye contact preferred during interactions
Use of interpreter: ☐ Family ☐ Friend ☐ Professional ☐ Other ☑ None
Overall communication style: ☑ Verbally loud and expressive ☐ Quiet, reserved ☐ Use of silence
Meaning of common signs—O.K., got ya nose, index finger summons, V sign, thumbs up
Understands above signs except "got ya nose"
Determine any familial colloquialisms used by individuals or families that may impact on assessment, treatment, or other interventions. _None noted_

Social orientation (culture, race, ethnicity, family role function, work, leisure, church, and friends)
Subjective data
Country of birth? _Haiti_ Years in this country? _3_
(If an immigrant or a refugee, how long has the patient lived in this country? —You are not questioning citizen status.)
What setting did you grow up in? ☐ Urban ☐ Suburban ☑ Rural
What is your ethnic identity? _Haitian_
What is your race? _Black_
Who are the major support people: ☑ Family members ☐ Friends ☐ Other _____
Who are the dominant family members? _Husband, grandparents_
Who makes major decisions for the family? _A family meeting is held_
Occupation in native country: _None_ Present occupation: _None_
Education? _Finished 6th grade_
Is religion important to you? _Yes_
What is your religious affiliation? _Catholic_ Would you like a chaplain visit? ☐ Yes ☑ No
Any cultural/religious practices/restrictions? If yes, describe _Balancing "hot" and "cold," believes in some voodoo passed down from mother and grandmother_

IDENTIFYING YOUR PATIENT'S CULTURAL NEEDS *(continued)*

Social orientation *(continued)*

Objective data

Interaction with family/significant other — describe   *Animated, physically close, frequent touch, eye contact with family members*

Age and life cycle factors must be considered in interactions with individuals and families (for example, high value placed on the decision of elders, the role of the eldest man or woman in families, or roles and expectation of children within the family).   *Elders highly respected, children expected to be obedient and respectful*

Religious icons on person or in room?   *Wearing cross*

Space (comfort in conversation, proximity to others, body movement, perception of space)
  Use of touch, kissing, and close proximity with family

Subjective data

  Distance maintained from nurse and doctor

Do you have any plans for the future?   *No, believes God will guide her*

What do you consider a proper greeting?   *Kissing and touch with family*

Objective data

☑ Tactile relationships, affectionate & embracing
☐ Non-contact
Personal space?   *Very close with family, maintains 2–3 foot distance from RN*

Biological variations (skin color, body structure, genetic and enzymatic patterns, nutritional preferences and deficiencies)

Subjective data

What type of food do you prefer?   *Rice, beans, plantains*

What type of food do you dislike?   *Yogurt, cottage cheese*

What do you believe promotes health?   *Good spiritual habits, balancing "hot and "cold," and eating well*

Family history of disease?   *Malaria, high blood pressure, "sugar"*

Objective data

Skin color *Deep brown*   Hair type *Coarse*

Environmental control (health practices, values, definitions of health and illness)

Subjective data

What do you think caused your problem? *"Ate wrong foods."*

Do you have an explanation for why it started when it did? *"No."*

What does your sickness do to you; how does it work? *"I don't think anything is wrong, but the doctor does."*

How severe is your sickness? How long do you expect it to last? *"It will go away soon."*

(continued)

IDENTIFYING YOUR PATIENT'S
CULTURAL NEEDS *(continued)*

Environmental control *(continued)*

Subjective data *(continued)*

What problems has your sickness caused you? *"The doctor says my baby is big. But, a big baby is a strong baby."*

What fears do you have about your sickness? *"I have no fear. I will have a healthy baby."*

What kind of treatment do you think you should receive? *"Eating healthy."*

What are the most important results you hope to receive from this treatment? *"A healthy baby."*

What are the health and illness beliefs and practices of the family? *Uses home remedies such as herbs to treat sickness*

What are the most important things you do to keep healthy? *"Eat well."*

Any concerns about health and illness? *"No."*

What types of healing practices do you engage in (hot tea and lemon for cold, copper bracelet for arthritis, magnets)? *"Avoiding spices because they bother the baby, balancing hot and cold"*

Objective data

Describe patient's appearance and surroundings *Patient is clean and neatly groomed. Appears slightly overweight.*

What diseases/disorders are endemic to the culture or country of origin? *Intestinal problems, malnutrition, STDs, TB, sickle cell anemia, htn, cancer, AIDs*

What are the customs and beliefs concerning major life events? *"Pregnant women are treated special. Father of the baby doesn't participate in the birth experience; this is "women's business.""*

Time (use of measures, definitions, social and work time, time orientation — past, present, and future)

Subjective data

Preventative health measures? ☐ Yes ☑ No

Objective data

Time orientation ☐ Present ☑ Past

History of noncompliance, missed appointments? *Often misses appts or arrives late*

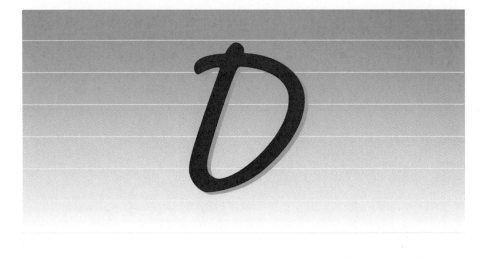

DEATH OF A PATIENT

After a patient dies, care includes preparing him for family viewing, arranging transportation to the morgue or funeral home, and determining the disposition of the patient's belongings. In addition, postmortem care entails comforting and supporting the patient's family and friends and providing them with privacy.

Postmortem care usually begins after a doctor certifies the patient's death. If the patient died violently or under suspicious circumstances, postmortem care may be postponed until the medical examiner completes an examination.

ESSENTIAL DOCUMENTATION

Document the date and time of the patient's death and the name of the doctor (or, in some states, the nurse) who pronounced the death. If resuscitation was attempted, indicate the time it started and ended, and refer to the code sheet in the patient's medical record. Note whether the case is being referred to the medical examiner. Include all postmortem care given, noting whether medical equipment was removed or left in place. List all belongings and valuables and the name of the family member who accepted and signed the appropriate valuables or belongings list. Record any belongings left on the patient. If the patient has dentures, note whether they were left in the patient's mouth or given to a family member. (If given to a family member, include the family member's name.) Document the disposition of the patient's body and the name, telephone number, and address of the funeral home. List the names of family members who were present at the time of death. If the family wasn't present, note the name of the family member notified and who viewed the body. Be sure to include any care, emotional support, and education given to the family.

8/22/05	1420	Called to room by pt.'s daughter, Mrs. Helen Jones, stating pt. not breathing. Pt. found unresponsive in bed at 1345, not breathing, no pulse, no heart or breath sounds auscultated. No code called because pt. has advance directive and DNR order signed in chart. Case not referred to medical examiner. Death pronounce- ment made by Dr. Holmes at 1350. NG tube, Foley catheter, and I.V. line in Ⓛ forearm removed and dressings applied. Pt. bathed and given oral care, dentures placed in mouth, hair combed, and fresh linens and gown applied. Belongings checked off on belongings list and signed by Mrs. Jones, who will take belongings home with her. Body tagged and sent to morgue at 1415. Mrs. Jones is making arrangements with Restful Funeral Home, 123 Main St., Pleasantville, NY (123) 456-7890. Daughter states she's glad her dad isn't suffering any more. Stayed with daughter throughout her visit. Stated she was OK to drive home. Declined visit by chaplain. Said she'll notify other family members who live out of state and won't be viewing body in hospital. ———————————— Jeanne Ballinger, RN

DEHYDRATION, ACUTE

Dehydration refers to the loss of water in the body with a shift in fluid and electrolytes, which can lead to hypovolemic shock, organ failure, and even death. Dehydration may be isotonic, hypertonic, or hypotonic. Common causes of dehydration are fever, diarrhea, and vomiting. Other causes include hemorrhage, excessive diaphoresis, burns, excessive wound or nasogastric drainage, and ketoacidosis. Prompt intervention is necessary to prevent complications, which can include death.

ESSENTIAL DOCUMENTATION

Record the date and time of your entry. Record the results of your physical assessment and any subjective findings. Include laboratory values and the results of any diagnostic tests (such as stool culture to identify the cause of excessive diarrhea). Closely monitor and record intake and output on an intake-output flow sheet. (See "Intake and output," page 230.) Record the name of the doctor notified, the time of notification, and any orders given. Document your interventions, such as I.V. therapy, and the patient's response. Record your actions to prevent complications, such as monitoring for I.V. infiltration and auscultating for breath sounds to detect fluid volume overload. Be sure to document patient education.

| 5/25/05 | 1300 | Pt. admitted to unit from nursing home with increasing lethargy and diarrhea X3 days. Pt. is drowsy, doesn't answer questions, occasionally moans. Skin and mucous membranes dry; tenting occurs when pinched. P 118, BP 92/58, RR 28, rectal T 101.2° F, wt. 102 lb (family reports this is down 3 lb in 3 days). Breath sounds clear, normal heart sounds. Peripheral pulses palpable but weak. No edema. Foley catheter inserted to monitor urine output. Urine sample sent to lab for UA and C&S. Urine color dark amber, specific gravity 1.001. Blood drawn for CBC with diff., BUN, creatinine, and electrolytes. Had approx. 300 ml of liquid stool, guaiac neg., sample sent for C&S. Dr. Holmes in to see pt. and orders written. Pt. placed on cardiac monitor, no arrhythmias noted. Administering O₂ at 2L via NC. I.V. infusion started in ℚ upper forearm with 18G catheter. Infusing NSS at 100 ml/hr. See I/O record and frequent vital signs assessment sheet for hourly VS and hourly I/O. ———————— Michelle Pressman, RN |

DEMENTIA

Dementia, which is also referred to as *senile dementia* or *chronic brain syndrome,* is considered a syndrome rather than a distinctive disease process. It's a progressive deterioration of intellectual performance characterized by memory loss, inability to perform abstract analysis, lack of judgment, and decline in language skills. Changes in personality and the inability to perform activities of daily living (ADLs) progress slowly until they become obvious and devastating over time.

Nursing interventions are focused on helping the patient maintain an optimal level of cognitive performance, preventing physical injury, decreasing anxiety and agitation, increasing communication skills, and promoting the patient's ability to perform ADLs.

ESSENTIAL DOCUMENTATION

Perform a neurologic assessment, as appropriate, including level of consciousness, appearance, behavior, speech, and cognitive function. If appropriate, record the patient's exact responses. Record measures taken to ensure patient safety, meet personal needs, and promote independence, and document the patient's response.

3/3/05	0900	Noted pt. leaving the unit at 0840. When asked where he
		was going, he stated, "To the store. We need groceries."
		While assisting pt. back to room, he kept insisting he had
		to go the store and resisted efforts to bring him back to
		his room. Pt. oriented to name only. Gait steady. Pt.'s
		shirt buttoned wrong, shoes mismatched, hair uncombed.
		Pt. resisting any further neurologic assessment. Dr. New-
		mann notified at 0850 of pt.'s wandering, spoke with
		family and obtained permission for use of wanderguard
		alarm. Alarm band placed on pt.'s wrist. Staff will check
		on pt. q15min and will reorient and redirect pt. as
		needed. ———————————— Charles Bricker, RN

DIABETIC KETOACIDOSIS

Characterized by severe hyperglycemia, diabetic ketoacidosis (DKA) is a potentially life-threatening condition that occurs most commonly in people with type 1 diabetes (formerly known as insulin-dependent diabetes). An acute insulin deficiency precedes DKA, causing glucose to accumulate in the blood. At the same time, the liver responds to energy-starved cells by converting glycogen to glucose, further increasing blood glucose levels. Because the insulin-deprived cells can't utilize glucose, they metabolize protein, which results in the loss of intracellular potassium and phosphorus and excessive liberation of amino acids. The liver converts these amino acids into urea and glucose. The result is grossly elevated blood glucose levels and osmotic diuresis, leading to fluid and electrolyte imbalances and dehydration. Moreover, the absolute insulin deficiency causes cells to convert fats to glycerol and fatty acids for energy. The fatty acids accumulate in the liver, where they're converted to ketones. The ketones accumulate in blood and urine. Acidosis leads to more tissue breakdown, more ketosis and, eventually, shock, coma, and death.

When your assessment reveals signs and symptoms of DKA, you'll need to act quickly to prevent a fatal outcome. Document your frequent assessments and interventions as they occur. Avoid charting in blocks of time. Although frequent notes take time, events will be fresh in your memory. Block charting looks vague, implies inattention to the patient, and makes it hard to determine when specific events occurred.

ESSENTIAL DOCUMENTATION

Record the date and time of your entry. Frequently record your patient's blood glucose levels, intake and output, urine glucose levels, mental status, ketone levels, and vital signs, according to patient condition or unit policy. Depending on the facility, these parameters may be documented on a frequent assessment flow sheet. Record the clinical manifestations of DKA assessed, such as polyuria, polydipsia, polyphagia, Kussmaul's respirations, fruity breath odor, changes in level of consciousness, poor skin turgor, hypotension, hypothermia, and warm, dry skin and mucous membranes. Document all interventions, such as fluid and electrolyte replacement and insulin therapy, and record the patient's response. Record any procedures, such as arterial blood gas analysis, blood samples sent to the laboratory, cardiac monitoring, or insertion of an indwelling urinary catheter. Record results, the names of persons notified, and the time of notification. Include emotional support provided and patient education in your note.

7/11/05	0810	Mr. Jones admitted at 0730 with serum blood glucose
		level of 900. Pt. c/o thirst, nausea, vomiting, and excessive urination. Urine positive for ketones. P 112, BP 94/58, RR 28 deep and rapid, oral T 96.8° F. Skin warm, dry, with tenting when pinched. Mucous membranes dry. Resting with eyes closed. Confused to time and date. Pt. states, "I didn't take my insulin for 2 days because I ran out." Dr. Bernhart notified and came to see pt. Blood sample sent to lab for ABG, electrolytes, BUN, creatinine, serum glucose, CBC. Urine obtained and sent for UA. O₂ 2 L via NC started with O₂ sat. 94% by pulse oximetry. 1000 ml of NSS being infused over 1 hr through I.V. line in ® forearm. 100 units I.V. bolus of regular insulin infused through I.V. line in ① antecubital followed by a cont. infusion of 100 units regular insulin in 100 ml NSS at 5 units/hr. Monitoring blood glucose with q1hr fingersticks. Next due at 0900. See frequent parameter flow sheet for I/O, VS, and blood glucose results. Notified diabetes educator, Teresa Mooney, RN, about pt.'s admission and the need for reinforcing diabetes regimen. ———— Louise May, RN

DIAGNOSTIC TESTING

Before receiving a diagnosis, most patients undergo testing, which could be as simple as a blood test or as complicated as magnetic resonance imaging.

ESSENTIAL DOCUMENTATION

Begin documenting diagnostic testing by making notes about any preliminary assessments you make of a patient's condition. For example, if your patient is pregnant or has certain allergies, record this information because it might affect the test or test result. If the patient's age, illness, or disability requires special preparation for the test, enter this information in his chart as well.

Always prepare the patient for the test, and document any teaching you've done about the test and any follow-up care associated with it. Be sure to document the administration or withholding of drugs and preparations, special diets, food or fluid restrictions, enemas, and specimen collection.

3/18/05	0700	24-hour urine test for creatinine clearance started. Pt. taught purpose of the test and how to collect urine. Sign placed on pt.'s door and in bathroom. Urine placed on ice in bathroom. ———————— Paul Steadman, RN

DIETARY RESTRICTION NONCOMPLIANCE

All mentally competent adults may legally refuse treatment, including following dietary restrictions. The patient or family may tell you about noncompliance, or you may suspect noncompliance based on test results, such as blood glucose levels or blood pressure readings. The patient may be noncompliant with diet for many reasons, including lack of motivation; lack of understanding; high cost of fresh fruits, vegetables, and specially prepared foods; lack of support; incompatibility with lifestyle, religion, or culture; lack of transportation to stores; unfamiliarity with new food preparation and cooking techniques; and diminished sense of taste.

Assess your patient to determine his reasons for not complying with dietary restrictions. Help him develop a plan that will be compatible with his needs and cognitive ability. Explain the relationship between proper nutrition and health. Teach about the consequences of not complying with dietary restrictions. Refer the patient to the dietitian for consultation and teaching. He may need a social services consult if finances are a problem. The home care department may be able to arrange for a home delivery meal service, such as Meals On Wheels, if the patient can't shop or prepare meals. Arrange for follow-up care and provide the patient with the names and telephone numbers of people to call with questions and concerns.

ESSENTIAL DOCUMENTATION

Document noncompliance objectively. Use the patient's own words, if appropriate, or describe the data that suggest noncompliance. Record the reasons for the noncompliance. Document your teaching about the diet, its relationship to the patient's medical problem, and the consequences of noncompliance. Include the patient's response to the teaching. Record the date and time of health care referrals made and the names of agencies and persons to whom the patient was referred.

5/15/05	1500	Pt. found in room eating a large piece of chocolate cake. Pt. is on 1800-calorie ADA diet. Discussed with Mr. Jones the importance of proper nutrition in the treatment of diabetes. Pointed out that his blood glucose levels by fingerstick have been elevated. Mr. Jones states, "I understand the importance of diet, but I'm frustrated with the food I'm getting in the hospital. I usually have a small dessert and sugar-free soda with my meals. They haven't been giving this to me here." Dietitian Pam Walker, RD, notified and will make changes in diet to provide for these items in caloric intake. She made an appt. to see Mr. and Mrs. Jones tomorrow at 1000 to review pt.'s diet and reinforce teaching. Dr. Benton called and approved diet changes. ———————————— May Brown, RN

DIFFICULT PATIENT

No doubt you've cared for dissatisfied patients and heard remarks like the following: "I've been ringing and ringing for a nurse. I could have died before you got here!" or "I've never seen such filth in my life. What kind of a hospital is this, anyway?" These are the sounds of unhappy patients. If you dismiss them, you may be increasing your risk of a lawsuit.

The first step in defusing a potentially troublesome situation is to recognize that it exists. Note the following signs of a difficult patient: constant grumpiness, endless complaints, no response to friendly remarks, and journaling of situations he views as wrong or causing him unnecessary distress. Use statements such as "You seem angry. Let's talk about what's bothering you." After acknowledging the situation, continue to reach out to the patient, even if you don't get a positive response. Never argue with the patient or try to convince him that a situation didn't happen the way he thinks it did. Don't make judgments, and don't become defensive. Your patient just needs reassurance that you'll try your best to improve the situation.

ESSENTIAL DOCUMENTATION

Document the patient's complaints using his own words in quotes. Record the specific care given to your patient in direct response to complaints. If the patient threatens to file suit against you or the hospital, document this and notify your nursing supervisor or your facility's legal department. Record details of your contacts with the patient. Update your care plan to include more frequent contact with the patient.

| 10/16/05 | 1500 | Pt. stated, "No one comes when I ask for pain medication or when I put on my call light to go to the bathroom. Doesn't anyone work around here?" Calmly reminded pt. that she couldn't receive pain medication any earlier because it wasn't 4 hours since last dose. Administered morphine sulfate 2 mg I.V. at 1445 for c/o incisional pain rated as 8 on a scale of 0 to 10, w/ 10 being worst pain imaginable. At 1500 pt. reported pain as 2 out of 10. Reassured pt. that nurse will assess pain and administer pain medication on time if needed. Also assisted pt. to the bathroom and told her a nurse would check on her every 1½ hours or at a time specified by her. Nursing care plan updated accordingly. ———— Sue Stiles, RN |
| | 1630 | Pt. reports pain is 4/10, states she doesn't want any pain medication as this time. Reassured pt. that nurse will continue to reassess pain and administer pain medication on time as needed. Assisted pt. to more comfortable position on Ⓛ side. Pt. responded to interaction by thanking nurse for checking in. Pt. reports not needing assistance to the bathroom at this time. ———————— Sue Stiles, RN |

DISCHARGE INSTRUCTIONS

Hospitals today commonly discharge patients earlier than they did in years past. As a result, the patient and his family must change dressings; assess wounds; deal with medical equipment, tube feedings, and I.V. lines; and perform other functions that a nurse traditionally performed.

To perform these functions properly, the patient and his home caregiver must receive adequate instruction. The nurse is usually responsible for these instructions. If a patient receives improper instructions and injury results, you could be held liable.

Many hospitals distribute printed instruction sheets that adequately describe treatments and home care procedures. The patient's chart should indicate which materials were given and to whom. Generally, the patient or responsible person must sign that he received and understood the discharge instructions.

Courts typically consider these teaching materials evidence that instruction took place. However, to support testimony that instructions were given, the materials should be tailored to each patient's specific needs and refer to any verbal or written instructions that were provided. If caregivers practice procedures with the patient and family in the hospital, this should be documented, too, along with the results.

ESSENTIAL DOCUMENTATION

Many facilities combine discharge summaries and patient instructions in one form. This form contains sections for recording patient assessment, patient education, detailed special instructions, and the circumstances of discharge. (See *The discharge summary form,* page 100.)

When writing a narrative note about discharge instructions, include the following information:

- date and time of discharge
- family members or caregivers present for teaching
- treatments, such as dressing changes, or use of medical equipment
- signs and symptoms to report to the doctor
- patient, family, or caregiver understanding of instructions or ability to give a return demonstration of procedures
- whether a patient or caregiver requires further instruction
- doctor's name and telephone number
- date, time, and location of any follow-up appointments or the need to call the doctor for a follow-up appointment
- details of instructions given to the patient, including medications, activity, and diet (include any written instructions given to patient).

12/1/05	1530	Pt. to be discharged today. Reviewed discharge instructions with pt. and wife. Reviewed all medications, including drug name, purpose, doses, administration times, routes, and adverse effects. Drug information sheets given to pt. Pt. able to verbalize proper use of medications. Wife will be performing dressing change to pt.'s Ⓛ foot. Wife was able to change dressing properly using sterile technique. Pt. and wife were able to state signs and symptoms of infections to report to doctor. Also reinforced low-cholesterol, low-sodium diet and progressive walking guidelines. Wife has many questions about diet and will meet with dietitian before discharge. Pt. understands he's to follow up with Dr. Carney in his office on 12/8/05 at 1400. Wrote doctor's phone number on written instructions. Written discharge instructions given to pt. ———————— Marcy Smythe, RN

THE DISCHARGE SUMMARY FORM

By combining the patient's discharge summary with instructions for care after discharge, you can fulfill two requirements with a single form. When using this documentation method, be sure to give one copy to the patient and keep one for the legal record.

DISCHARGE INSTRUCTIONS

1. Summary *Tara Nicholas is a 55-year-old woman admitted with complaints of severe headache and hypertensive crisis.*
Treatment: Nitroprusside gtt for 24 hours
Started Lopressor for hypertension
Recommendation: Lose 10–15 lb
Follow low-sodium, low-cholesterol diet

2. Allergies *penicillin*

3. Medications (drug, dose time) *Lopressor 25 mg at 6 a.m. and 6 p.m.*
temazepam 15 mg at 10 p.m.

4. Diet *Low-sodium, low-cholesterol*

5. Activity *As tolerated*

6. Discharged to *Home*

7. If questions arise, contact Dr. *James Pritchett*   **Telephone No.** *(233) 555-1448*

8. Special instructions *Call doctor with headaches, dizziness*

9. Return visit Dr. *Pritchett*   **Place** *Health Care Clinic*

On Date *12/15/05*   **Time** *0845 a.m.*

Tara Nicholas
Signature of patient or person responsible for receipt of instructions from doctors

JE Pritchett, MD
Signature of doctor or nurse reviewing instructions

DO-NOT-RESUSCITATE ORDER

When a patient is terminally ill and death is expected, his doctor and family (and the patient if appropriate) may agree that a do-not-resuscitate (DNR), or no-code, order is appropriate. The doctor writes the order, and the staff carries it out if the patient goes into cardiac or respiratory arrest.

Because DNR orders are recognized legally, you'll incur no liability if you don't try to resuscitate a patient and that patient later dies. You may, however, incur liability if you initiate resuscitation on a patient who has a DNR order.

Every patient with a DNR order should have a written order on file. The order should be consistent with the facility's policy, which commonly requires that such orders be reviewed every 48 to 72 hours.

Increasingly, patients are deciding in advance of a crisis whether they want to be resuscitated. Health care facilities must provide written information to patients concerning their rights under state law to make decisions regarding their care, including the right to refuse medical treatment and the right to formulate an advance directive.

This information must be provided to all patients upon admission. You must also document that the patient received this information and whether he brought a written advance directive with him. (See "Advance directive," page 9.) In some instances, you can file a photocopy of the directive in the patient's record.

ESSENTIAL DOCUMENTATION

If a terminally ill patient without a DNR order tells you that he doesn't want to be resuscitated in a crisis, document his statement as well as his degree of awareness and orientation. Then contact the patient's doctor and your nursing supervisor and ask for assistance from administration, legal services, or social services.

As a nurse, you have a responsibility to help the patient make an informed decision about continuing treatment. If the patient's wishes differ from those of his family or doctor, make sure the discrepancies are thoroughly recorded in the chart. Then document that you notified your nursing supervisor, legal services, or social services.

6/19/05	1700	Pt. stated, "If my heart should stop or if I stop breathing, just let me go. I've suffered with this cancer long enough. I've lived a full life and have no regrets." Pt.'s wife was present for this conversation and stated, "I don't want to see him in pain anymore. If he feels he doesn't want any heroic measures, then I stand by his decision." Pt. is alert and oriented to time, place, and person. Dr. Patel notified of pt.'s wishes concerning resuscitation and stated he'll be in this evening to discuss DNR status with pt. and wife and write DNR orders. Elizabeth Sawyer, nursing supervisor, notified of pt.'s wishes for no resuscitation. —— Joan Byers, RN

DOCTOR'S ORDERS, CLARIFICATION OF

Although unit secretaries may transcribe orders, the nurse is ultimately responsible for the accuracy of the transcription. Only you have the authority and knowledge to question the validity of orders and to spot errors.

Follow your health care facility's policy for clarifying orders that are vague, ambiguous, or possibly erroneous. If you don't have a policy to cover a particular situation, contact the prescribing doctor and always document your actions. Then ask your nurse administrator for a step-by-step policy to follow so you'll know what to do if the situation ever recurs.

An order may be correct when issued but improper later because of changes in the patient's status. When this occurs, delay treatment until you've contacted the doctor and clarified the situation. Follow your facility's policy for clarifying an order.

Document your efforts to clarify the order, and document whether the order was carried out.

ESSENTIAL DOCUMENTATION

When you question a doctor's order, document your assessment and other data leading you to question the order. Record your conversation with the doctor and whether the order was carried out. Also, note whether the order was clarified or rewritten. If you refuse to carry out an order you believe to be written in error, record your refusal, your reasons for refusing, the names of the doctor and nursing supervisor you notified, the time of notification, and their responses.

9/7/05	1235	Order written by Dr. Corrigan at 1155 for Darvocet N 1
		tab P.O. q4hr prn incision pain. Called Dr. Corrigan at 1210
		to clarify Darvocet dose. Order should read Darvocet N
		100 P.O. q4hr prn incision pain. Clarification written on
		dr.'s orders and faxed to pharmacy. Dose changed on
		MAR. ————————————— Penelope Green, RN

DOCTOR'S ORDERS, FAXING

The doctor may use a facsimile, or fax, machine to transmit patient orders. Faxing has two main advantages: It speeds transmittal of the doctor's orders, and it reduces the likelihood of errors. When you receive a doctor's order by fax, place the fax in the patient's medical record, and transcribe the order onto the doctor's order sheet if your facility requires this. The order is then carried out like any other order.

ESSENTIAL DOCUMENTATION

Record the faxed order on the doctor's order sheet as soon as possible. Note the date and time, and then copy the order as written on the fax. On the next line, write "faxed order." Then write the doctor's name, and sign your name. Draw lines through blank spaces in the order.

12/14/05	1300	Ferrous sulfate 300 mg P.O. b.i.d. ———————
		——————— Faxed order Dr. Beastly/Holly Ivers, RN

DOCTOR'S ORDERS, ILLEGIBLE

Doctors have a responsibility to write orders that are medically correct, complete, and legible. If you can't read a doctor's order, don't guess what it says. This puts your patient at risk for harm and makes you vulnerable to a lawsuit.

When you can't read a doctor's order, contact him immediately to clarify the order. If you can't reach the doctor, notify your nursing supervisor. Ideally, you should review a doctor's orders with him before he leaves the unit.

ESSENTIAL DOCUMENTATION

Date your entry. Record the time of each attempt you made to contact the doctor for clarification of the illegible order. Note how you attempted to reach the doctor, such as placing a call to the office, answering service, or pager. Document clarification of the order with the doctor. After you clarify the order, transcribe it. Note that it's a clarification of a previous order.

| 8/2/05 | 1810 | Unable to read handwriting in order written by Dr. Bellows at 1800. Paged doctor for clarification. ——— ———————————————————— Tina Miota, RN |
| | 1820 | Received telephone call from Dr. Bellows clarifying order written at 1800. Order should read: gentamicin 6.5 mg I.V. q 12hr. ——————————— Tina Miota, RN |

| 8/2/05 | 1900 | Clarification of order by Dr. Bellows for gentamicin ordered 8/2/05 at 1800. Gentamicin 6.5 mg I.V. q 12 hr. ——————————— T.O. order Dr. Bellows/Tina Miota, RN |

DOCTOR'S ORDERS, PREPRINTED

Many health care facilities use preprinted order forms to make doctor's orders easier to read and interpret. Such forms are especially useful for commonly performed procedures such as cardiac catheterization. As with other standardized documents, blanks are used for information that must be individualized according to the patient's needs.

If your facility uses these forms, don't assume they're flawless just because they're preprinted. You may still need to clarify an order by discussing it with the doctor who gave it. (See *Guidelines for using preprinted order forms.*)

ESSENTIAL DOCUMENTATION

Before transcribing orders from a preprinted order form, make sure the doctor has written in the date, time, the patient's full name, and any allergies. Check that all blanks are filled in and individualized to the patient. After you've reviewed the orders and determined that they're complete, record the date and time, and sign your full name and credentials.

Review *Preprinted orders,* page 106, for an example of documentation.

GUIDELINES FOR USING PREPRINTED ORDER FORMS

When documenting the execution of a doctor's preprinted order, make sure that you've interpreted and carried out the order correctly. Even though these forms aim to prevent problems (caused by illegible handwriting, for example), they may still be misread. Here are some considerations for using preprinted forms.

INSIST ON APPROVED FORMS

Use only preprinted order forms that have your health care facility's approval and the seal of approval of the medical records committee. Most facilities stamp or print an identification number or code on the form. When in doubt, call the medical records department—the doctor may be using a form he developed or one provided by a drug manufacturer.

REQUIRE COMPLIANCE WITH POLICIES

To enhance communication and continuity, a preprinted order form needs to comply with facility policies and other regulations. For example, a postoperative preprinted order form shouldn't say "Renew all previous orders" if facility policy requires specific orders. It also shouldn't allow you to select a drug dose from a range ("meperidine 50 to 100 mg I.M. q 4 hr," for example) if that's prohibited in your state. Alert your nurse-manager if any order form requires you to perform duties that are outside your scope of practice.

MAKE SURE THE FORM IS COMPLETED CORRECTLY

Many preprinted order forms list more orders than the doctor wants you to follow, so he'll need to indicate which specific interventions he's ordering. For example, he may check the appropriate orders, put his initials next to them, or cross out those he doesn't want.

ASK FOR CLARITY AND PRECISION

Make sure that the doctor orders drug doses in the unit of measure in which they're dispensed. For example, make sure that the form uses the metric system instead of the error-prone apothecary system. Report any errors to your nurse-manager.

PROMOTE PROPER NOMENCLATURE

Ask doctors to use generic drug names, especially when more than one brand of a generic drug is available (for example, "acetaminophen" instead of "Tylenol"). If only one brand of a drug is available, its name can be included in parentheses after the generic name—for example, "dobutamine (Dobutrex)."

TAKE STEPS TO AVOID MISINTERPRETATION

Unapproved, potentially dangerous abbreviations and symbols—such as q.d., U, and q.o.d.—don't belong on preprinted order forms. Improper spacing between a drug name and its dosage can also contribute to medication errors. For example, a 20-mg dose of Inderal written as "Inderal20 mg" could be misinterpreted as 120 mg. (See "Abbreviations to avoid," page 478.)

ENSURE THAT THE COPY IS READABLE

If your facility uses a no-carbon-required form, make sure that the bottom copy contains an identical set of preprinted orders; this is the copy that goes to the pharmacy. All lines on the bottom copy should also appear on the top copy—extra lines on the pharmacy copy can hide decimal points (making 1.5 look like 15, for example) and the tops of numbers (making 7 look like 1 and 5 look like 3).

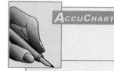

PREPRINTED ORDERS

The following is an example of a preprinted form for charting doctor's orders. This form specifies the treatment for a patient who's about to undergo cardiac catheterization.

DOCTOR'S ORDERS

Name: *Thomas Smith*

ID number: *0135461*

Allergies: *None known*

Date/Time	PRECARDIAC CATHETERIZATION ORDERS:
12/7/05 1330	1. NPO after *midnight* except for medications.
	2. Shave and prep right and left groin areas.
	3. Premedications:
	Benadryl *25* mg ⎫
	Xanax *0.5* mg ⎭ P.O. on call to Cath lab
	4. Have ECG, PT, PTT, creatinine, Hgb, HCT, and platelet count
	on chart before sending the patient to the Cath lab.
	5. Have patient void before leaving for the Cath lab.
	——————————————————— *Mona Jones, MD*
12/7/05 1400	——————————————————— *Susan Smith, RN*

DOCTOR'S ORDERS, QUESTIONABLE

Most nurse practice acts state that you have a legal duty to carry out a doctor's orders. Yet, as a licensed professional, you also have an ethical and legal duty to use your own judgment when providing patient care. If a doctor's order seems vague or even wrong, follow your facility's policy for clarifying the order. If there's no policy, contact the prescribing doctor and discuss your concerns. If you can't resolve the problem, notify your nursing supervisor. (See *Questioning a doctor's order.*)

ESSENTIAL DOCUMENTATION

Record the name of the doctor you notified and the date and time of notification. Document your concerns, the doctor's response, and whether

QUESTIONING A DOCTOR'S ORDER

An order may be correct when issued but incorrect later because of changes in the patient's status. When this occurs, delay the treatment until you've contacted the doctor and clarified the situation.

FAILURE TO QUESTION

In *Poor Sisters of Saint Francis Seraph of the Perpetual Adoration, et al. v. Catron (1982)*, a hospital was sued for negligence because a nurse failed to question a doctor's order regarding an endotracheal tube.

The doctor ordered that the tube be left in place for 5 days instead of the standard 2 to 3 days. The nurse knew that 5 days was exceptionally long but, instead of questioning the doctor's order and documenting her actions, she followed the order. As a result, the patient's larynx was irreparably damaged, and the court ruled the hospital negligent.

you carried out the order. If you refuse to carry out an order, document your refusal, including the reasons you refused, your communications with the doctor, the name of the nursing supervisor you notified of your refusal, and her response.

| 1/22/06 | 1330 | Dr. Howard ordered Tylenol 650 mg P.O. q4hr around the clock for pain. Pt. also taking Allerest for allergy symptoms, exceeding the maximum daily dosage of 4 g acetaminophen. Notified Dr. Howard of excess dosage. Orders given to stop Tylenol and start ibuprofen 300 mg P.O. q6hr. Orders transcribed and faxed to pharmacy. —— Joan Roberts, RN |

DOCTOR'S ORDERS, REFUSAL TO CARRY OUT

If you believe a doctor's order is inappropriate, contact the doctor and communicate your concerns along with your rationales. You may discuss the medical soundness of the order and the scientific rationale with a trusted colleague before contacting the doctor. If you and the doctor can't resolve the conflict, contact your nursing supervisor to discuss the situation. If you and the nursing supervisor agree that the order is inappropriate, contact the doctor to request clarification of the order. If the order remains unchanged, tell the doctor that you refuse to carry out the order. You or the nursing supervisor may consult the chief of service or medical director about your concerns. The chief of service or medical director commonly has the responsibility to contact the doctor to discuss the order. The goal is resolution of the conflict with written orders that are medically sound and appropriate for the patient's condition.

ESSENTIAL DOCUMENTATION

Many facilities have a form that's used to document a nurse's refusal to carry out a doctor's order. On this form, or in a letter to your nursing supervisor, document the order in question, your rationale for refusing to carry out the order (including patient data and assessments), and discussions with the doctor. Include the time, the names of the nursing supervisor and the chief of service or medical director notified, and their responses. This form or letter should be reviewed with the risk management department or legal services.

Documentation in the medical record should be confined to interventions that directly affect the patient's care. Discussions and conferences regarding the clarification of orders aren't necessary in the patient's medical record unless they're relevant to the care that the patient received or an order that wasn't implemented.

TO: Lauren Peachy, RN
FROM: Susan Smith, RN
At 1200 on 9/4/05
I received an order for Amy Kratz for "Gentamicin 100 mg I.V. every 12 hours."
The infant's weight is 4 kg. The drug literature states that the dosage for an infant is 5 mg/kg/day. Based on this information, the infant should receive 10 mg I.V. every 12 hours. Doctor phoned and order clarified that, based on drug literature information, the infant should receive 10 mg not 100 mg. Doctor stated "Administer the gentamicin as I ordered it." I replied that I wouldn't carry out the order and that I'm referring it to my supervisor.
    I called supervisor, Ms. Burke, at 1215 and reported concerns about the gentamicin order. Supervisor calculated drug requirement and determined that, based on the infant's weight, the dosage should be 10 mg I.V. Supervisor stated that she would phone the doctor and, if necessary, the chief of service. ———— Susan Smith, RN

DOCTOR'S ORDERS, TELEPHONE

Ideally, you should accept only written orders from a doctor. However, when your patient needs immediate treatment and the doctor isn't available to write an order, telephone orders are acceptable. Telephone orders may also be taken to expedite care when new information, such as laboratory data, is available that doesn't require a physical examination. Keep in mind that telephone orders are for the patient's well-being and not strictly for convenience. They should be given directly to you, rather than through a third party. Carefully follow your facility's policy on accepting and documenting a telephone order. When you receive a telephone order, write it down immediately and then read it back to the person who gave you the order for verification.

ESSENTIAL DOCUMENTATION

Record the telephone order on the doctor's order sheet while the doctor is still on the telephone. Note the date and time. Write the order verbatim. On the next line, write "T.O." for telephone order. (Don't use "P.O." for phone order; that abbreviation could be misinterpreted to mean "by mouth.") Note that you read the order back and received confirmation that it's correct. Write the doctor's name and sign your name. If another nurse listened to the order with you, have her sign the order, too. Draw lines through any blank spaces in the order.

Make sure the doctor countersigns the order within the set time limits. Without his signature, you may be held liable for practicing medicine without a license.

12/4/05	0900	Demerol 75 mg and Vistaril 50 mg I.M. now for pain.
		Order read back to Dr. White, who confirmed it.
		———————— T.O. Dr. White/Cathy Phillips, RN

DOCTOR'S ORDERS, VERBAL

Errors made interpreting or documenting verbal orders can lead to mistakes in patient care and liability problems for you. Clearly, verbal orders can be a necessity, especially if you're providing home health care. However, in a health care facility, try to take verbal orders only in an emergency, and according to facility policy, when the doctor can't immediately attend to the patient.

In most cases, do-not-resuscitate and no-code orders shouldn't be taken verbally. Carefully follow your facility's policy for documenting a verbal order, and use a special form if one exists.

ESSENTIAL DOCUMENTATION

If possible, write the order out while the doctor is still present. Read the order back for verification and note it in the chart. Note the date and time, and record the order verbatim. On the following line, write "V.O."

for verbal order. Write the doctor's name and the name of the nurse who read the order back to the doctor. Sign your name, and draw a line for the doctor to sign. Draw lines through any spaces between the order and your verification of the order. Record the type of drug, dosage, time you administered it, and any other information your facility's policy requires.

Make sure the doctor countersigns the order within the time limits set by your facility's policy. Without this countersignature, you may be held liable for practicing medicine without a license.

| 3/23/05 | 1500 | V.O. by Dr. Blackstone taken for Digoxin 0.125 mg P.O. now and daily in a.m. Furosemide 40 mg P.O. now and daily starting in a.m. Order read back and confirmed. ———————————— Judith Schilling, RN & ———————————— Carla Roy, RN ———————————— Doctor's signature |

DOCTOR'S ORDERS, WRITTEN

No matter who transcribes a doctor's orders — a registered nurse, licensed practical nurse, or unit secretary — a second person needs to double-check the transcription for accuracy. Your unit should also have some method of checking for transcription errors, such as performing 8-hour or 24-hour chart checks.

When checking a patient's order sheet, always make sure the orders were written for the intended patient. Occasionally, an order sheet stamped with one patient's identification plate will inadvertently be placed in another patient's chart. By double-checking, you'll avert potential mistakes.

ESSENTIAL DOCUMENTATION

Night-shift nurses usually do the 24-hour check by placing a line across the order sheet to indicate that all orders above the line have been checked. They also sign and date the sheet to verify that they've done the 24-hour medication check. The nurse caring for the patient will perform the 8-hour check.

1/12/06	1520	Digoxin 0.125 mg P.O. daily Dr. Johnson ———————— ———————————— Mary Bookbinder, RN
1/12/06	1945	Lasix 40 mg I.V. X 1 now, Dr. Johnson ———— Thomas Colley, RN
1/13/06	0020	24-hour order check. ———————— Tanya Fielding, RN

DRUG ADMINISTRATION

Your employer probably includes a medication administration record (MAR) in your documentation system. Commonly included in a card file (a medication Kardex) or on a separate medication administration sheet, the MAR is the central record of medication orders and their execution and is part of the patient's permanent record.

ESSENTIAL DOCUMENTATION

When using the MAR, follow these guidelines:
- Know and follow your facility's policies and procedures for recording drug orders and charting drug administration.
- Make sure all drug orders include the patient's full name; the date; and the drug's name, dosage, administration route or method, and frequency. When appropriate, include the specific number of doses given or the stop date.
- Be sure to include drug allergy information.
- Write legibly.
- Use only standard abbreviations approved by your facility. When doubtful about an abbreviation, write out the word or phrase.
- After administering the first dose, sign your full name, licensure status, and initials in the appropriate space on the MAR.
- Record drugs immediately after administration so that another nurse doesn't give the drug again.
- If you document by computer, chart your information for each drug immediately after you administer it. This is particularly important if you don't use printouts as a backup. By keying in information immediately, you ensure that all health care team members have access to the latest drug administration data for the patient.
- If a specific assessment parameter must be monitored during administration of a drug, document this requirement on the MAR. For example, when digoxin is administered, the patient's pulse rate needs to be monitored and charted on the MAR.

See *The medication Kardex,* pages 112 and 113, for proper documentation of medications.

(Text continues on page 114.)

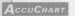

THE MEDICATION KARDEX

One type of Kardex is the medication Kardex. It contains a permanent record of the patient's medications. The medication Kardex may also include the patient's diagnosis and information about allergies and diet. Routine and p.r.n. drugs may be on separate forms. A sample form is shown below.

NAME: *Jack Lemmons*   MEDICAL RECORD #: *1234567*

NURSE'S FULL SIGNATURE, STATUS, AND INITIALS					
Roy Charles, RN	INIT. *RC*		INIT.		INIT.
Theresa Hopkins, RN	*TH*				

DIAGNOSIS: *Heart failure, atrial flutter, COPD*

ALLERGIES: *ASA*   DIET: *Cardiac*

ROUTINE/DAILY ORDERS.			DATE: *1/24*		DATE: *1/25*		DATE: *1/26*		DATE: *1/27*		DATE: *1/28*		DATE: *1/29*		DATE: *1/30*	
ORDER DATE	MEDICATIONS DOSE, ROUTE, FREQUENCY	TIME	SITE	INT.	SITE	INT.	SITE	INT.	SITE	INT.	SITE	INT.	SITE	INT.	SITE	INT.
1/24/06	*digoxin 0.125 mg*	*0900*	℞ *subclavian*	*RC*		℞⃝										
RC	*I.V. daily*	*HR*	*68*		*52*											
1/24/06	*furosemide 40 mg*	*0900*	℞ *subclavian*	*RC*	℞ *subclavian*	*RC*										
RC	*I.V. q12hr*	*2100*	℞ *subclavian*	*TH*												
1/24/06	*enalaprilat 1.25 mg*	*0511*	℞ *subclavian*	*TH*	℞ *subclavian*	*TH*										
RC	*I.V. q6hr*	*1100*	℞ *subclavian*	*RC*												
		1700	℞ *subclavian*	*RC*												

THE MEDICATION KARDEX *(continued)*

					P.R.N. MEDICATION			
	Addressograph			ALLERGIES: ASA				
INITIAL	SIGNATURE & STATUS	INITIAL	SIGNATURE & STATUS	INITIAL	SIGNATURE & STATUS	INITIAL	SIGNATURE & STATUS	
RC	Roy Charles, RN							
TH	Theresa Hopkins, RN							

YEAR 20 06 — P.R.N. MEDICATIONS

ORDER DATE: 1/24	RENEWAL DATE: /	DISCONTINUED DATE: /	DATE	1/24								
MEDICATION: acetaminophen		DOSE: 650 mg	TIME GIVEN	0930								
DIRECTION: p.r.n. mild pain		ROUTE: P.O.	SITE	P.O.								
			INIT.	RC								

ORDER DATE: 1/24	RENEWAL DATE: 1/26	DISCONTINUED DATE: /	DATE	1/24								
MEDICATION: morphine sulfate		DOSE: 2 mg	TIME GIVEN	0930								
DIRECTION: 15 min prior to changing ® heel dressing		ROUTE: I.V.	SITE	® subclavian								
			INIT.	RC								

ORDER DATE: 1/24	RENEWAL DATE: /	DISCONTINUED DATE: /	DATE	1/24								
MEDICATION: Milk of Magnesia		DOSE: 30 ml	TIME GIVEN	2115								
DIRECTION: q6hr p.r.n.		ROUTE: P.O.	SITE	® subclavian								
			INIT.	TH								

ORDER DATE: 1/25	RENEWAL DATE: /	DISCONTINUED DATE: 1/25	DATE	1/25	1/25							
MEDICATION: prochlorperazine		DOSE: 5 mg	TIME GIVEN	1100	2230							
DIRECTION: q8hr p.r.n.		ROUTE: P.O.	SITE	® glut.	® glut.							
p.r.n. nausea and vomiting			INIT.	RC	TH							

ORDER DATE: 1/25	RENEWAL DATE: /	DISCONTINUED DATE: 1/25	DATE	1/25								
MEDICATION: fluzone		DOSE: 0.5 ml	TIME GIVEN	1100								
DIRECTION: x1 dose only		ROUTE: I.M.	SITE	® delt.								
			INIT.	RC								

ORDER DATE: 1/25	RENEWAL DATE: /	DISCONTINUED DATE: 1/25	DATE	1/25								
MEDICATION: furosemide		DOSE: 40 mg	TIME GIVEN	1300								
DIRECTION: stat now		ROUTE: I.V.	SITE	® subclavian								
			INIT.	RC								

ORDER DATE: /	RENEWAL DATE: /	DISCONTINUED DATE: /	DATE									
MEDICATION:		DOSE:	TIME GIVEN									
DIRECTION:		ROUTE:	SITE									
			INIT.									

DRUG ADMINISTRATION, ADVERSE EFFECTS OF

Also called a *side effect,* an adverse drug effect is an undesirable response that may be mild, severe, or life-threatening. Any clinically useful drug can cause an adverse effect.

As a nurse, you play a key role in reporting adverse drug effect events. Reporting adverse effects helps ensure the safety of drugs regulated by the Food and Drug Administration (FDA). The FDA's Medical Products Reporting Program supplies health care professionals with MedWatch forms on which they can report adverse events.

Complete a MedWatch form when you suspect that a drug is responsible for:

- death
- life-threatening illness
- initial or prolonged hospitalization
- disability
- congenital anomaly
- need for any medical or surgical intervention to prevent a permanent impairment or an injury.

Also, promptly inform the FDA of product quality problems, such as:

- defective devices
- inaccurate or unreadable product labels
- packaging or product mix-ups
- intrinsic or extrinsic contamination or stability problems
- particulates in injectable drugs
- product damage.

ESSENTIAL DOCUMENTATION

When filing a MedWatch form, keep in mind that you aren't expected to establish a connection between the drug and the problem. You don't have to include a lot of details; you only have to report the adverse event or the problem with the drug.

What's more, you don't even have to wait until the evidence seems compelling. FDA regulations protect your identity and the identities of your patient and employer. Send completed forms to the FDA by using the fax number or mailing address on the form. For voluntary reporting,

AccuChart

MEDWATCH FORM FOR
REPORTING ADVERSE DRUG REACTIONS

MEDWATCH
THE FDA MEDICAL PRODUCTS REPORTING PROGRAM

For **VOLUNTARY** reporting by health professionals of adverse events and product problems

Page ___ of ___

Form Approved: OMB No. 0910-0291 Expires: 4/30/96
See OMB statement on reverse

FDA Use Only
Triage unit sequence #

A. Patient information

1. Patient identifier	2. Age at time of event:	3. Sex	4. Weight
01234	or _____	☑ female	_____ lbs
In confidence	Date of birth: 3/11/58	☐ male	59 kgs

B. Adverse event or product problem

1. ☐ Adverse event and/or ☑ Product problem (e.g., defects/malfunctions)

2. Outcomes attributed to adverse event (check all that apply)
   - ☐ death ____ (mo/day/yr)
   - ☐ life-threatening
   - ☐ hospitalization – initial or prolonged
   - ☐ disability
   - ☐ congenital anomaly
   - ☐ required intervention to prevent permanent impairment/damage
   - ☐ other:

3. Date of event (mo/day/yr) 3/8/05	4. Date of this report (mo/day/yr) 3/8/05

5. Describe event or problem

After reconstituting 100-mg vial with 10 ml of bacteriostatic water, the drug crystallized and turned yellow.

Drug wasn't given.

6. Relevant tests/laboratory data, including dates

7. Other relevant history, including preexisting medical conditions (e.g., allergies, race, pregnancy, smoking and alcohol use, hepatic/renal dysfunction, etc.)

PLEASE TYPE OR USE BLACK INK

C. Suspect medication(s)

1. Name (give labeled strength & mfr/labeler, if known)
   #1 *Leucovorin calcium for*
   #2 *Injection — 100-mg vial*

2. Dose, frequency & route used	3. Therapy dates (if unknown, give duration) from/to (or best estimate)
#1 *100 mg IV X1*	#1 3/8/05
#2	#2

4. Diagnosis for use (indication)	5. Event abated after use stopped or dose reduced
#1 *Megaloblastic anemia*	#1 ☐ yes ☐ no ☐ doesn't apply
#2	#2 ☐ yes ☐ no ☐ doesn't apply

6. Lot # (if known)	7. Exp. date (if known)	8. Event reappeared after reintroduction
#1 #891	#1	#1 ☐ yes ☐ no ☐ doesn't apply
#2	#2	#2 ☐ yes ☐ no ☐ doesn't apply

9. NDC # (for product problems only)
   — — —

10. Concomitant medical products and therapy dates (exclude treatment of event)

D. Suspect medical device

1. Brand name

2. Type of device

3. Manufacturer name & address

4. Operator of device
☐ health professional
☐ lay user/patient
☐ other: _____

5. Expiration date (mo/day/yr)

6.
model # _____
catalog # _____
serial # _____
lot # _____
other #

7. If implanted, give date (mo/day/yr)

8. If explanted, give date (mo/day/yr)

9. Device available for evaluation? (Do not send to FDA)
   ☑ yes ☐ no ☐ returned to manufacturer on _____ (mo/day/yr)

10. Concomitant medical products and therapy dates (exclude treatment of event)

E. Reporter (see confidentiality section on back)

1. Name & address   phone # (123) 456-7890
   Patricia Cohen
   987 Elm Ave.
   Cincinnati, Ohio

2. Health professional?	3. Occupation	4. Also reported to
☑ yes ☐ no	RN	☐ manufacturer
		☐ user facility
5. If you do NOT want your identity disclosed to the manufacturer, place an " X " in this box. ☐		☑ distributor

Mail to: MEDWATCH
5600 Fishers Lane
Rockville, MD 20852-9787
or FAX to:
1-800-FDA-0178

FDA Form 3500 (1/96)   Submission of a report does not constitute an admission that medical personnel or the product caused or contributed to the event.

nurses can also report adverse events online using the MedWatch Voluntary Reporting Online Form (3500). The mandatory reporting MedWatch form (3500a) may be downloaded, but can't be submitted online.

File a separate MedWatch form for each patient, and attach additional pages if needed. Also, remember to comply with your health care facility's protocols for reporting adverse events associated with drugs.

Product lot numbers are used in product identification, tracking, and product recall; therefore, the lot number should be retained and your supervisor should keep a copy of the report on file.

The FDA will report back to you on the actions it takes and will continue to work to instruct health care professionals about adverse events.

See *MedWatch form for reporting adverse drug reactions,* page 115, for an example of a completed form.

DRUG ADMINISTRATION, ONE-TIME DOSE

Single-dose medications, which can include a supplemental dose or a stat dose, should be documented not only in the medication administration record, but also in the progress notes.

When transcribing a one-time order to be given on another shift, be sure to communicate information to the next shift during report, or use a medication alert sticker to flag the order.

ESSENTIAL DOCUMENTATION

Your documentation should include the name of the person who gave the drug order, why the order was given, and the patient's response to the drug. Frequent monitoring and documentation show that you monitored the patient for adverse effects, other potential outcomes, and changes in condition.

6/5/05	1100	Pt. agreed to influenza virus vaccine after Dr. Moore explained that she was in the high-risk category because of her advanced age and long history of COPD. Dr. Moore also explained risks of vaccine to pt. Pt. denies allergic reaction to eggs, chicken, or chicken feathers or dander. Pt. is afebrile, oral T 97.2° F, and has no active infections. Fluzone 0.5 ml I.M. injected in ℞ deltoid. Explained fever, malaise, and myalgia may occur up to 2 days after vaccination and site may feel tender. ——————————— Angela Casale, RN

DRUG ADMINISTRATION, OPIOID

Whenever you administer an opioid, you must follow stringent federal, state, and institutional regulations concerning administration and documentation. Government regulations are strict and carry heavy penalties for the institution when they're breached. These regulations require opioid drugs to be counted after each nursing shift to ensure an accurate drug count. They also require that a second nurse document your activity and observe you if an opioid or part of a dose must be wasted.

Many facilities now use an automated storage system for opioids that eliminates the need for counting the opioids at the end of a shift. This system allows the nurse easy access (via an ID and password or fingerprint) to medications, including other drugs and floor stocks for nursing units. Nurses may remove one or more medications by selecting the patient, medication, and amount needed on the keypad. The nurse must then count the amount of the drug remaining in the system and enter it. Each transaction is recorded and copies are sent to the pharmacy and billing department.

ESSENTIAL DOCUMENTATION

Whenever you give an opioid, you must document it according to federal, state, and facility regulations. Use the special control sheets provided by the pharmacy and follow these procedures:
- Sign out the drug on the appropriate form.
- Verify the amount of drug in the container before giving it.
- Have another nurse document your activity and observe you if you must waste or discard part of an opioid dose.

At the end of your shift:
- Record the amount of each opioid on the opioid control sheet while the nurse beginning her shift counts the opioids out loud.
- Sign the opioid control sheet only if the count is correct. Have the other nurse countersign.
- Identify and correct any discrepancies before any nurse leaves the unit. If the discrepancy can't be resolved, follow your employer's policy for reporting this and file an incident report. An investigation will follow. (See *Opioid control sheet,* page 118.)

AccuChart

OPIOID CONTROL SHEET

The sample opioid control sheet demonstrates proper documentation of opioids and an end-of-shift opioid count.

Unit ___45___   Date ___1/5/06___

CITY HOSPITAL

**24-HOUR RECORD
CONTROLLED SUBSTANCES**

7 a.m. INVENTORY		CODEINE 30 MG TAB	PERCOCET TAB	TYLENOL #3 TAB	VALIUM 2 MG TAB	VALIUM 5 MG TAB	TEMAZEPAM 15 MG TAB	DEMEROL 50MG INJ	DEMEROL 75MG INJ	DEMEROL 100MG INJ	DILAUDID 2 MG INJ	MORPHINE 2MG INJ	MORPHINE 10MG INJ	VERSED 2ML INJ	DOSE	AMOUNT WASTED	Signature	Witness
		25	20	18	15	16	10		10	8	5	10	15	13	3				
Patient name	**Patient number**																		
0915 Orr, Carl	555112												12		5mg	5mg	M. Stevens, RN	D. Bozon, RN
1000 Davis, Donna	555161			16											ii̅		M. Koller, RN	
1115 McGowen, John	555111					15									i̅		K. Collins, RN	

DRUG ADMINISTRATION, STAT ORDER

A drug that's ordered stat is to be administered to the patient immediately for an urgent medical problem. This single-dose medication should be documented in the medication administration record (MAR) and in the progress notes.

ESSENTIAL DOCUMENTATION

Your documentation should include the name of the person who gave the order, why the order was given, and the patient's response to the drug. In the MAR, write the drug's name, dosage, route, and time given.

| 2/3/05 | 0900 | Pt. SOB with crackles auscultated bilaterally in the bases and O₂ sat. decreased to 89% on room air. P 104, BP 92/60, RR 32 and labored. Lasix 40 mg P.O. given as per Dr. Singh's order ———————— Ann Barrow, RN |
| | 1000 | Pt. responded with urine output of 1500 ml, decreased SOB, and O₂ sat. increased to 97% on room air. P 98, BP 94/60, and RR 28. ———————— Ann Barrow, RN |

DRUG ADMINISTRATION, WITHHOLDING ORDERED DRUG

Under certain circumstances, a prescribed drug can't or shouldn't be given as scheduled. For example, you may decide to withhold a stool softener in a patient with diarrhea. A patient may be scheduled for a test that requires him to not take a certain drug, or a change in the patient's condition may make the drug inappropriate to give. For example, an antihypertensive drug may have been prescribed for a patient who now has low blood pressure. In some circumstances, a patient may refuse a drug. For example, a patient may refuse to take his cholestyramine because he believes it's causing abdominal upset. If a drug is withheld, notify the doctor.

ESSENTIAL DOCUMENTATION

In your note, document the date and time the drug was withheld, the reason for withholding the drug, the name of the doctor notified, and the doctor's response. If the doctor changed a drug order, record and document the new order and the time it was carried out. Document any actions taken to safeguard your patient.

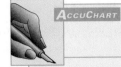

WITHHOLDING AN
ORDERED MEDICATION

When withholding an ordered medication, it's necessary to document it on the medication administration record as indicated below. This is usually indicated by circling your initials.

NAME: *Jack Lemmons*   MEDICAL RECORD #: *987654*

NURSE'S FULL SIGNATURE, STATUS, AND INITIALS

	INIT.		INIT.		INIT.
Roy Charles, RN	RC				
Theresa Hopkins, RN	TH				

DIAGNOSIS: *Heart failure, atrial flutter, COPD*

ALLERGIES: ASA   DIET: *Cardiac*

ORDER DATE	MEDICATIONS DOSE, ROUTE, FREQUENCY	TIME	DATE: 1/24 SITE	INT.	DATE: 1/25 SITE	INT.	DATE: 1/26 SITE	INT.	DATE: 1/27 SITE	INT.	DATE: 1/28 SITE	INT.	DATE: 1/29 SITE	INT.	DATE: 1/30 SITE	INT.
1/24/06	digoxin 0.125 mg	0900	@ subclavian	RC		(RC)										
RC	I.V. daily	HR	68		52											
1/24/06	furosemide 40 mg	0900	@ subclavian	RC	@ subclavian	RC										
RC	I.V. q12hr	2100	@ subclavian	TH												
1/24/06	enalaprilat 1.25 mg	0511	@ subclavian	TH	@ subclavian	TH										
RC	I.V. q6hr	1100	@ subclavian	RC												
		1700	@ subclavian	RC												
		2300	@ subclavian	TH												

On the medication administration record (MAR) or medication Kardex, initial the appropriate box as usual but circle your initials to indicate the drug was not given. (See *Withholding an ordered medication.*) Record the correct code indicating why the drug wasn't given, or fill in the appropriate section on the MAR with the date, time, name and dose of the drug withheld, and the reason for withholding the drug.

3/3/05	1800	Digoxin 0.125 mg P.O. not given due to pulse less than
		60. Dr. Miller notified that medication was witheld. ——
		——————————————————————— Betty Griffin, RN

DRUGS, ILLEGAL

If you observe that your patient has illegal drugs or drug paraphernalia in his possession, follow your facility's policy and notify your nursing supervisor, security, and the patient's doctor. (See "Evidence collection, suspected criminal case," page 142.) Depending on your state's guidelines, you may be obligated to report the patient to the police. (See *Conducting a drug search,* page 122.)

ESSENTIAL DOCUMENTATION

If you discover evidence of drugs in your patient's room or on his person, document the circumstances of the discovery. Document that you told the patient about the facility's policy on contraband and the patient's response. Record the names and departments of the people you notified, instructions given, and your actions. Document whether a search was performed, who was present during the search, and what was found. When describing what you suspect are illegal drugs, document the form (such as pills, liquid, or powder) as well as the amount, color, and shape. Fill out an incident report, according to your facility's policy.

CONDUCTING A DRUG SEARCH

If you suspect your patient is abusing drugs, you have a duty to do something about it. If such a patient harms himself or anyone else, resulting in a lawsuit, the court may hold you liable for his actions.

WHEN YOU KNOW ABOUT DRUG ABUSE

Suppose you know for certain that a patient is abusing drugs—if you're an emergency department nurse, you may find drugs in a patient's clothes or handbag while looking for identification. Your hospital policy may obligate you to confiscate the drugs and take steps to ensure that the patient doesn't acquire more.

WHEN YOU SUSPECT DRUG ABUSE

When a patient's erratic or threatening behavior makes you suspect he's abusing drugs, consult your hospital's policy, which may require that you conduct a search. Is your search legal? As a rule of thumb, if you strongly believe the patient poses a threat to himself or others and you can document your reasons for searching his possessions, you're probably safe legally.

GUIDELINES FOR SEARCHES

Before you conduct a search, review your hospital's guidelines on the matter. Then follow the guidelines carefully. Most hospital guidelines will first direct you to contact your supervisor and explain why you have legitimate cause for a search. If she gives you her approval, ask a security guard to help you. Besides protecting you, he'll serve as a witness if you do find drugs. When you're ready, confront the patient, tell him you intend to conduct a search, and tell him why.

Depending on your hospital's guidelines, you can search a patient's belongings as well as his room. If you find illegal drugs during your search, confiscate them. Remember, possession of illegal drugs is a felony. Depending on your hospital's guidelines, you may be obligated to report the patient to the police.

MAINTAINING WRITTEN RECORDS

After you've completed your search, record your findings in your nurse's note and in an incident report. Your written records will be an important part of your defense (and your hospital's) if the patient decides to sue.

| 9/1/05 | 1000 | Clear plastic bag containing white powdery substance, approx. 3 tbsp, with odd odor found in pt.'s bedside stand while retrieving his wash basin at 0930. Upon questioning, pt. stated, "That stuff is none of your business." Told pt. that drugs not prescribed by the doctor aren't allowed in the hospital. Security director, Michael Daniels; nursing supervisor, Stacey McLean, RN; and Dr. Phillips notified at 0940. Mr. Daniels and Mrs. McLean visited pt. in his room and reinforced hospital policy on contraband. Pt. flushed powder down toilet. Witnessed by Mr. Daniels, Mrs. McLean, and myself. Dr. Phillips will see pt. at 1030 to discuss situation. ———— Greg Little, RN |

DRUGS, INAPPROPRIATE USE OF

You may suspect that your patient is taking opioids or other drugs when his behavior suddenly changes after he has visitors. If you suspect your patient is abusing drugs, you have a duty to do something about it. If the patient harms himself or anyone else, resulting in a lawsuit, the court may hold you liable for his actions. Follow your facility's policy when you suspect drug abuse.

ESSENTIAL DOCUMENTATION

Record the date and time of your entry. Document how the patient appeared before and after the visitors came to see him. Record your observations and physical assessment findings. Chart the name of the doctor and the nursing supervisor notified, the time of notification, their instructions, and your actions.

1/2/06	1125	Upon entering room, pt. found in bed lethargic. Pupils constricted, speech slurred. P 68, BP 102/58, RR 16. Pt. stated, "My friend gave me something to help with the pain." Dr. Ettingoff and Ron Howell, RN, nursing supervisor, notified at 1130 and told of lethargy, slurred speech, pinpoint pupils, and pt.'s explanation. Dr. Ettingoff will be here immediately to see pt. ———————————————— Eileen Sullivan, RN
	1130	Dr. Ettingoff in to see pt. Orders written for Narcan. Narcan given as ordered. P 72, BP 114/60, RR 20. Speech less slurred, oriented to person, place, and day but not time. Pupils still constricted. ——— Eileen Sullivan, RN

DRUGS, PATIENT HIDING

Your patient may hide drugs for a variety of reasons: He may think they aren't working, he may be saving them for double-dosing at night if they're pain medications, or he may be collecting them for a suicide attempt or to sell. If your patient is hiding medications, you must confront him, talk about the situation, and discover his reason for doing it. He may need some education regarding the function of the medications. If your patient believes the medications are ineffective, discuss that with his doctor. If you believe the patient is suicidal, call the doctor and stay with the patient or have another nurse stay with the patient until the doctor arrives.

ESSENTIAL DOCUMENTATION

Record the date and time of your entry. Document how you found the drugs. If you discovered drugs that weren't prescribed, describe the type of drug, such as pills or powders, the amount, and its appearance, such as the color and shape. If you discovered prescribed drugs, record the type of drug and the amount. Record your discussion with the patient about why he's hiding medications. Use the patient's own words in quotes whenever possible. Document your interventions, such as patient teaching; rescheduling of doses if the patient takes medication at a different time at home; and, if appropriate, removing medications from the patient's room and storing them per your facility's policy. Record the name of the doctor notified, the time of notification, and any actions taken. Make sure you describe events in chronological order and note the time.

5/21/05	0900	While assisting pt. with her bath at 0800, noted pills in
		her makeup case. When asked what they were, pt. stated
		"just some pills." I stated that they looked like her mor-
		phine sulfate and she said they were. After some dis-
		cussion, pt. stated, "My pain is so severe at night, and I
		want to get a good night's sleep, so I save my daytime
		dose for the evening." Discussed with pt. the importance of
		taking morphine sulfate as prescribed, the dangers of an
		overdose, and the importance of allowing her health care
		team to assist in relieving her pain by changing her dose as
		needed according to her reports of pain relief. Morphine
		sulfate pills sent to pharmacy for identification at 0830.
		Dr. Smith notified and came to see pt. Dosage changed with
		patient input. Pt. instructed to report relief per pain
		scale and given information sheet on morphine sulfate.
		Adverse reactions reviewed. Pt. agreed to comply with
		medication plan and verbalized an understanding of the
		importance of doing so. ————— Phillip Stevens, RN

DRUGS, PATIENT REFUSAL TO TAKE

If a patient refuses to take his prescribed drugs, notify his doctor and describe the event in his chart. By documenting the refusal, you avoid the misinterpretation that you omitted the drug by mistake.

ESSENTIAL DOCUMENTATION

Record the date and time of your entry. Document that your patient refused to take his prescribed drugs and the reason, assuming he tells you. Record the name of the refused drugs and the time they were due.

Include any explanations given on the indications for the drugs and why they were ordered for the patient.

2/15/05	1015	*Pt. refused K-Dur tabs scheduled for 1000, stating that*
		they were too big for her to swallow. Dr. Boyle notified.
		K-Dur tabs discontinued. KCL elixir ordered and given.
		——————————————— *Kathy Collins, RN*

DYSPNEA

Commonly a symptom of cardiopulmonary dysfunction, dyspnea is the sensation of difficult or uncomfortable breathing. Usually, it's reported as shortness of breath. Dyspnea may arise suddenly or slowly and may subside rapidly or persist for years. Most people usually experience dyspnea when they overexert themselves, and its severity depends on their physical condition. In the healthy person, dyspnea is quickly relieved by rest. Pathologic causes of dyspnea include pulmonary, cardiac, neuromuscular, and allergic disorders. In addition, anxiety may cause shortness of breath.

Whatever the cause of dyspnea, place the patient in an upright position, unless contraindicated, and perform a rapid respiratory assessment. Prepare to administer oxygen by nasal cannula, mask, or endotracheal tube. Start an I.V. infusion and begin cardiac monitoring to detect arrhythmias. Anticipate interventions, such as inserting a chest tube for pneumothorax, giving a morphine injection to treat pulmonary edema, or administering breathing treatments for acute asthma.

ESSENTIAL DOCUMENTATION

Record the date and time of your entry. State the problem in the patient's own words, if he can communicate. If it's appropriate, question the patient about the following:

- what he was doing when the dyspnea started
- whether it began gradually or suddenly
- if it occurs at rest or with activity
- what aggravates or alleviates the dyspnea
- presence of a productive or nonproductive cough
- history of recent trauma or disease
- whether he smokes
- accompanying symptoms, such as orthopnea, paroxysmal nocturnal dyspnea, or progressive fatigue.

Document your cardiopulmonary examination, including vital signs; respiratory rate, depth, and effort; breath and heart sounds; use of accessory muscles; skin color; presence of edema; mental status; and chest pain.

Record the name of the doctor notified, the time of notification, and any orders given. Include any diagnostic tests and results, if available, such as chest X-ray, pulse oximetry, arterial blood gas analysis, hemoglobin level, hematocrit, pulmonary function tests, and ECG. Describe your interventions and results, such as cardiac monitoring, administering oxygen, I.V. infusions, medications, breathing treatments, and positioning. Document patient education, such as how to perform coughing and deep breathing, pursed-lip breathing, relaxation techniques, and incentive spirometry. Also include emotional support given.

| 1/3/06 | 0900 | Pt. c/o SOB after walking from bathroom to bed, approx. 25'. Assisted pt. back to bed, placed him in high Fowler's position, reattached to O_2 at 2 L/min by NC. Lungs with scattered rhonchi, bilaterally. P 118, BP 132/90, RR 40 labored with use of accessory muscles, axillary T 97.4° F., O_2 sat. by pulse oximetry 87%. Nl heart sounds. Skin pale, +1 edema of both ankles. Alert and oriented to time, place, and person. No c/o chest pain. Pt. states he's been having increasing SOB at home with less and less activity due to worsening heart failure. He said he's been discussing the use of O_2 at home with his doctor. Dr. Smith called and came to see pt. Ordered O_2 to be used when out of bed and ambulating. Carla Moore, in respiratory therapy, notified. Pt. instructed to cough and deep-breathe q1hr while awake. Coughed up moderate amount of white sputum. —————————— Sally Jones, RN |
| 1/3/06 | 0920 | Pt. states he's no longer SOB. P 102, BP 130/88, RR 20, with less effort. O_2 sat. by pulse oximetry 97%. Maintaining O_2 at 2 L/min by NC. ————— Sally Jones, RN |

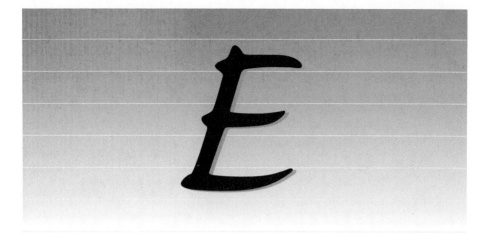

ELOPEMENT FROM A HEALTH CARE FACILITY

If you discover that a patient is missing or has left the health care facility without having said anything about leaving (called "elopement"), look for him on your unit immediately and notify the nurse-manager, the patient's physician, and his family. Notify the police if the patient is at risk for harming himself or others.

The legal consequences of a patient leaving the facility without medical permission can be particularly severe, especially if he's confused, mentally incompetent, or injured or if he dies of exposure as a result of his absence.

ESSENTIAL DOCUMENTATION

Document the time that you discovered the patient missing, your attempts to find him, and the people you notified.

3/25/05	0800	Entered pt.'s room to administer his medication and
		discovered pt. wasn't in his room. Pt.'s bathroom and
		unit were searched. Hospital security; Janice Welsh,
		nurse-manager; and Dr. Parone notified. Pt.'s family
		called and informed that he was missing. ———
		——————————————————— Valerie Stelatto, RN

EMERGENCY TREATMENT, PATIENT REFUSAL OF

A competent adult has the right to refuse emergency treatment. His family can't overrule his decision, and his doctor isn't allowed to give the expressly refused treatment, even if the patient becomes unconscious.

In most cases, the health care personnel who are responsible for the patient can remain free from legal jeopardy as long as they fully inform the patient about his medical condition and the likely consequences of refusing treatment. The courts recognize a competent adult's right to refuse medical treatment, even when that refusal will clearly result in his death. If the patient understands the risks but still refuses treatment, notify the nursing supervisor and the patient's doctor.

The courts recognize several circumstances that justify overruling a patient's refusal of treatment. These include instances when refusing treatment endangers the life of another, when a parent's decision threatens the child's life, or when, despite refusing treatment, the patient makes statements to indicate he wants to live. If none of these grounds exist, then you have an ethical duty to defend your patient's right to refuse treatment. Try to explain the patient's choice to his family. Emphasize that the decision is his as long as he's competent.

ESSENTIAL DOCUMENTATION

When your patient refuses care, document that you have explained the care and the risks involved in not receiving it. Document your patient's understanding of the risks, using his own words. Record the names of the nursing supervisor and doctor you notified and the time of notification. Document that the doctor saw the patient and explained the risks of refusing emergency treatment.

Ask the patient to complete a refusal of treatment form. (See *Refusal of treatment form.*) The signed form indicates that appropriate treatment would have been given had the patient consented. If the patient refuses to sign the release form, document this in your nurse's note by writing "refused to sign" on the patient's signature line. Initial it with your own initials and date it. For additional protection, your facility may require you to get the patient's spouse or closest relative to sign a refusal of treatment form. In the same manner as you did for the patient, document whether the spouse or relative does this.

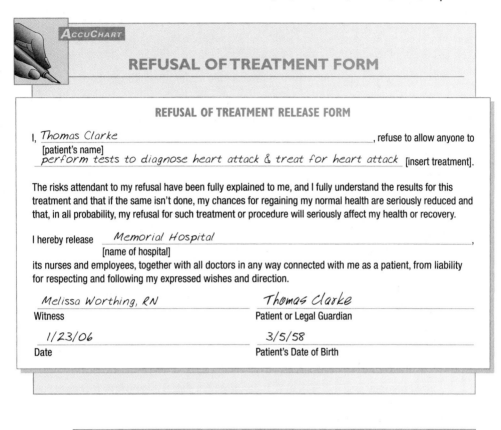

AccuChart

REFUSAL OF TREATMENT FORM

REFUSAL OF TREATMENT RELEASE FORM

I, _Thomas Clarke_ _____ , refuse to allow anyone to
  [patient's name]
  perform tests to diagnose heart attack & treat for heart attack [insert treatment].

The risks attendant to my refusal have been fully explained to me, and I fully understand the results for this
treatment and that if the same isn't done, my chances for regaining my normal health are seriously reduced and
that, in all probability, my refusal for such treatment or procedure will seriously affect my health or recovery.

I hereby release _____ _Memorial Hospital_ _____ ,
                          [name of hospital]
its nurses and employees, together with all doctors in any way connected with me as a patient, from liability
for respecting and following my expressed wishes and direction.

Melissa Worthing, RN	_Thomas Clarke_
Witness	Patient or Legal Guardian
_1/23/06_	_3/5/58_
Date	Patient's Date of Birth

1/23/06	1300	Pt. brought to ED by ambulance with chest pain, radiating
		to Ⓛ arm. Pt. sitting up in bed, not in acute distress.
		Skin pale, RR 28, occasionally rubbing Ⓛ arm. Pt. refusing
		physical exam, blood work, and ECG. States "I didn't want
		to come to the hospital. My coworkers called an am-
		bulance without telling me. I'm fine, my arm's just sore
		from raking leaves. I'm leaving." Explained to pt. that
		chest and arm pain may be symptoms of a heart attack
		and explained the risks of leaving without treatment,
		including death. Pt. stated, "I told you, I'm not having a
		heart attack. I want to leave." Notified Mary Colwell,
		RN, nursing supervisor, and Dr. Lowell. Dr. Lowell ex-
		plained the need for diagnostic tests to r/o MI and
		the risks involved in not having treatment. Pt. still
		refusing treatment but did agree to sign refusal of
		treatment release form. Explained signs and symptoms
		of MI to pt. Encouraged pt. to seek treatment and
		call 911 if symptoms persist. Pt. discharged with ED #
		to call with questions. ———— Melissa Worthing, RN

END-OF-LIFE CARE

Nurses must meet the physical and emotional end-of-life needs of both the dying patient and his family. The dying patient may experience a variety of physical symptoms, including pain, respiratory distress, loss of appetite, nausea and vomiting, and bowel problems. Emotional concerns may include confusion, depression, anxiety, sleep disturbances, and spiritual distress. Your nursing interventions should be individualized to the specific needs of the patient.

The nurse can also make the death more comfortable and meaningful for the family. Tell the family what to expect, if they want to hear about it. Encourage them to talk to and touch the patient. Allow them to help with care, if they desire. Provide them with a comfortable environment, encourage verbalization of concerns and feelings, and determine whether they would like a member of the clergy to visit.

ESSENTIAL DOCUMENTATION

Record the time and date of your entry. Document your interventions related to pain assessment and management, relief of respiratory distress, administration or withholding of nutrition and hydration, control of nausea and vomiting, and management of bowel problems. Describe measures taken to meet the patient's emotional needs and his response. If you call the doctor, include the time and date of notification, orders given, and whether the doctor saw the patient. Include the names of other people or departments you notified (such as pastoral care, respiratory therapy, or nutritional support), the time you called, the reason for your telephone call, and the response.

Also, record your interventions to meet the physical and emotional needs of the family, the names of family members present, and their responses. Document any teaching you provided the patient and his family and their responses to teaching. In some facilities, teaching may be documented on a patient-teaching record.

2/22/05	0920	Pt. alert and oriented to time, place, and person.
		Lethargic, but easily arousable. States he feels like he
		didn't sleep at all last night. Requesting to see
		chaplain this morning. Called chaplain's office at 0910.
		Father Smith will be by to see pt. around noon. Pt.
		rates pain as 3 on a scale of 0 to 10, w/ 10 being the
		worst pain imaginable; doesn't want pain med at this
		time. Lungs clear, RR 22, unlabored, shallow in semi-
		Fowler's position. BP 98/62, P 74, oral T 97.2° F. Ate
		two spoonfuls of scramble eggs with a few sips of
		orange juice for breakfast. Stated he "just wasn't
		hungry." No c/o nausea, no abdominal distention noted,
		bowel sounds diminished and hypoactive in all 4
		quadrants. Wife, Patty Linden, trying to get pt. to eat
		"just one more spoonful." Explained to wife that
		forcing pt. to eat could lead to nausea, vomiting, and
		abdominal distention or pain and that reduced intake
		may produce endorphins, which have a pain-relieving
		effect. Wife states she understands this but that "it's
		hard to watch him waste away." ———— Bonnie Little, RN

ENDOTRACHEAL EXTUBATION

When your patient no longer requires endotracheal (ET) intubation, the airway can be removed. Explain the procedure to your patient and obtain another nurse's assistance to prevent traumatic manipulation of the tube when it's untaped or unfastened. Teach the patient to cough and deep-breathe after the ET tube is removed, and assess him frequently for signs of respiratory distress.

ESSENTIAL DOCUMENTATION

Record the date and time of extubation, presence or absence of stridor or other signs of upper airway edema, breath sounds, type of supplemental oxygen administered, any complications and required subsequent therapy, and the patient's tolerance of the procedure. Document patient teaching and support given.

5/26/05	1700	Explained extubation procedure to pt. Pt. acknowledged
		understanding by nodding his head "yes." Placed pt. in
		high Fowler's position and suctioned for scant amount
		of thin white secretions. ETT removed at 1630. No
		stridor or respiratory distress noted, breath sounds
		clear. RR 22, P 92, BP 128/82, oral T 98.4° F. Pulse
		oximetry 97% on O_2 2 L by NC. Pt. states he's happy to
		have tube out. Instructed pt. on importance of coughing
		and deep breathing every hr. Pt. was able to give proper
		return demonstration. Cough nonproductive.
		———————————— Margie Egan, RN

ENDOTRACHEAL INTUBATION

Endotracheal (ET) intubation involves the oral or nasal insertion of a flexible tube through the larynx into the trachea for the purpose of controlling the airway and mechanically ventilating the patient. Performed by a doctor, anesthetist, respiratory therapist, or nurse educated in the procedure, ET intubation usually occurs in emergencies such as cardiopulmonary arrest, or in diseases such as epiglottiditis. However, ET intubation may also occur under more controlled circumstances; for example, just before surgery. In these instances, ET intubation requires teaching and preparing the patient.

ET intubation establishes and maintains a patent airway, protects against aspiration by sealing off the trachea from the digestive tract, permits removal of tracheobronchial secretions in patients who can't cough effectively, and provides a route for mechanical ventilation.

ESSENTIAL DOCUMENTATION

Document that the doctor explained the procedure, risks, complications, and alternatives to the patient or person responsible for making decisions concerning the patient's health care. Indicate that the patient or health care proxy consented to the procedure. Record the date and time of intubation and the name of the person performing the procedure. Include indications for the procedure and success or failure. Chart the type and size of tube, cuff size, amount of inflation, and inflation technique. Indicate whether drugs were administered. Document the initiation of supplemental oxygen or ventilation therapy. Record the results of chest auscultation and chest X-ray. Note the occurrence of any complications, necessary interventions, and the patient's response. Describe the patient's reaction to the procedure. Also, document any teaching done before and after the procedure.

3/16/05	1015	Pt. informed by Dr. Eagan of the need for intubation,
		the risks, potential complications, and alternatives. Pt.
		consented to the procedure. Pt. given 2 mg morphine
		sulfate by I.V. and intubated by Dr. Langley at 0945
		with size 8 oral cuffed ETT. Tube taped in place in
		right corner of mouth. Cuff inflated with 5 ml of air.
		Pt. on ventilator set at TV 750, FIO_2 45%, 5 cm PEEP,
		AC of 12. RR 20, nonlabored. Portable CXR confirms
		proper placement. ® lung with basilar crackles and
		expiratory wheezes. Ⓛ lung clear. Pt. opening eyes when
		name is called. When asked if he's comfortable and in
		no pain, pt. nods head yes. ———————— Jim Hanes, RN

ENDOTRACHEAL TUBE, PATIENT REMOVAL OF

Because an endotracheal (ET) tube is used to provide mechanical ventilation and maintain a patent airway, the removal of an ET tube by a patient is an emergency situation. The patient may not have spontaneous respirations, may be in severe respiratory distress, or may suffer trauma to the larynx or vocal cords.

If your patient removes his ET tube, stay with him and call for help. Assign someone to notify the doctor while you assess the patient's respiratory status. If the patient is in distress, perform manual ventilation while others prepare for reinsertion of the ET tube and monitor vital signs. If your patient is alert, speak calmly and explain the reintubation procedure. If the patient isn't in distress, provide oxygen therapy. If the decision is made not to reintubate the patient, monitor his respiratory status and vital signs every 15 minutes for 2 to 3 hours, or as ordered by the doctor.

ESSENTIAL DOCUMENTATION

Record the date and time of your entry. Note how you discovered the ET tube was removed by the patient. Record your respiratory assessment. Record the name of the doctor notified and the time of notification. Document your actions, such as oxygen therapy and mechanical ventilation, and the patient's response. If the patient required reinsertion of the ET tube, follow the procedure for documenting endotracheal intubation. (See "Endotracheal intubation.") Record any patient education provided.

1/30/06	0400	Summoned to room by ventilator alarms at 0330.
		Found pt. in bed with ETT in hand. P 86 and regular,
		BP 140/70, RR 32 regular and deep. No use of
		accessory muscles, skin warm, dry, and pink, O_2 sat. by
		pulse oximetry 94%. Lungs clear to auscultation
		bilaterally. Pt. oriented to time, place, and person. Pt.
		stated in a raspy voice, "I must have been dreaming. And
		when I woke up, the tube was in my hand." Administered
		O_2 at 4 L by NC with O_2 sat. 97%. Stayed with pt. while
		another nurse notified Dr. Smith at 0335. Dr. Smith
		came to see pt. at 0345 and, after assessing pt., made
		decision to keep ETT out. Plan is to maintain O_2 at 4 L
		by NC and monitor pt.'s respiratory status q 15 min for
		2 hr. Instructed pt. on the use of incentive spirometer
		q/hr while awake. Pt. was able to give proper return
		demonstration and verbalized understanding that it
		should be performed every hour. ——— Amy Young, RN

END-TIDAL CARBON DIOXIDE MONITORING

Monitoring end-tidal carbon dioxide ($ETCO_2$) determines the CO_2 concentration in exhaled gas. In this technique, a photodetector measures the amount of infrared light absorbed by airway gas during inspiration and expiration. A monitor converts this information to a CO_2 value and a corresponding waveform or capnogram.

$ETCO_2$ monitoring provides information about the patient's pulmonary, cardiac, and metabolic status, which aids patient management and helps prevent clinical compromise. This technique has become standard during anesthesia administration and mechanical ventilation. It may be used to help wean a patient with a stable acid-base balance from mechanical ventilation. It also reduces the need for frequent arterial blood gas (ABG) measurements, especially when combined with pulse oximetry. Other uses for $ETCO_2$ monitoring include assessing resuscitation efforts and identifying the return of spontaneous circulation. Because no CO_2 is exhaled when breathing stops, this technique also detects apnea. When used during endotracheal (ET) intubation, $ETCO_2$ monitoring can avert neurologic injury and even death by confirming correct ET tube placement and, because CO_2 isn't normally produced by the stomach, by detecting accidental esophageal intubation.

When a patient requires ET intubation, an $ETCO_2$ detector or monitor is usually applied immediately after the tube is inserted. For a nonintubated patient, the adapter is placed near the patient's airway. If a

ACCUCHART

DOCUMENTING ETco_2
ON A FLOW SHEET

		0001	0100	0200	0300	0400	0500	0600	0700
							DATE 10/13/05		
PULMONARY	Ventilator settings	CMV/2 TV 800							
	Peak pressures	/	/	/	/	/	/	/	/
	O$_2$ /delivery system	35%							
	Oximetry	97%							
	ETco_2	35%							

patient is alert, with or without ET intubation, explain the purpose and expected duration of the monitoring.

ESSENTIAL DOCUMENTATION

Record the date and time of your entry. Document the initial ETco_2 value and all ventilator settings. Describe the waveform if one appears on the monitor. If the monitor has a printer, you may want to print out a sample waveform and include it in the patient's medical record. Document ETco_2 values at least as often as vital signs, whenever significant changes in waveform or patient status occur, and before and after weaning, respiratory, and other interventions. Periodically obtain samples for ABG analysis as the patient's condition dictates, and document the corresponding ETco_2 values. Some facilities may document ETco_2 values on a flow sheet for easy assessment of changes in a patient's condition.

See *Documenting ETco_2 on a flow sheet* for an example of documenting ETco_2 values.

ENEMA ADMINISTRATION

An enema is a solution introduced into the rectum and colon. Enemas are used to administer medication, clean the lower bowel in preparation for diagnostic or surgical procedures, relieve distention and promote expulsion of flatus, lubricate the rectum and colon, and soften hardened stool for removal. Enema solutions and methods vary to suit your patient's condition or treatment requirements.

ESSENTIAL DOCUMENTATION

Record the date and time of enema administration. Include any special equipment used. Write down the type and amount of solution used, the retention time, and approximate amount returned. Describe the color, consistency, amount of the return, and any abnormalities with the return. Record complications that occurred, actions taken, and the patient's response. Document the patient's tolerance of the procedure.

Depending on your facility's policy, you may also need to document the enema on the medication Kardex or treatment record.

2/28/05	0900	Pt. c/o constipation. States she hasn't had a BM for 2 days. Dr. Martin notified and ordered Fleet enema 1 daily p.r.n. constipation. Procedure, risks, and alternatives explained to pt. and she consented. Received Fleet enema, 100 ml, at 0830 and held for 20 minutes. Pt. had large amount of brown, solid stool. No c/o abd. pain; no abd. distention noted. ———— Sue Smith, RN

EPIDURAL ANALGESIA

Epidural analgesia improves pain relief, causes less sedation, and allows patients to do coughing and deep-breathing exercises and to walk earlier after surgery. It's also useful in patients with chronic pain that is not relieved by less invasive methods of pain relief. An epidural catheter is placed by an anesthesiologist in the epidural space outside the spinal cord between the vertebrae. Pain relief with minimal adverse effects is the result of drug delivery so close to the opiate receptors.

Opioids, such as preservative-free morphine (Duramorph) and fentanyl, are administered through the catheter and move slowly into the cerebrospinal fluid to opiate receptors in the dorsal horn of the spinal cord. The opioids may be administered by bolus dose, continuous infusion by pump, or patient-controlled analgesia. They may be administered alone or in combination with bupivacaine (a local anesthetic).

Adverse effects of epidural analgesia include sedation, nausea, urinary retention, orthostatic hypotension, itching, respiratory depression, headache, back soreness, leg weakness and numbness, and respiratory depression. The nurse must monitor the patient for these adverse reactions and notify the doctor or anesthesiologist if they occur. Most facilities have policies or standards of care that address interventions for adverse effects and monitoring parameters.

ESSENTIAL DOCUMENTATION

Record the date and time of your entry. Document the type and dose of the drug administered. Include the patient's level of consciousness, pain level (using a 0-to-10 scale, with 0 being no pain and 10 being the worst pain imaginable), and respiratory rate and quality. Also record the amount of drug received per hour and the number of dose attempts by the patient if the analgesia is patient-controlled. Be sure to include site assessment, dressing changes, infusion bag changes, tubing changes, and patient education. Document complications, such as numbness, leg weakness, and respiratory depression, your interventions, and the patient's response.

Most facilities use a flow sheet to document drug dosage, rate, route, vital signs, respiratory rate, pulse oximetry, pain scale, and sedation scale. Follow your facility's policy; however, these parameters should be monitored frequently for the first 12 hours, and then every 4 hours after that. If you don't have a specific flow sheet for epidural documentation, use your regular flow sheet and document in the progress notes other assessments, as needed, or unusual circumstances.

5/22/05	1500	Pt. received from PACU with epidural catheter in place.
		Dressing covering site clean, dry, and intact. Pt. receiv-
		ing bupivacaine 0.125% and fentanyl 5 mcg/ml in 250
		ml NSS at rate of 2 ml/hr. Respiratory rate 20 and
		deep, level of sedation 0 (alert), O₂ sat. by pulse oxime-
		try on O₂ 2L by NC 99%, BP 120/80, P 72. Pt. reports
		pain as 2 on a scale of 0 to 10, w/ 10 being worst pain
		imaginable. No c/o nausea, itching, H/A, leg weakness,
		back soreness. Pt. voided 300 ml yellow urine. Bladder
		scan shows no residual after void. Told pt. to report
		any pain greater than 3 out of 10, inability to void, and
		numbness in legs. Epidural infusion label applied to
		catheter, infusion tubing, and infusion pump. See flow
		sheet for frequent monitoring of drug dose, rate, VS,
		resp. rate, pulse ox., level of pain, and sedation level.
		———— Mary Holmes, RN

EPIDURAL HEMATOMA

Your patient who is receiving or has recently received epidural analgesia is at risk for epidural hematoma, a complication that can lead to lower extremity paralysis. This risk is increased if the patient has received anticoagulants or traumatic or repeated epidural punctures. Frequently assess for diffuse back pain or tenderness, paresthesia, and bowel and bladder dysfunction, according to unit protocol or doctor's orders, to detect signs of epidural hematoma. Your prompt assessments and interventions are necessary to avoid paralysis in your patient receiving epidural analgesia.

ESSENTIAL DOCUMENTATION

Document your frequent assessments. Record the date and time of these assessments, avoiding block charting. If your assessments suggest epidural hematoma, record the name of the doctor notified, the time of notification, orders given, your actions, and the patient's response. Record patient education and emotional support.

2/23/05	0925	Called to room by pt. at 0910 for c/o lower back
		discomfort and numbness in right leg. When asked to
		point to pain, pt. moved hand around general region
		of lower back. Pedal pulses palpable with capillary refill
		less than 3 sec bilaterally. ® foot weaker than left
		when asked to dorsiflex and plantar flex foot against
		resistance. Unable to raise ® foot off bed. Pt. alert
		and oriented to time, place, and person. No difficulty
		urinating, voided 350 ml on bedpan at 0830. Told pt.
		to remain in bed, placed call bell within reach, and
		verified that pt. knows how to use it. Dr. Hoffman,
		anesthesiologist, notified at 0920 of pt.'s symptoms and
		will be here to see pt. at 0930. —— Julie Robbins, RN

EQUIPMENT MALFUNCTION

When providing care, make sure the equipment you use is in good working order. When equipment is defective, assess the patient to determine whether there's a change in his condition. If the patient isn't in distress or immediate danger, call the doctor and obtain and carry out his orders. If the patient is in distress or immediate danger, call for help, assign some-

PROTECTING THE PATIENT FROM FAULTY EQUIPMENT

You're responsible for making sure that the equipment used for patient care is free from defects. You also need to exercise reasonable care in selecting equipment for a specific procedure and patient and then helping to maintain the equipment. Your patient care must reflect what the reasonably well-qualified and prudent nurse would do in the same or similar circumstances. This means that if you know a specific piece of equipment isn't functioning properly, you must take steps to correct the defects and document the steps you took. If you don't, and a patient is injured because of the defective equipment, you may be sued for malpractice.

one to call the doctor, and intervene immediately, starting with airway, breathing, and circulation.

Remove malfunctioning or defective equipment from the patient's room. Attach a note stating "NEEDS REPAIR," and briefly describe the problem. Report the incident to the nurse-manager, risk manager, and engineering, and complete an incident report. Obtain new equipment and reassure the patient by checking out the new equipment to make sure it's functioning properly. Make sure the steps you take reflect your facility's policy and procedures. (See *Protecting the patient from faulty equipment*.)

ESSENTIAL DOCUMENTATION

On the incident report, record the time and date and describe how you discovered the equipment malfunction. Document your assessment of the patient's condition and the steps you took to ensure his safety and prevent further injury. Note the name of persons notified, such as the doctor, nursing supervisor, and risk manager, and the time of notification. Record doctor's orders given, your actions, and the patient's response. Outline the steps you took to troubleshoot or remove the faulty equipment. Include the name of the equipment, model, and serial number. Describe how the replacement equipment was checked to make sure it was functioning properly. Include your patient's response to the situation, patient education provided, and measures you took to reassure and calm the patient.

Faulty medical equipment may also need to be reported on a MedWatch form to the Food and Drug Administration.

4/1/05	2215	While performing hourly check at 2130, noted from
		time-tape of tube-feeding bag that 300 ml of tube
		feeding had been infused over past hour, despite the
		pump being set at 60 ml/hr. Calculated and counted
		drip rate of feeding and noted that it was running at
		300 ml/hr, rather than the ordered rate of 60 ml/hr.
		Immediately stopped tube feeding, flushed tube with
		30 ml of tap water, and capped tube. Placed pt. in high
		Fowler's position, breath sounds clear, abdomen soft
		and slightly distended, bowel sounds active in all 4
		quadrants. No c/o nausea, abdominal cramping or pain.
		P 92, BP 122/64, RR 24, oral T 98.0° F. Fresh urine
		sample neg for glucose. Blood glucose level by finger-
		stick 126. Dr. Rogers notified of incident at 2145.
		Ordered tube feeding to be held for next 5 hours and
		then restarted at 60 ml/hr. Blood glucose level to be
		added to morning blood work. Lab notified. Nursing
		supervisor, Michael Connor, RN, notified of incident at
		2150. Message left on answering machine of risk
		manager, Paula Brown, RN. Infusion Tech pump model
		230A, serial # 1234 removed from pt.'s room and
		placed in soiled utility room with note indicating that
		pump needs repair because of improper rate. Work
		order filled out, engineering called, and message left
		to notify of malfunctioning pump. Obtained new
		feeding pump, time-taped feeding bag. Will check drip
		rate q15min for first hour. Explained pump problem to
		pt. and that assessment revealed that pump malfunction
		hasn't caused him any problems. In answer to his
		questions, explained that a new pump is being used and
		that rate will be checked q15min for first hour, then
		hourly. Told pt. to report any abdominal cramps,
		bloating, pain, constipation, or diarrhea. ————
		———————————————— Peter Swanziger, RN

ESOPHAGEAL TUBE INSERTION

Used to control hemorrhage from esophageal or gastric varices, an esophageal tube is inserted nasally or orally by a doctor and advanced into the esophagus or stomach. A gastric balloon exerts pressure on the cardia of the stomach, securing the tube and controlling bleeding varices. Most tubes also contain an esophageal balloon to control esophageal bleeding. Usually, gastric or esophageal balloons are deflated after 24 to 36 hours, according to facility policy, to reduce the risk of pressure necrosis.

ESSENTIAL DOCUMENTATION

Document that the patient understands the procedure and that a consent form has been signed. Make sure your documentation includes the date and time that you assisted with the insertion of the esophageal tube and the name of the doctor who performed the procedure. Include the type of tube used. As applicable, record the type of sedation administered. Record vital signs before, during, and after the procedure. Document the patient's tolerance of the insertion procedure.

Document the intraesophageal balloon pressure (for Sengstaken-Blakemore and Minnesota tubes), the intragastric balloon pressure (for the Minnesota tube), or the amount of air injected (for Linton and Sengstaken-Blakemore tubes). Include the amount of any fluid used for gastric irrigation and the color, consistency, and amount of gastric return before and after lavage.

Because intraesophageal balloon pressure varies with respirations and esophageal contractions, be sure to record the baseline pressure, which is the most important pressure.

2/11/05	1210	Procedure explained to pt. by Dr. Fisher. Pt. verbalized
		understanding of procedure and consent signed. Before
		procedure P 102, BP 90/60, RR 22, oral T 97.0° F.
		Sengstaken-Blakemore tube placed w/o difficulty by Dr.
		Fisher via ® nostril. 50 ml air injected into gastric
		balloon. Abdominal X-ray obtained to confirm placement.
		Gastric balloon inflated with 500 ml air. Tube secured
		to football helmet traction. P 102, BP 98/52, RR 28.
		Large amt. bright red bloody drainage noted. Tube
		irrigated with 1800 ml of NSS until clear. NG tube
		placed in Ⓛ nostril by Dr. Fisher and attached to
		continuous suction. Esophageal balloon inflated to
		30 mm Hg and clamped. Equal breath sounds bilaterally.
		No SOB. After procedure P 98, BP 92/58, RR 24, oral T
		97.0° F. Stayed with pt. throughout procedure and held
		his hand. Directed pt. to take slow deep breaths to
		maintain RR and HR WNL. ———— Evelyn Sutcliffe, RN

ESOPHAGEAL TUBE REMOVAL

After gastric or esophageal bleeding has been controlled, the doctor will remove the esophageal tube by first deflating the esophageal balloon. Then, if bleeding doesn't recur, traction from the gastric tube is removed and the gastric balloon is deflated.

ESSENTIAL DOCUMENTATION

Make sure you document the date and time you assisted with removal of the esophageal tube and the name of the doctor who performed the procedure. Record whether bleeding recurred after deflation of the esophageal balloon. Record deflation of the gastric balloon. Document vital signs before and after the tube removal. Include the patient's tolerance of the procedure and any mouth or nasal care performed.

2/12/05	1100	Assisted Dr. Fisher with removal of Sengstaken–
		Blakemore tube. Before removal P 84, BP 102/68, RR 18,
		oral T 99.1° F. No bleeding noted after deflation of
		esophageal tube. Gastric balloon deflated. No resistance
		noted with removal of esophageal tube. After removal
		P 86, BP 110/68, RR 20, oral T 99.2° F. Pt. stated he
		was "happy to have the tube out." Assisted pt. to brush
		teeth and rinse with mouthwash. Cleaned crusted nasal
		secretions with cotton-tipped applicators and warm
		water. ———————————————— Evelyn Sutcliffe, RN

EVIDENCE COLLECTION, SUSPECTED CRIMINAL CASE

Suppose you're asked to care for an injured suspect who's accompanied by the police. Because the police need evidence, they ask you to give them the patient's belongings and also a sample of his blood. If you're ignorant of the law and fail to follow proper protocol, the evidence you turn over to the police may not be admissible in court. Worse still, the patient may later be able to sue you for invasion of privacy. However, if an accused

LEGAL CASEBOOK

TO SEARCH OR NOT TO SEARCH

The Fourth Amendment to the U.S. Constitution provides that "the right of the people to be secure in their persons, houses, papers, and effects, against unreasonable searches and seizures shall not be violated, and no warrants shall be issued, but upon probable cause." This means that every individual, even a suspected criminal, has a right to privacy, including a right to be free from intrusions that are made without search warrants. However, the Fourth Amendment doesn't absolutely prohibit all searches and seizures, only the unreasonable ones.

In general, searches that occur as part of medical care don't violate a suspect's rights. However, searches made for the sole purpose of gathering evidence — especially if done at police request — very well may. Several courts have said that a suspect subjected to an illegal private search has a right to seek remedy against the unlawful searcher in a civil lawsuit.

---

person consents to a search, any evidence found is considered admissible in court. (See *To search or not to search.*)

Opinions differ as to whether a blood test, such as an alcohol blood test, is admissible in court if the person refused consent for the test. A doctor or nurse who does blood work without the patient's consent may be liable for committing battery, even if the patient is a suspected criminal and the blood work is medically necessary. (See *Collecting blood as evidence,* page 144.)

Because the laws of search and seizure are complex and subject to change by new legal decisions, consult an administrator or hospital attorney before complying with a police request to turn over a patient's personal property.

ESSENTIAL DOCUMENTATION

Be careful and precise in documenting all medical and nursing procedures. Note any blood work done. List all treatments and the patient's response to them. Record anything you turn over to the police or administration and the name of the person you gave it to. Statements made by the patient should be recorded only if they're directly related to his care. If your patient keeps a journal during his stay, document this in your note. Document the presence of a police officer and your interactions

LEGAL CASEBOOK

COLLECTING BLOOD AS EVIDENCE

Opinions differ as to whether a blood test, such as a blood alcohol test, is admissible in court if the person refused consent for the test. In *Schmerber v. California (1966)*, the U.S. Supreme Court said that a blood extraction obtained without a warrant, incidental to a lawful arrest, isn't an unconstitutional search and seizure and is admissible evidence. Many courts have held this to mean that a blood sample must be drawn after the arrest to be admissible.

Further, the blood sample must be drawn in a medically reasonable manner. In *People v. Kraft (1970)*, a suspect was pinned to the floor by two police officers while a doctor drew a blood sample. In *State v. Riggins (1977)*, a suspect's fractured arm was twisted while a police officer sat on him to force consent to a blood test. In both cases, the courts ruled the test results inadmissible. The courts have also ruled as inadmissible—and as a violation of due process rights—evidence gained by the forcible and unconsented insertion of a nasogastric tube into a suspect to remove stomach contents *(Rochin v. California [1952])*.

Courts have admitted blood tests as evidence when the tests weren't for medically necessary purposes such as blood typing *(Commonwealth v. Gordon [1968])*. Some courts have also allowed blood work to be admitted as evidence when it was drawn for nontherapeutic reasons and voluntarily turned over to the police.

Be careful, though. A doctor or nurse who does blood work without the patient's consent may be liable for committing battery, even if the patient is a suspected criminal and the blood work is medically necessary.

with the officer. Document the name of the administrator or hospital attorney with whom you consulted before turning anything over to the police.

If you discover evidence, use your facility's chain of custody form to document the identity of each person handling the evidence as well as the dates and times it was in their possession. If your facility doesn't have a chain of custody form, keep careful notes of exactly what was taken, by whom, and when. Give this information to the administrator when you deliver the evidence. Until such time as the evidence can be turned over, it should be kept in a locked area.

6/7/05	2300	Mr. Piper was escorted by a police officer to the ED
		with four lacerations on Ⓛ leg. Pt. smelled of alcohol
		and cigarette smoke. He was calm but easily agitated.
		While cutting his pant leg to remove his pants, a ziplock
		bag with a white powder fell to the floor. In addition,
		a pocketknife, $6.87, and a pen were collected. Officer
		Smitts requested the knife and bag of white powder.
		After discussing the request with Arnold Beckwith, Chief
		Administrator, the knife and bag of powder were
		turned over to Officer Smitts. The remaining items
		and clothing, which consisted of pen, brown belt, and
		lightweight blue jacket, were bagged and left with pt. Pt.
		states he had tetanus shot last year. Lacerations of Ⓛ
		leg were irrigated with sterile NSS, stitched by Dr.
		Rogers after administering local anesthetic injections,
		antibiotic ointment applied, and covered with dry sterile
		dressings. Mr. Piper reports only minimal discomfort at
		laceration site. Explained care of lacerations and signs
		and symptoms of infection to report. Pt. verbalized
		understanding. Written ED guidelines for care of
		stitches given to pt. —————————— L. Salamon RN

EXPERIMENTAL PROCEDURES

At times, you may participate in administering experimental drugs or procedures to patients or administering established drugs in new ways or at experimental dosage levels. Follow the experimental protocol – not your usual sources, such as policies and procedures. Obtain information on the project and attempt to reach the research coordinator. Another resource is your institutional review board or human subjects committee, who review and accept the protocol before it's instituted. Ensure that the patient has provided informed consent.

If you work in a facility that uses investigational drugs or engages in research, your policies and procedures must state that the patient or surrogate receives a clear explanation of experimental treatment. This includes the procedures to be followed, a clear description of potential discomforts and risks, a list of alternative treatments, and a clear explanation that patients may refuse to participate in the research project without compromising their access to care and treatment.

ESSENTIAL DOCUMENTATION

Document that the patient has given informed consent for the drug or procedure. Obtain a copy of the consent form, if possible. Record the purpose of the drug or procedure, carefully describing the rationale for its use. Obtain a copy of the protocol, if possible, and follow the protocol precisely. Obtain a doctor's order permitting the continuation of the drug or treatment. Note deviations to the protocol and the addition of other treatments or medications. Record concerns or questions that the patient may have about the protocol, who you notified about the concerns, their response, and the patient's response. Likewise, describe possible adverse effects, who you notified, their response, your actions, and the patient's response.

10/03/05	1400	Pt. admitted to unit at 1315. States she's enrolled in a study for an experimental chemotherapy drug and that she wishes to continue with her treatment during this admission. Dr. Marks notified of pt.'s admission and participation in a drug trial at 1330. Informed consent for drug trial, name of drug, drug information, study protocol, and contact information faxed to unit and placed in pt.'s chart. Verbal and faxed orders obtained to continue drug protocol. Drug information and orders faxed to pharmacy. Nursing supervisor, Colleen Begacki, RN, notified of situation at 1335. ———————————————————— Lisa Mendocino, RN

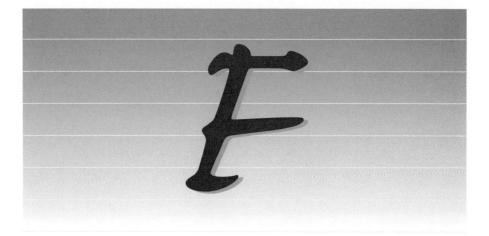

FAILURE TO PROVIDE INFORMATION

You may occasionally encounter a patient who refuses to provide accurate or complete information about his health history, current medications, or treatments. He may be uncooperative for various reasons: He thinks too many caregivers have asked him the same questions too many times, he doesn't understand the significance of the information, he's fearful or disoriented, or he's suspicious of why you want him to divulge personal information. Alternatively, he may have severe pain, a psychiatric problem, or a language barrier. In such situations, try to obtain the information from other sources or forms.

ESSENTIAL DOCUMENTATION

Clearly document any trouble you've had communicating with the patient. Record his responses using his own words. Include your interventions or explanations of the importance of this information in order to provide the patient with the best possible care. Document the name of the doctor you notified about the patient's refusal to share information and the time of notification. Write down other sources of information, such as family members or previous records.

2/5/05	0830	When asked for a list of his current medications, the pt. said, "Why do you want to know? What business is it of yours? I don't know why I have to answer that question." Explained reasons for needing to know about medications, but pt. still refused to share this information. No previous records available. No family members in to visit pt. Pt. won't share names or telephone numbers of family members. Called Dr. Traynor at 0815 to report pt. failure to provide information. Dr. will speak with pt. on his rounds this a.m. ——————————————— Nora Martin, RN

FALLS, PATIENT

Falls are a major cause of injury and death among elderly people. In fact, the older the person, the more likely he'll die due to a fall or its complications. In acute care hospitals, 85% of all inpatient incident reports are related to falls; of those who fall, 10% fall more than once and 10% experience a fatal fall. In nursing homes, approximately 60% of residents fall every year and about 40% of those residents experience more than one fall.

If your patient falls despite your preventative measures, stay with him and don't move him until you've performed a head-to-toe assessment and checked his vital signs. Assign another person to notify the doctor. Provide any emergency measures necessary, such as securing an airway, controlling bleeding, or stabilizing a deformed limb. Ask the patient or a witness what happened. Ask the patient if he's in pain or hit his head. If you don't detect any problems, return the patient to bed with the help of another person.

ESSENTIAL DOCUMENTATION

If a patient falls despite precautions, be sure to file an incident report and chart the event. (See "Incident report," page 219.) Record how the patient was found and the time he was discovered. Stick to your objective assessment, avoiding any judgments or opinions. Assess the patient and record any bruises, lacerations, or abrasions. Describe any pain or deformity in the extremities, particularly the hip, arm, leg, or lumbar spine. Record vital signs, including orthostatic blood pressure. Document your patient's neurologic assessment. Include slurred speech, weakness in the extremities, or a change in mental status. Record the name of the doctor and other persons notified, such as family members, and the time of notification. Include instructions or orders given. Also document any patient education.

11/6/05	1400	Pt. found on floor between bed and chair on left side
		of bed at 1330. Pt. c/o pain in her ℞ hip area and
		difficulty moving ℞ leg. No abrasions or lacerations
		noted. BP elevated at 158/94. Didn't move pt. to
		determine orthostatic changes, P 94, RR 22, oral T
		98.2° F. Pt states, "I was trying to get into the chair
		when I fell." Pt. alert and oriented to time, place, and
		person. Speech clear and coherent. Hand grasps strong
		bilaterally. ℞ leg externally rotated and shorter than Ⓛ
		leg. Dr. Dayoub notified at 1338. Pt. assisted back to bed
		with assist of 3, maintaining ℞ hip and leg in alignment.
		Hip X-ray ordered and showed ℞ hip fracture. Dr.
		Dayoub aware and family notified. Pt. to be evaluated by
		orthopedic surgeon. Pt. medicated for pain with Demerol
		50 mg I.M. Maintaining bed rest at present time.
		Explaining all procedures to pt. Call bell in hand and
		understands to call for help with moving. ———
		————————————— Beverly Kotsur, RN

FALLS, PRECAUTIONS

Patient falls resulting from slips, slides, knees giving way, fainting, or tripping over equipment can lead to prolonged hospitalization, increased hospital costs, and liability problems. Because falls raise so many problems, your facility may require you to assess each patient for his risk of falling and to take measures to prevent falls. (See *Reducing the risk of falls,* page 150.) If your facility requires a risk assessment form for patients, complete it and keep it in the patient's chart. (See *Risk assessment for falls,* page 151.) Those at risk require a care plan reflecting interventions to prevent falls. (See *Reducing your liability in patient falls,* page 152.)

ESSENTIAL DOCUMENTATION

Record the time and date of your entry. Describe the reasons for implementing fall precautions for your patient, such as a high score on a risk for falls assessment tool. Document your interventions, such as frequent toileting, reorienting the patient to his environment, and placing needed objects within his reach. Include the patient's response to these interventions. Note measures taken to alert other health care workers of the risk for falls, such as placing a band on the patient's wrist and communicating

(Text continues on page 152.)

REDUCING THE RISK OF FALLS

There are no foolproof ways to prevent a patient from falling, but the Joint Commission on Accreditation of Healthcare Organizations recommends the following steps to reduce the risks of falls and injuries. Be sure to document your safety interventions in the appropriate place in the medical record.

PHYSICAL MEASURES
- Provide adequate exercise and ambulation.
- Offer frequent food and liquids.
- Provide regular toileting.
- Evaluate medications (hypnotics, sedatives, analgesics, psychotropics, antihypertensives, laxatives, diuretics, and polypharmacy increase the risk of falling).
- Assess and manage pain.
- Promote normal sleep patterns.

PSYCHOLOGICAL MEASURES
- Reorient the patient to his environment.
- Communicate with the patient and his family about the risk for falls and the need to call for help before getting up on his own.
- Teach relaxation techniques.
- Provide companionship, such as sitters or volunteers.
- Provide diversionary activities.

ENVIRONMENTAL MEASURES
- Orient the patient to his environment.
- Use appropriate lighting and noise control.
- Consider a bed alarm.
- Provide a safe space layout (long-term care), such as a low-lying bed or mattress or pads on the floor.
- Place assistive devices within the patient's reach at all times.
- Provide bed adaptations (long-term care).
- Provide accessibility to needed objects at all times.
- Ensure frequent observation of any patient at risk, such as moving the patient closer to the nurses' station and involving family.
- Provide side rail adaptations and alternatives.
- Use appropriate seating and equipment.
- Provide identifiers of high-risk status, such as an arm band or an identifier on the patient's bed or door.

EDUCATION
- Provide staff, patient, and family education on identifying and reducing the risk of falls.

| 1/26/06 | 1000 | Score of 13 on admission Risk Assessment for Falls form. High risk for falls communicated to pt. and family. Risk for falls ID placed on pt.'s L wrist, high-risk for falls checked off on care plan and Kardex. Pt. alert and oriented to time, place, and person. Oriented pt. and family to room and call bell system. Told pt. to call for help before getting out of bed or up from chair on his own. Pt. demonstrated proper use of call bell and verbalized when to use it. Personal items and call bell placed within reach. ———— Betty Floyd, RN |

AccuChart

RISK ASSESSMENT FOR FALLS

Because falls raise so many problems, your facility may require an all-out risk assessment and prevention effort. If so, you'll need to document your role in this activity. For example, if your facility requires a risk assessment form for patients, complete it and keep it in the patient's chart.

Certain patients have a greater risk of falling than others. Using a chart such as the one below, which was developed for use with older patients, can help you determine the extent of the risk. To use the chart, check each applicable item and total the number of points. A score of 10 or more indicates a risk of falling.

DETERMINING A PATIENT'S RISK OF FALLING

Points	Patient category
	Age
1	80 or older
2 ✓	70 to 79 years old
	Mental state
0	Oriented at all times or comatose
2	Confused at all times
4 ✓	Confused periodically
	Duration of hospitalization
0 ✓	Over 3 days
2	0 to 3 days
	Falls within the past 6 months
0	None
2 ✓	1 or 2
5	3 or more
	Elimination
0 ✓	Independent and continent
1	Uses catheter, ostomy, or both
3	Needs help with elimination
5	Independent and incontinent
1 ✓	**Visual impairment**
3	**Confinement to chair**
2	**Blood pressure** Drop in systolic pressure of 20 mm Hg or more between lying and standing positions

Points	Patient category
	Gait and balance Assess gait by having the patient stand in one spot with both feet on the ground for 30 seconds without holding onto something. Then have him walk straight ahead and through a doorway. Next, have him turn while walking.
1	Wide base of support
1	Loss of balance while standing
1 ✓	Balance problems when walking
1	Diminished muscle coordination
1	Lurching or swaying
1	Holds on or changes gait when walking through a doorway
1	Jerking or instability when turning
1	Needs an assistive device such as a walker
	Medications How many different drugs is the patient taking?
0	None
1	1
2 ✓	2 or more

___ Alcohol	___ Cathartics
___ Anesthetics	___ Diuretics
___ Antihistamines	___ Opioids
✓ Antihyperten-sives	___ Psychotropics
___ Antiseizure drugs	___ Sedative-hypnotics
___ Antidiabetics	___ Other drugs
✓ Benzodiazepines	(specify)

1 ✓   Check if the patient has changed drugs, dosage, or both in the past 5 days.

13   **TOTAL**

REDUCING YOUR LIABILITY
IN PATIENT FALLS

Patient falls are a very common area of nursing liability. Patients who are elderly, infirm, sedated, or mentally incapacitated are the most likely to fall. The case of *Stevenson v. Alta Bates (1937)* involved a patient who had a stroke and was learning to walk again. As two nurses, each holding one of the patient's arms, assisted her into the hospital's sunroom, one of the nurses let go of the patient and stepped forward to get a chair for her. The patient fell and sustained a fracture. The nurse was found negligent: The court said she should have anticipated the patient's need for a chair and made the appropriate arrangements before bringing the patient into the sunroom.

this risk on the patient's Kardex. Record any patient and family teaching and their level of understanding. In some facilities, patient and family education may be documented on an education flow sheet.

FALLS, VISITOR OR OTHER

Despite your best efforts to maintain a safe environment, falls may occur. Not only can your patient fall, but family members and other visitors may slip, slide, have knees give way, faint, or trip over equipment as well. When a visitor falls, document the event on an incident report. If the visitor requires medical attention, he should be seen in the emergency department.

ESSENTIAL DOCUMENTATION

Document a fall by a visitor on an incident report, not in the medical record of the patient he was visiting. Include the date and time in the incident report, and record the name, address, and telephone number of the visitor. Also, record the exact location of the fall and the visitor's report of how the fall occurred. Describe only what you saw and heard and what actions you took to provide care at the scene. Unless you saw the fall, write "found on floor." Record the name of the doctor and any other persons, such as the nursing supervisor, who were notified and the time of notification.

Assess the visitor and record any bruises, lacerations, or abrasions. Describe any pain or deformity in the extremities, particularly the hip, arm, leg, or lumbar spine. Record vital signs, including orthostatic blood pressure. Document your visitor's neurologic assessment. Include slurred speech, weakness in the extremities, or a change in mental status.

8/3/05	1215	Visitor Arlene Smith was observed being lowered to the floor by a second visitor, Jacob Smith, in the hallway outside room 402. Mrs. Smith bumped her ® elbow on the edge of the hallway railing and there is a 1" laceration with minimal bleeding. Mrs. Smith stated that she "felt dizzy" and asked her husband to help her. BP 100/58 lying, 98/60 standing, P 50, RR 22. Laceration cleaned with sterile NSS and 4" X 4" dressing applied. Assisted visitor into a wheelchair and taken to the ED for further evaluation. ———— Karen Cummings, RN

FIREARMS AT BEDSIDE

If you observe or have reason to believe that your patient has a firearm in his possession, follow your facility's policy and contact security and your nursing supervisor immediately. Keep other patients, staff, and visitors away from the area and let security handle the situation.

ESSENTIAL DOCUMENTATION

Record the date and time of your entry. Describe the circumstances of the discovery of the weapon and its appearance, including distinguishing marks, color, and approximate size. Record the name of the security guard and nursing supervisor notified, the time of notification, their instructions, and your actions. Record the visits of security and the nursing supervisor to the patient's room and their outcome. You'll also need to complete an incident report. (See "Incident report," page 219.)

8/23/05	1000	When reaching in bedside table at 0930 to retrieve
		basin to assist pt. with a.m. care, noted black gun,
		approx. 6" long. Closed bedside table door, pushing table
		back out of reach of bed, left room and closed door.
		Called security at 0931 and reported gun in bedside
		table of Rm. 312 to Officer Halliday, who responded
		that a security guard would be sent up immediately, to
		keep out of pt.'s room, and to keep staff, visitors, and
		other patients away from area. Called Mary Delaney, RN,
		nursing supervisor, at 0933, who reported she's on her
		way to the floor immediately. Security officer Moore
		spoke with pt., who produced license to carry gun and
		turned unloaded gun over to the officer to be locked
		in hospital safe until discharge. Ms. Delaney reinforced
		hospital policy on firearms to pt. who stated he under-
		stood. ——————————————— Tom O'Brien, RN

FIREARMS IN THE HOME

Weapons in the home, especially firearms, present a real and frightening threat to the safety and well-being of the patient, his family, and the home care team. Follow your agency's policies and procedures for dealing with firearms in the home

Above all, don't allow your patient or his family to keep a loaded firearm in the same room where you're delivering care. If a patient refuses to remove a loaded gun from the room, preferably to a locked location, don't continue your visit. Make it clear why you're leaving. Then call your supervisor and the patient's doctor and let them know about the firearm danger. Your agency may have an incident report in which you should document the problem.

In addition to considering your own safety in the presence of a loaded gun, you must also consider the safety of your patient and his family. If you become aware of a gun, assess the patient's home situation. Does the gun pose a threat to children in the home? Does anyone in the home have a mental illness? Do any family members have a history of violence? If you feel that a gun creates an unacceptable risk for someone in your patient's home, talk with your supervisor about which actions are appropriate.

ESSENTIAL DOCUMENTATION

Record your observations of weapons in the home, including location, ownership, and whether a gun is loaded. Document a history of mental illness in the patient or family members. Record whether the weapon is kept under lock and key. Note whether anyone in the family has a history of violence. If you discontinue your visit and leave the home because of a firearm, describe your reasons for leaving and include the name of the supervisor and doctor you notified. If you feel the home is unsafe for children or other family members, objectively document your reasons and record the name of the supervisor you notified, the directions given, and your actions taken.

4/10/05	1015	During visit to pt.'s home to assess abdominal wound,
		observed a firearm on the bedside table. Pt. stated it
		was his weapon and was unloaded. When asked, pt.
		agreed to remove gun and place it in a locked cabinet.
		Pt. denies personal or family history of mental illness
		or suicide attempts. States no problems with violence in
		family members. No children live in the home, although
		grandchildren occasionally visit. Pt. verbally agreed to
		lock up gun in cabinet before home health visits and
		when grandchildren visit. Supervisor, John Bellamy, RN,
		and Dr. Roche alerted to gun in home and pt.'s
		agreement to lock up gun before home visits. ————
		————————————————————— Sonja Tjaer, RN

FIREARMS ON FAMILY MEMBER OR VISITOR

If you observe that a family member or visitor has brought a gun to your facility, follow your facility's policy on dealing with firearms. Immediately contact your security department and nursing supervisor, and calmly divert all other visitors, staff, and patients away from the area.

ESSENTIAL DOCUMENTATION

Document the occurrence on an incident report. Record the visitor's name and relationship to the patient, if known. Describe the circumstances of the discovery of the weapon and its appearance, including distinguishing marks, color, and approximate size. Record the names of the security guard and nursing supervisor notified, the time of notification, their instructions, and your actions. Record the visits of security and the nursing supervisor to the patient's room and their outcome.

9/30/05	1445	While pt.'s brother, John Long, was visiting pt., noticed a
		gun in a holster under arm of his jacket when he bent
		over. Security officer, John Nelson, and nursing super-
		visor, Betty O'Leary, RN, notified immediately. ————
		————————————————————— Colleen Berry, RN

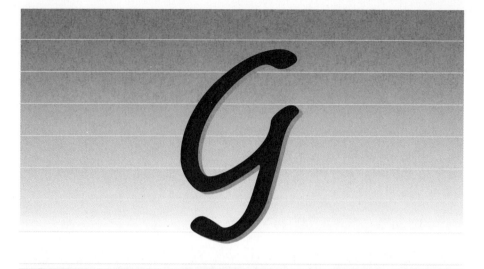

GASTRIC LAVAGE

After poisoning or a drug overdose, especially in patients who have central nervous system depression or an inadequate gag reflex, gastric lavage is used to flush the stomach and remove ingested substances through a gastric lavage tube. For patients with gastric or esophageal bleeding, a lavage with normal saline solution may be used to stop bleeding. Gastric lavage is contraindicated after ingestion of a corrosive substance, such as lye, ammonia, or mineral acids, because the lavage tube may perforate the already compromised esophagus.

Typically, a doctor, gastroenterologist, or nurse performs this procedure in the emergency department or intensive care unit. Correct lavage tube placement is essential for patient safety because accidental misplacement (in the lungs, for example) followed by lavage can be fatal.

Essential documentation

If possible, note the type of substance ingested, when the ingestion occurred, and how much substance was ingested. Obtain and record pre-procedure vital signs and level of consciousness (LOC). Record the date and time of lavage, the size and type of nasogastric tube used, the volume and type of irrigant, and the amount of drained gastric contents, including the color and consistency of drainage. Document the amount of irrigant solution instilled and gastric contents drained on the intake and output record sheet. Note whether drainage was sent to the laboratory for analysis. Also record any drugs instilled through the tube. Assess and record vital signs every 15 minutes on a frequent vital signs assessment sheet and LOC on a Glasgow Coma Scale sheet until the patient is stable. (See "Intake and output," page 230; "Level of consciousness, changes in," page 251; and "Vital signs, frequent," page 442.) Indicate the time that the tube was removed and how the patient tolerated the procedure.

4/22/05	2300	Single lumen #30 Fr. Ewald tube placed by Dr. Jones at
		2230, without difficulty, for gastric lavage following
		ingestion of unknown quantity of diazepam. Prelavage
		P 56, BP 90/52, RR 14 and shallow, rectal T 97.0° F. Pt.
		lethargic, unresponsive to verbal stimuli, but responsive
		to painful stimuli, gag reflex present but diminished,
		reflexes hypoactive, PEARL. Lavage performed with 250
		ml NSS, returned contents liquid green with small blue
		flecks and some undigested food. Sample collected and
		sent to lab for analysis. Postprocedure P 58, BP 90/54,
		RR 15, LOC unchanged. ———— Lisa Greenwald, RN
	2315	Lavage repeated x2 with 500 ml NSS each. Gastric
		return clear after third lavage. Total return 1375 ml.
		P 60, BP 94/52, RR 15. Lethargic but responsive to
		verbal stimuli, reflexes still sluggish. q15min VS and LOC
		documented on frequent vital signs and Glasgow Coma
		Scale sheets. Gastric tube left in place until pt. alert.
		———— Lisa Greenwald, RN

GI HEMORRHAGE

The loss of a large amount of blood from the GI tract is referred to as a GI hemorrhage. Bleeding in the upper GI tract is caused primarily by ulcers, varices, or tears within the GI system, whereas lower GI bleeding may be caused by diverticulitis, polyps, ulcerative colitis, or cancer. Your immediate lifesaving interventions focus on stabilizing the cardiovascular system, identifying the bleeding source, and stopping the bleeding.

ESSENTIAL DOCUMENTATION

Question your patient, if possible, and document how long blood has been noted in stool or vomitus and the amount and color of blood (for example, frank red blood, coffee-ground vomitus, or dark-colored or black stool). Record the results of your cardiovascular and GI assessments. Document your immediate interventions such as placing the vomiting patient on his side with the head of the bed elevated. Frequent vital signs and intake and output may be charted on the frequent vital signs assessment and intake and output sheets, respectively. (See "Intake and output," page 230; "Vital signs, frequent," page 442.) Record the name of the doctor that you notified, the time of notification, orders given, your actions, and the patient's response. Document patient education and emotional support given.

5/11/05	1315	Upon answering bathroom call light, found pt. sitting on commode, pale, c/o abdominal pain and reporting "The toilet is filled with blood." Toilet was filled with large amount of bright red blood. Assisted pt. to bed. BP 90/50, P 114 weak and regular, RR 28, oral T 99° F. Skin diaphoretic, cool. Pt. c/o dizziness but alert and oriented to time, place, and person. Abdomen slightly distended and tender to palpation in right upper and lower quadrants. Bowel sounds hyperactive. Noted blood seeping from rectum. Dr. Cooper notified at 1310 and will be here immediately to evaluate pt. ———————————————————————— L. Michelson, RN
	1330	Dr. Cooper in to see pt. and new orders written. Administering O₂ at 2 L/min via NC. Lab in to draw blood for CBC and electrolytes. I.V. infusion started with 20G catheter in ⓁU antecubital. 1000 ml NSS running at 125 ml/hr. Informed consent obtained by Dr. Cooper for colonoscopy. Reinforced with pt. what to expect before, during, and after the procedure. Pt. transported to the GI lab for colonoscopy via stretcher and escorted by medical resident. ——— L. Michelson, RN

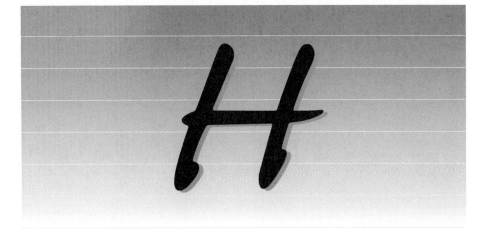

HEALTH INSURANCE PORTABILITY AND ACCOUNTABILITY ACT

The Health Insurance Portability and Accountability Act (HIPAA) of 1996 went into effect in the spring of 2003 to strengthen and protect patient privacy. Health care providers (such as doctors, nurses, pharmacies, hospitals, clinics, and nursing homes), health insurance plans, and government programs (such as Medicare and Medicaid) must notify patients about their right to privacy and how their health information will be used and shared. This includes information in the patient's medical record, conversations about the patient's care between health care providers, billing information, health insurers' computerized records, and other health information. Employees must also be taught about privacy procedures.

Under HIPAA, the patient also has the right to access his medical information, know when health information is shared, and make changes or corrections to his medical record. Patients also have the right to decide if they want to allow their information to be used for certain purposes, such as marketing or research. Patient records with identifiable health information must be secured so that the records aren't accessible to those who don't have a need for them. Identifiable health information may include the patient's name, Social Security number, identification number, birth date, admission and discharge dates, and health history.

When a patient receives health care, he will need to sign an authorization form before protected health information can be used for purposes

AccuChart

DOCUMENTING PATIENT AUTHORIZATION TO USE PERSONAL HEALTH INFORMATION

Your agency probably has an authorization form similar to the one below to be used for release of a patient's personal health information for reasons other than routine treatment or billing. Make sure all the required information is completed before having the patient or legal guardian sign the form.

AUTHORIZATION FORM

By signing, I authorize Community Hospital to use and/or disclose certain protected health information (PHI) about me to ___Dr. Bedarnz___. This authorization permits Community Hospital to use and/or disclose the following individually identifiable health information about me (specifically describe the information to be used or disclosed, such as dates(s) of services, type of services, level of detail to be released, origin of information, etc.):

X-ray films and report, notes on care from 2/6/05 Emergency Department visit

The information will be used or disclosed for the following purpose:

f/u care with Dr. Bedarnz

(If disclosure is requested by the patient, purpose may be listed as "at the request of the individual.")

The purpose(s) is/are provided so that I can make an informed decision whether to allow release of the information. This authorization will expire on ___2/7/05___.
The practice _____ will __X__ will not receive payment or other remuneration from a third party in exchange for using or disclosing the PHI.
I do not have to sign this authorization in order to receive treatment from Community Hospital. In fact, I have the right to refuse to sign this authorization. When my information is used or disclosed pursuant to this authorization, it may be subject to redisclosure by the recipient and may no longer be protected by the federal HIPAA Privacy Rule. I have the right to revoke this authorization in writing except to the extent that the practice has acted in reliance upon this authorization. My written revocation must be submitted to the Privacy Office at:

Community Hospital
123 Main Street
Oakwood, PA

Marcy Thayer	2/6/05	*self*
Signed by:	Date:	Relationship to patient:

Marcy Thayer	
Print patient's name	Print name of Legal Guardian, if applicable

other than routine treatment or billing. The form should be placed in the patient's medical record. (See *Documenting patient authorization to use personal health information.*)

ESSENTIAL DOCUMENTATION

Use your agency's HIPAA authorization form to document your patient's consent for the use and disclosure of protected health information. An authorization form must include a description of the health information that will be used and disclosed, the person authorized to use or disclose the information, the person to whom the disclosure will be made, an expiration date, and the purpose for sharing or using the information. The form is to be signed by the patient or legal guardian and placed in the patient's medical record.

HEARING IMPAIRMENT

Hearing loss occurs in varying degrees that range from the loss of only certain tones to total deafness. Hearing loss is most commonly classified by the cause of the impairment. Conductive loss results from the failure of sound waves to be transmitted through the external ear, middle ear, or both. Sensorineural loss results from pathologic changes in the inner ear, 8th cranial nerve, auditory centers of the brain, or all three. Mixed loss is a combination of conductive and sensorineural loss. Central hearing loss is a result of damage to the brain's auditory pathways or auditory center. Gross or precise assessment can be done to determine the extent of the hearing loss.

ESSENTIAL DOCUMENTATION

Determine the length of time that your patient has had the hearing loss. Describe the patient's degree of hearing loss and whether it's unilateral or bilateral. Note if the increased hearing loss is more significant in one ear. Record whether any hearing aids are being used. Include the effectiveness of hearing aids and the use of secondary modes of communication. Determine what additional methods are currently being used to compensate for the loss, such as lip-reading, sign language, picture boards, or writing pads. Update the nursing care plan to reflect alternative forms of communication with your patient.

8/06/05	1000	Pt. states he has had a gradual loss of hearing to both
		ears caused by many years of working in steel mills. He
		states he has used bilateral hearing aids for 6 years but
		has used only the ® aid for the last 2 months because the
		Ⓛ aid isn't fitting well and he hasn't replaced it. He's able
		to follow conversations and respond appropriately to
		questions. He states that lip-reading enhances compre-
		hension. Care plan amended to include facing pt. when
		speaking, no gum chewing while speaking with pt., and using
		a normal tone of voice. Dr. Peters notified of ill-fitting
		hearing aid. Audiologist will meet with pt. tomorrow at
		1000 to assess hearing aid fit and function. ————
		———————————————— Kimberly Sigfried, RN

HEART FAILURE, DAILY ASSESSMENT

A syndrome characterized by myocardial dysfunction, heart failure leads to impaired pump performance (reduced cardiac output) or to frank heart failure and abnormal circulatory congestion. Congestion of systemic venous circulation in right-sided heart failure may result in peripheral edema or hepatomegaly; congestion of pulmonary circulation in left-sided heart failure may cause pulmonary edema, an acute, life-threatening emergency.

Although heart failure may be acute (as a direct result of myocardial infarction), it's generally a chronic disorder associated with the retention of sodium and water by the kidneys. Care for a patient with heart failure centers on symptom management, fluid balance, and prevention and management of complications.

ESSENTIAL DOCUMENTATION

Record the date and time of your entry. Record your patient's subjective symptoms, such as shortness of breath, cough, activity intolerance, chest pain, orthopnea, and fatigue. Document your assessment of the respiratory system (adventitious breath sounds, use of accessory muscles, respiratory rate, pulse oximetry, and signs and symptoms of hypoxia) and cardiovascular system (jugular vein distention, abnormal heart sounds, heart rate, blood pressure, pallor, diaphoresis, cool, clammy skin, hemodynamic monitoring results, arrhythmias, the degree and location of edema, urine output, and mental status). Include any new laboratory data, ECG findings, and chest X-rays.

Record interventions, such as daily weight measurements, fluid restriction, I.V. therapy, and oxygen therapy, and the patient's response. Chart drugs given during your shift on the medication administration record or medication Kardex. Daily intake and output are recorded on the intake and output record. (See "Intake and output," page 230.) Record patient education on such topics as energy conservation, disease process, nutrition, fluid restrictions, daily weights, drugs and other treatments, and signs and symptoms to report to the nurse or doctor. Some facilities may use a patient education record to document any teaching you provide (See "Patient teaching," page 297.)

7/8/05	1500	Pt. is alert and oriented to time, place, and person. BP
		136/80, P 88 and regular, RR 20, oral T 98.6° F. O₂ sat.
		94% by pulse oximetry on 2 L by NC. Pt. reports SOB with
		ambulation to the bathroom, approx. 25' each way. Denies
		SOB at rest, no c/o cough or chest pain. Sleeps with 2
		pillows. Lungs with scattered rhonchi to posterior fields
		bilaterally, no use of accessory muscles. Skin is warm and
		dry, +2 pedal and ankle edema bilaterally, no JVD, S₃ heart
		sound on auscultation. Reports being compliant with 1500
		ml fluid restriction with 900 ml taken on this shift.
		Output this shift 1000 ml clear yellow urine. Wt. #132.5,
		unchanged from yesterday. Encouraged pt. to perform
		ADLs with rest periods as needed. Reviewed 2 gm Na diet
		and 1500 ml fluid restriction with pt. and wife. They
		asked many questions and verbalized understanding. See
		flowsheets for documentation of frequent VS, I10.
		———————————— June Lockhart, RN

HEAT APPLICATION

Heat applied directly to the patient's body raises tissue temperature and enhances the inflammatory process by causing vasodilation and increasing local circulation. This promotes leukocytosis, suppuration, drainage, and healing. Heat also increases tissue metabolism, reduces pain caused by muscle spasm, and decreases congestion in deep visceral organs. Moist heat softens crusts and exudates and penetrates deeper than dry heat.

ESSENTIAL DOCUMENTATION

Record the date and time of the application; the reason for the use of heat; the site of application; the type of heat used, such as dry or moist; the type of device, such as a hot-water bottle, electric heating pad, K pad, chemical hot pack, or warm compresses; the temperature or heat setting; measures taken to protect the patient's skin; and the duration of time the heat was applied. Include the condition of the skin before and after the application of heat, signs of complications, and the patient's response to the treatment. Record any patient education provided.

11/4/05	0900	Warm moist compress (128° F by bath thermometer)
		applied to lumbar region of the back for 20 min. for
		c/o stiffness and discomfort. Skin pink, warm, dry, and
		intact before application. Told pt. to lay compress over
		back and not to lie directly on compress. Instructed pt.
		to call for nurse if he experienced any pain. Skin pink,
		warm, dry, and intact after the procedure. Pt. reports
		decrease in stiffness and discomfort. — Brian Petry, RN

HEMODYNAMIC MONITORING

Continuous pulmonary artery pressure (PAP) and intermittent pulmonary artery wedge pressure (PAWP) measurements provide important information about left ventricular function and preload. This information is useful not only for monitoring, but also for aiding diagnosis, refining your assessment, guiding interventions, and projecting patient outcomes.

Nearly all acutely ill patients are candidates for PAP monitoring – especially those who are hemodynamically unstable, who need fluid management or continuous cardiopulmonary assessment, or who are receiving multiple or frequently administered cardioactive drugs. PAP monitoring is also crucial for patients with shock, trauma, pulmonary or cardiac disease, or multiorgan disease. It's also used before some major surgeries to obtain baseline measurements.

Current pulmonary artery (PA) catheters have up to six lumens. In addition to distal and proximal lumens used to measure pressures, a balloon inflation lumen inflates a balloon for PAWP measurement and a thermistor connector lumen allows cardiac output measurement. Some catheters also have a pacemaker wire lumen that provides a port for pacemaker electrodes and measures continuous mixed venous oxygen saturation.

The PA catheter is inserted into the heart's right side with the distal tip lying in the pulmonary artery. Fluoroscopy may not be required during catheter insertion because the catheter is flow directed, following venous blood flow from the right heart chambers into the pulmonary artery.

ESSENTIAL DOCUMENTATION

Document the date and time of catheter insertion. Include the name of the doctor who performed the procedure. Identify the number of catheter lumens, catheter insertion site, the pressure waveforms and values of the various heart chambers, and the balloon inflation volume required to obtain a wedge tracing. Note whether any arrhythmias occurred during or after the procedure. Document any solution infusing through the catheter ports. Record the type of flush solution used and its heparin concentration (if any). Describe the type of dressing applied and the patient's tolerance of the procedure. Chart all site care, dressing changes, tubing, and solution changes.

8/19/05	1300	PA catheter insertion procedure and need for hemo-dynamic monitoring explained to pt. and informed consent obtained by Dr. Monroe. Four-lumen thermo-dilution catheter inserted via the ® subclavian vein. Pressures on insertion: RV 30/5 mm Hg, PAP 24/10 mm Hg, PAWP 10 mm Hg, and CVP 6 mm Hg. Wedge tracing obtained with 1.5 ml of air for balloon inflation. Portable CXR completed to confirm place-ment. Standard flush solution infusing into distal port. NS infusing at 30 ml/hr into proximal port. Cardiac monitor shows sinus tachycardia with rate of 102; no arrhythmias noted during insertion. Site covered with sterile occlusive dressing. Pt. resting comfortably in bed with HOB at 30°, no c/o pain; breathing unlabored. ———— Kathy Osborne RN

HOME CARE, HOME CARE AIDE NEEDS

Home care aides provide hands-on personal care to the patient or services needed to maintain the patient's health or facilitate his medical treatment. Aides also provide respite to family members. Remember that Medicare will reimburse only for care provided by a certified level III home care aide.

You're responsible for developing the aide's care plan and supervising her activities in the patient's home. Most agencies use a standard care plan or duty assignment sheet for this purpose that can be adapted to fit each patient's needs.

To maintain state licensure and certification from Medicare and the Joint Commission on Accreditation of Healthcare Organizations, your agency must require the home care aide to follow the patient's care plan

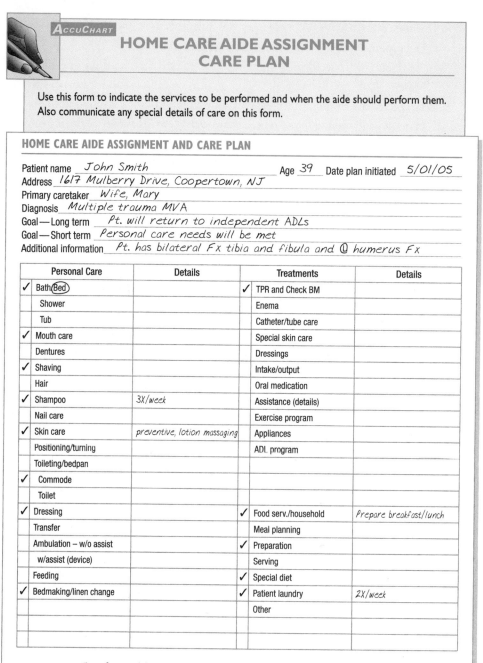

AccuChart

HOME CARE AIDE ASSIGNMENT
CARE PLAN

Use this form to indicate the services to be performed and when the aide should perform them.
Also communicate any special details of care on this form.

HOME CARE AIDE ASSIGNMENT AND CARE PLAN

Patient name *John Smith*   Age *39*   Date plan initiated *5/01/05*
Address *1617 Mulberry Drive, Coopertown, NJ*
Primary caretaker *Wife, Mary*
Diagnosis *Multiple trauma MVA*
Goal — Long term   *Pt. will return to independent ADLs*
Goal — Short term *Personal care needs will be met*
Additional information   *Pt. has bilateral Fx tibia and fibula and ① humerus Fx*

	Personal Care	Details		Treatments	Details
✓	Bath (Bed)		✓	TPR and Check BM	
	Shower			Enema	
	Tub			Catheter/tube care	
✓	Mouth care			Special skin care	
	Dentures			Dressings	
✓	Shaving			Intake/output	
	Hair			Oral medication	
✓	Shampoo	*3X/week*		Assistance (details)	
	Nail care			Exercise program	
✓	Skin care	*preventive, lotion massaging*		Appliances	
	Positioning/turning			ADL program	
	Toileting/bedpan				
✓	Commode				
	Toilet				
✓	Dressing		✓	Food serv./household	*Prepare breakfast/lunch*
	Transfer			Meal planning	
	Ambulation – w/o assist		✓	Preparation	
	w/assist (device)			Serving	
	Feeding		✓	Special diet	
✓	Bedmaking/linen change		✓	Patient laundry	*2X/week*
				Other	

RN signature ___*Jane Forman, RN*___

and to complete a separate home care aide note or entry in the patient's clinical record for every visit.

ESSENTIAL DOCUMENTATION

On the home care aide assignment and care plan form, you must itemize every activity that the aide is permitted to provide. This form may consist of a checklist of services and should include the date that the plan was initiated. (See *Home care aide assignment care plan.*) If the care plan was revised, this date must also be included. The patient's name, identifying information, doctor's name, diagnosis, and short- and long-term goals are also included on the plan.

HOME CARE, INITIAL ASSESSMENT

After you have received a referral and orders to begin home care, you need to perform a thorough assessment of the patient and his home environment to set reasonable goals and tailor the care to the patient's specific needs. Assessments vary slightly from agency to agency, but the basic information required for completion is the same.

The proposed Conditions of Participation for Home Health Agencies requires that Medicare-certified agencies complete a comprehensive assessment of home care patients using a standardized data set called the Outcome and Assessment Information Set (OASIS). OASIS was developed specifically to measure outcomes for adults who receive home care. Using this instrument, you'll collect data to measure changes in your patient's health status over time. Typically, you'll need to collect OASIS data when a patient starts home care, at the 60-day recertification point, and when the patient is discharged or transferred to another health care facility, such as a hospital or subacute care facility. (See *OASIS – Be careful how you chart,* page 168.)

ESSENTIAL DOCUMENTATION

Use your agency's form to thoroughly and specifically document your assessment of the patient's:
- nutritional status
- home environment in relation to safety and supportive services and groups, such as family, neighbors, and community

OASIS—BE CAREFUL HOW YOU CHART

The Outcome and Assessment Information Set (OASIS) was first implemented in 1999 to measure outcomes in home health care. In October of 2000, the OASIS format changed because of the new Medicare payment system for home health care called Prospective Payment System (PPS). What you document can have a significant impact on services your patient receives and the reimbursement your agency collects.

A point system is established for certain questions on the OASIS form, and it determines the reimbursement your agency will receive. For example, if your patient has had coronary artery bypass graft surgery and has two wounds, you must document each wound in the appropriate sections of the OASIS form. Failure to document one or both of the wounds could potentially cost your agency a significant amount of money. Wounds are just one of the indicators that govern how much your agency will be reimbursed for patient care.

Problems can also occur when your assessment on the OASIS form is inconsistent with the doctor's orders. For example, if the doctor has ordered gait training and transfers but you document on the OASIS form that your patient can transfer and ambulate independently, the entire claim may be denied because physical therapy isn't needed if the patient is independent.

These OASIS tools will be used by Medicare to compare information and review claims. If you have any questions about how to correctly answer OASIS questions in a given circumstance, contact your supervisor or continuous quality improvement nurse. Keep in mind that what you document has significant impact on your patient and your agency. Read the questions carefully and be sure of your answers. You do make a difference!

- knowledge of his disease or current condition, prognosis, and treatment plan
- potential for complying with the treatment plan.

When completing the OASIS data set, you'll fill in or check off information on more than 80 topics, including:

- sociodemographic data
- physiologic data
- functional data
- service utilization data
- mental, behavioral, and emotional data.

Refer to the OASIS-B1 form for an example of a completed data set. (See *Using the OASIS-B1 form,* pages 169 to 185.)

(Text continues on page 186.)

AccuChart

USING THE OASIS-B1 FORM

The Oasis-B1 form includes more than 80 topics, such as socioeconomic, physiologic, and functional data; service utilization information; and mental, behavioral, and emotional data.

OUTCOME AND ASSESSMENT INFORMATION SET (OASIS-B1)

START OF CARE Assessment (also used for Resumption of Care Following Inpatient Stay)	Client's Name: *Terry Elliot* Client Record No. *541234*

The Outcome and Assessment Information Set (OASIS) is the intellectual property of The Center for Health Services and Policy Research. Copyright ©2000 Used with Permission.

DEMOGRAPHIC/GENERAL INFORMATION

1. (M0010) Agency Medicare Provider Number:

2. (M0012) Agency Medicaid Provider Number:

> **Branch Identification** *(Optional, for Agency Use)*
> 3. (M0014) Branch State: _____
> 4. (M0016) Branch ID Number:
>
> Agency-assigned

5. (M0020) Patient ID Number:
   QCB/811757

6. (M0030) Start of Care Date: *07 / 02 / 2005*
   month   day   year

7. (M0032) Resumption of Care Date:
   ____ / ____ / ____   ☒ NA - Not Applicable
   month   day   year

8. (M0040) Patient Name:
   Terry   *S*
   First   MI
   Elliot   *Mr.*
   Last   Suffix

   Patient Address:
   11 Second Street
   Street, Route, Apt. Number
   Hometown
   City
   (M0050) Patient State of Residence: *PA*
   (M0060) Patient Zip Code: *10981 - 1234*
   Phone: (*881*) *555* - *2937*

9. (M0063) Medicare Number:
   134765482 A
   including suffix
   ☐ NA - No Medicare

10. (M0064) Social Security Number:
    111 - *22* - *3333*
    ☐ UK - Unknown or Not Available

11. (M0065) Medicaid Number:

    ☐ NA - No Medicaid

12. (M0066) Birth Date: *07 / 08 / 1926*
    month   day   year

13. (M0069) Gender:
    ☒ 1 - Male   ☐ 2 - Female

14. (M0072) Primary Referring Physician ID:
    222222   (UPIN#)
    ☐ UK - Unknown or Not Available
    Name *Dr. Kyle Stevens*
    Address *10 State St.*
    Hometown, PA 10981
    Phone: (*881*) *555* - *6900*
    FAX: (*881*) *555* - *6974*

15. (M0080) Discipline of Person Completing Assessment:
    ☒ 1-RN   ☐ 2-PT   ☐ 3-SLP/ST   ☐ 4-OT

16. (M0090) Date Assessment Completed:
    07 / 02 / 2005
    month   day   year

(continued)

USING THE OASIS-BI FORM *(continued)*

17. (M0100) This Assessment is Currently Being Completed for the Following Reason:

Start/Resumption of Care

- [X] 1 - Start of care—further visits planned
- [ ] 2 - Start of care—no further visits planned
- [ ] 3 - Resumption of care (after inpatient stay)

Follow-Up

- [ ] 4 - Recertification (follow-up) reassessment [Go to *M0150*]
- [ ] 5 - Other follow-up [Go to *M0150*]

Transfer to an Inpatient Facility

- [ ] 6 - Transferred to an inpatient facility—patient not discharged from agency [Go to *M0150*]
- [ ] 7 - Transferred to an inpatient facility—patient discharged from agency [Go to *M0150*]

Discharge from Agency—Not to an Inpatient Facility

- [ ] 8 - Death at home [Go to *M0150*]
- [ ] 9 - Discharge from agency [Go to *M0150*]
- [ ] 10 - Discharge from agency—no visits completed after start/resumption of care assessment [Go to *M0150*]

18. Marital status:
- [ ] Not Married [X] Married [ ] Widowed
- [ ] Divorced [ ] Separated [ ] Unknown

19. (M0140) Race/Ethnicity (as identified by patient): (Mark all that apply.)
- [ ] 1 - American Indian or Alaska Native
- [ ] 2 - Asian
- [ ] 3 - Black or African-American
- [ ] 4 - Hispanic or Latino
- [ ] 5 - Native Hawaiian or Pacific Islander
- [X] 6 - White
- [ ] UK - Unknown

20. Emergency contact:

Name _Susan Elliot_

Address _11 Second St._

Hometown, PA 10981

Phone: (_881_) _555_ - _2937_

21. (M0150) Current Payment Sources for Home Care: (Mark all that apply.)
- [ ] 0 - None; no charge for current services
- [X] 1 - Medicare (traditional fee-for-service)
- [ ] 2 - Medicare (HMO/managed care)
- [ ] 3 - Medicaid (traditional fee-for-service)
- [ ] 4 - Medicaid (HMO/managed care)
- [ ] 5 - Workers' compensation
- [ ] 6 - Title programs (Title III, V, or XX)
- [ ] 7 - Other government (CHAMPUS, VA, etc.)
- [ ] 8 - Private insurance
- [ ] 9 - Private HMO/managed care
- [ ] 10 - Self-pay
- [ ] 11 - Other (specify) _____
- [ ] UK - Unknown

22. (M0160) Financial Factors limiting the ability of the patient/family to meet basic health needs: (Mark all that apply.)
- [X] 0 - None
- [ ] 1 - Unable to afford medicine or medical supplies
- [ ] 2 - Unable to afford medical expenses that are not covered by insurance/Medicare (copayments)
- [ ] 3 - Unable to afford rent/utility bills
- [ ] 4 - Unable to afford food
- [ ] 5 - Other (specify)

PATIENT HISTORY

23. (M0175) From which of the following **Inpatient Facilities** was the patient discharged *during the past 14 days*? (Mark all that apply.)
- [ ] 1 - Hospital
- [ ] 2 - Rehabilitation facility
- [ ] 3 - Skilled nursing facility
- [ ] 4 - Other nursing home
- [ ] 5 - Other (specify) _____
- [X] NA - Patient was not discharged from an inpatient facility [If NA, go to *M0200*]

24. (M0180) Inpatient Discharge Date (most recent):

_____ / _____ / _____
month day year

- [ ] UK - Unknown

USING THE OASIS-B1 FORM *(continued)*

25. **(M0190)** Inpatient Diagnoses and ICD code categories (three digits required; five digits optional) *for only those conditions treated during an inpatient facility stay within the last 14 days* (no surgical or V-codes):

Inpatient Facility Diagnosis	ICD
a._____	(_____ . ____)
b._____	(_____ . ____)

26. **(M0200)** **Medical or Treatment Regimen Change Within Past 14 Days:** Has this patient experienced a change in medical or treatment regimen (medication, treatment, or service change due to new or additional diagnosis) within the last 14 days?

☐ 0 - No [If No, go to *M0220*]

☒ 1 - Yes

27. **(M0210)** List the patient's **Medical Diagnoses** and ICD code categories (three digits required; five digits optional) *or those conditions requiring changed medical or treatment regimen* (no surgical or V-codes):

Changed Medical Regimen Diagnosis	ICD
a. *open wound @ ankle*	(*891* . ____)
b._____	(_____ . ____)
c._____	(_____ . ____)
d._____	(_____ . ____)

28. **(M0220)** **Conditions Prior to Medical or Treatment Regimen Change or Inpatient Stay Within Past 14 Days:** If this patient experienced an inpatient facility discharge or change in medical or treatment regimen within the past 14 days, indicate any conditions that existed *prior to* the inpatient stay or change in medical or treatment regimen. **(Mark all that apply.)**

☐ 1 - Urinary incontinence

☐ 2 - Indwelling/suprapubic catheter

☐ 3 - Intractable pain

☐ 4 - Impaired decision-making

☐ 5 - Disruptive or socially inappropriate behavior

☐ 6 - Memory loss to the extent that supervision required

☒ 7 - None of the above

☐ NA - No inpatient facility discharge *and* no change in medical or treatment regimen in past 14 days

☐ UK - Unknown

29. **(M0230/M0240)** **Diagnoses and Severity Index:** List each medical diagnosis or problem for which the patient is receiving home care and ICD code category (three digits required; five digits optional — no surgical or V-codes) and rate them using the following severity index. (Choose one value that represents the most severe rating appropriate for each diagnosis.)

0 - Asymptomatic, no treatment needed at this time

1 - Symptoms well controlled with current therapy

2 - Symptoms controlled with difficulty, affecting daily functioning; patient needs ongoing monitoring

3 - Symptoms poorly controlled, patient needs frequent adjustment in treatment and dose monitoring

4 - Symptoms poorly controlled, history of rehospitalizations

(M0230) Primary Diagnosis   **ICD**

a. *open wound @ ankle* (*891* . *00*)

Severity Rating ☐ 0 ☐ 1 ☒ 2 ☐ 3 ☐ 4

(M0240) Other Diagnoses   **ICD**

b. *Type 2 diabetes* (*250* . *72*)

Severity Rating ☐ 0 ☐ 1 ☒ 2 ☐ 3 ☐ 4

c. *PVD* (*443* . *89*)

Severity Rating ☐ 0 ☐ 1 ☐ 2 ☐ 3 ☐ 4

d._____ (_____ . ____)

Severity Rating ☐ 0 ☐ 1 ☐ 2 ☐ 3 ☐ 4

e._____ (_____ . ____)

Severity Rating ☐ 0 ☐ 1 ☐ 2 ☐ 3 ☐ 4

f._____ (_____ . ____)

Severity Rating ☐ 0 ☐ 1 ☐ 2 ☐ 3 ☐ 4

30. Patient/family knowledge and coping level regarding present illness:

Patient *Knowledgeable about disease process*

Family *anxious to assist in care*

31. Signifcant past health history:

PVD

Type 2 diabetes

® BKA

USING THE OASIS-B1 FORM *(continued)*

32. (M0250) **Therapies** the patient receives *at home*: **(Mark all that apply.)**

☐ 1 - Intravenous or infusion therapy (excludes TPN)

☐ 2 - Parenteral nutrition (TPN or lipids)

☐ 3 - Enteral nutrition (nasogastric, gastrostomy, jejunostomy, or any other artificial entry into the alimentary canal)

☒ 4 - None of the above

33. (M0260) **Overall Prognosis:** BEST description of patient's overall prognosis for *recovery from this episode of illness*.

☐ 0 - Poor: little or no recovery is expected and/or further decline is imminent

☒ 1 - Good/Fair: partial to full recovery is expected

☐ UK - Unknown

34. (M0270) **Rehabilitative Prognosis:** BEST description of patient's prognosis for *functional status*.

☒ 0 - Guarded: minimal improvement in functional status is expected; decline is possible

☐ 1 - Good: marked improvement in functional status is expected

☐ UK - Unknown

35. (M0280) **Life Expectancy:** (Physician documentation is not required.)

☒ 0 - Life expectancy is greater than 6 months

☐ 1 - Life expectancy is 6 months or fewer

36. **Immunization/screening tests:**

Immunizations:

Flu	☒ Yes ☐ No	Date	*10/04*
Tetanus	☒ Yes ☐ No	Date	*3/00*
Pneumonia	☒ Yes ☐ No	Date	*10/04*
Other _____		Date	

Screening:

Cholesterol level	☒ Yes ☐ No	Date	*1/05*
Mammogram	☐ Yes ☒ No	Date	
Colon cancer screen	☒ Yes ☐ No	Date	*1/03*
Prostate cancer screen	☒ Yes ☐ No	Date	*1/05*

Self-exam frequency:

Breast self-exam frequency _____

Testicular self-exam frequency _____

37. **Allergies:** *NKA* _____

38. (M0290) **High Risk Factors** characterizing this patient: **(Mark all that apply.)**

☒ 1 - Heavy smoking

☐ 2 - Obesity

☐ 3 - Alcohol dependency

☐ 4 - Drug dependency

☐ 5 - None of the above

☐ UK - Unknown

LIVING ARRANGEMENTS

39. (M0300) **Current Residence:**

☒ 1 - Patient's owned or rented residence (house, apartment, or mobile home owned or rented by patient/couple/significant other)

☐ 2 - Family member's residence

☐ 3 - Boarding home or rented room

☐ 4 - Board and care or assisted living facility

☐ 5 - Other (specify) _____

40. (M0310) **Structural Barriers** in the patient's environment limiting independent mobility: **(Mark all that apply.)**

☐ 0 - None

☒ 1 - Stairs inside home which *must* be used by the patient (to get to toileting, sleeping, eating areas)

☐ 2 - Stairs inside home which are used optionally (to get to laundry facilities)

☒ 3 - Stairs leading from inside house to outside

☐ 4 - Narrow or obstructed doorways

41. (M0320) **Safety Hazards** found in the patient's current place of residence: **(Mark all that apply.)**

☒ 0 - None

☐ 1 - Inadequate floor, roof, or windows

☐ 2 - Inadequate lighting

☐ 3 - Unsafe gas/electric appliance

☐ 4 - Inadequate heating

☐ 5 - Inadequate cooling

☐ 6 - Lack of fire safety devices

☐ 7 - Unsafe floor coverings

☐ 8 - Inadequate stair railings

☐ 9 - Improperly stored hazardous materials

☐ 10 - Lead-based paint

☐ 11 - Other (specify) _____

USING THE OASIS-BI FORM *(continued)*

42. **(M0330) Sanitation Hazards** found in the patient's current place of residence: **(Mark all that apply.)**

- ☒ 0 - None
- ☐ 1 - No running water
- ☐ 2 - Contaminated water
- ☐ 3 - No toileting facilities
- ☐ 4 - Outdoor toileting facilities only
- ☐ 5 - Inadequate sewage disposal
- ☐ 6 - Inadequate/improper food storage
- ☐ 7 - No food refrigeration
- ☐ 8 - No cooking facilities
- ☐ 9 - Insects/rodents present
- ☐ 10 - No scheduled trash pickup
- ☐ 11 - Cluttered/soiled living area
- ☐ 12 - Other (specify) _____

43. **(M0340) Patient Lives With: (Mark all that apply.)**

- ☐ 1 - Lives alone
- ☒ 2 - With spouse or significant other
- ☐ 3 - With other family member
- ☐ 4 - With a friend
- ☐ 5 - With paid help (other than home care agency staff)
- ☐ 6 - With other than above

Comments: _____

44. **Others living in household:** _____

Name *Susan* _____ Age *70* Sex *F*
Relationship *wife* Able/willing to assist ☒ Yes ☐ No
Name _____ Age _____ Sex _____
Relationship _____ Able/willing to assist ☐ Yes ☐ No
Name _____ Age _____ Sex _____
Relationship _____ Able/willing to assist ☐ Yes ☐ No
Name _____ Age _____ Sex _____
Relationship _____ Able/willing to assist ☐ Yes ☐ No
Name _____ Age _____ Sex _____
Relationship _____ Able/willing to assist ☐ Yes ☐ No
Name _____ Age _____ Sex _____
Relationship _____ Able/willing to assist ☐ Yes ☐ No

SUPPORTIVE ASSISTANCE

45. **Persons/Organizations providing assistance:**

_____
_____
_____

46. **(M0350) Assisting Person(s) Other than Home Care Agency Staff: (Mark all that apply.)**

- ☐ 1 - Relatives, friends, or neighbors living outside the home
- ☒ 2 - Person residing in the home (EXCLUDING paid help)
- ☐ 3 - Paid help
- ☐ 4 - None of the above
       [If None of the above, go to *Review of Systems*]
- ☐ UK - Unknown [If Unknown, go to *Review of Systems*]

47. **(M0360) Primary Caregiver** taking *lead* responsibility for providing or managing the patient's care, providing the most frequent assistance (other than home care agency staff):

- ☐ 0 - No one person [If No one person, go to *M0390*]
- ☒ 1 - Spouse or significant other
- ☐ 2 - Daughter or son
- ☐ 3 - Other family member
- ☐ 4 - Friend or neighbor or community or church member
- ☐ 5 - Paid help
- ☐ UK - Unknown [If Unknown, go to *M0390*]

48. **(M0370) How Often** does the patient receive assistance from the primary caregiver?

- ☒ 1 - Several times during day and night
- ☐ 2 - Several times during day
- ☐ 3 - Once daily
- ☐ 4 - Three or more times per week
- ☐ 5 - One to two times per week
- ☐ 6 - Less often than weekly
- ☐ UK - Unknown

USING THE OASIS-B1 FORM *(continued)*

49. (M0380) Type of Primary Caregiver Assistance: (Mark all that apply.)

☒ 1 - ADL assistance (bathing, dressing, toileting, bowel/bladder, eating/feeding)

☒ 2 - IADL assistance (meds, meals, housekeeping, laundry, telephone, shopping, finances)

☐ 3 - Environmental support (housing, home maintenance)

☒ 4 - Psychosocial support (socialization, companionship, recreation)

☒ 5 - Advocates or facilitates patient's participation in appropriate medical care

☐ 6 - Financial agent, power of attorney, or conservator of finance

☐ 7 - Health care agent, conservator of person, or medical power of attorney

☐ UK - Unknown

Comments: _____

_____

_____

REVIEW OF SYSTEMS

SENSORY STATUS

(Mark S for subjective, O for objectively assessed problem. If no problem present or if not assessed, mark NA.)

Head *NA* Dizziness

NA Headache (describe location, duration) _____

_____

Eyes *O* Glasses *NA* Cataracts *NA* Blurred/double vision

O PERRL ____ Other (specify) _____

50. (M0390) Vision with corrective lenses if the patient usually wears them:

☒ 0 - Normal vision: sees adequately in most situations; can see medication labels, newsprint.

☐ 1 - Partially impaired: cannot see medication labels or newsprint, but *can* see obstacles in path, and the surrounding layout; can count fingers at arm's length.

☐ 2 - Severely impaired: cannot locate objects without hearing or touching them *or* patient nonresponsive.

Ears *NA* Hearing aid *NA* Tinnitus

____ Other (specify) _____

51. (M0400) Hearing and Ability to Understand Spoken Language in patient's own language (with hearing aids if the patient usually uses them):

☒ 0 - No observable impairment. Able to hear and understand complex or detailed instructions and extended or abstract conversation.

☐ 1 - With minimal difficulty, able to hear and understand most multi-step instructions and ordinary conversation. May need occasional repetition, extra time, or louder voice.

☐ 2 - Has moderate difficulty hearing and understanding simple, one-step instructions and brief conversation; needs frequent prompting or assistance.

☐ 3 - Has severe difficulty hearing and understanding simple greetings and short comments. Requires multiple repetitions, restatements, demonstrations, additional time.

☐ 4 - *Unable* to hear and understand familiar words or common expressions consistently, *or* patient nonresponsive.

Oral *NA* Gum problems *NA* Chewing problems

O Dentures ____ Other (specify) _____

52. (M0410) Speech and Oral (Verbal) Expression of Language (in patient's own language):

☒ 0 - Expresses complex ideas, feelings, and needs clearly, completely, and easily in all situations with no observable impairment.

☐ 1 - Minimal difficulty in expressing ideas and needs (may take extra time; makes occasional errors in word choice, grammar or speech intelligibility; needs minimal prompting or assistance).

☐ 2 - Expresses simple ideas or needs with moderate difficulty (needs prompting or assistance, errors in word choice, organization or speech intelligibility). Speaks in phrases or short sentences.

☐ 3 - Has severe difficulty expressing basic ideas or needs and requires maximal assistance or guessing by listener. Speech limited to single words or short phrases.

☐ 4 - *Unable* to express basic needs even with maximal prompting or assistance but is not comatose or unresponsive (speech is nonsensical or unintelligible).

☐ 5 - Patient nonresponsive or unable to speak.

USING THE OASIS-B1 FORM *(continued)*

Nose and sinus
_N/A_ Epistaxis ____ Other (specify)_____

Neck and throat
_N/A_ Hoarseness _N/A_ Difficulty swallowing
____ Other (specify)_____

Musculoskeletal, Neurological

_N/A_ Hx arthritis	_N/A_ Joint pain	_N/A_ Syncope
_N/A_ Gout	_N/A_ Weakness	_N/A_ Seizure
_N/A_ Stiffness	_S_ Leg cramps	_N/A_ Tenderness
_N/A_ Swollen joints	_S_ Numbness	_N/A_ Deformities
_N/A_ Unequal grasp	_O_ Temp changes	_N/A_ Comatose
_N/A_ Tremor	_N/A_ Aphasia/inarticulate speech	

____ Paralysis (describe)_____
_X_ Amputation (location) _® BKA_
____ Other (specify)_____
Coordination, gait, balance (describe)
 Gait steady

Comments (Prosthesis, appliances)
 Uses a walker + ® prosthesis

Patient's perceived pain level: ___4___ (Scale 1-10)

53. (M0420) Frequency of Pain interfering with patient's activity or movement:
- [ ] 0 - Patient has no pain or pain does not interfere with activity or movement
- [ ] 1 - Less often than daily
- [x] 2 - Daily, but not constantly
- [ ] 3 - All of the time

54. (M0430) Intractable Pain: Is the patient experiencing pain that is *not easily relieved*, occurs at least daily, and affects the patient's sleep, appetite, physical or emotional energy, concentration, personal relationships, emotions, or ability or desire to perform physical activity?
- [x] 0 - No
- [ ] 1 - Yes
Comments (pain management)_____

INTEGUMENTARY STATUS
_O_ Hair changes (where) _balding_
_N/A_ Puritus ____ Other (specify)_____
Skin condition (Record type # on body area. Indicate size to right of numbered category.)

	Type	Size
1.	Lesions	
2.	Bruises	
3.	Masses	
4.	Scars	
5.	Stasis Ulcers	_1/2" round_
6.	Pressure Ulcers	
7.	Incisions	
8.	Other (specify)	

55. (M0440) Does this patient have a **Skin Lesion** or an **Open Wound**? This excludes "OSTOMIES."
- [ ] 0 - No [If No, go to *Cardio/respiratory status*]
- [x] 1 - Yes

56. (M0445) Does this patient have a **Pressure Ulcer**?
- [x] 0 - No [If No, go to *M0468*]
- [ ] 1 - Yes

(continued)

USING THE OASIS-B1 FORM *(continued)*

57. (M0450) **Current Number of Pressure Ulcers at Each Stage:** (Circle one response for each stage.)

Pressure Ulcer Stages	Number of Pressure Ulcers
a) Stage 1: Nonblanchable erythema of intact skin; the heralding of skin ulceration. In darker-pigmented skin, warmth, edema, hardness, or discolored skin may be indicators.	0 1 2 3 4 or more
b) Stage 2: Partial-thickness skin loss involving epidermis and/or dermis. The ulcer is superficial and presents clinically as an abrasion, blister, or shallow crater.	0 1 2 3 4 or more
c) Stage 3: Full-thickness skin loss involving damage or necrosis of subcutaneous tissue, which may extend down to, but not through, underlying fascia. The ulcer presents clinically as a deep crater with or without undermining of adjacent tissue.	0 1 2 3 4 or more
d) Stage 4: Full-thickness skin loss with extensive destruction, tissue necrosis, or damage to muscle, bone, or supporting structures (tendon, joint capsule)	0 1 2 3 4 or more

e) In addition to the above, is there at least one pressure ulcer that cannot be observed due to the presence of eschar or a nonremovable dressing, including casts?

☐ 0 - No
☐ 1 - Yes

58. (M0460) **Stage of Most Problematic (Observable) Pressure Ulcer:**

☐ 1 - Stage 1
☐ 2 - Stage 2
☐ 3 - Stage 3
☐ 4 - Stage 4
☐ NA - No observable pressure ulcer

59. (M0464) **Status of Most Problematic (Observable) Pressure Ulcer:**

☐ 1 - Fully granulating
☐ 2 - Early/partial granulation
☐ 3 - Not healing
☐ NA - No observable pressure ulcer

60. (M0468) Does this patient have a **Stasis Ulcer?**

☐ 0 - No [If No, go to *M0482*]
☒ 1 - Yes

61. (M0470) **Current Number of Observable Stasis Ulcer(s):**

☐ 0 - Zero
☒ 1 - One
☐ 2 - Two
☐ 3 - Three
☐ 4 - Four or more

62. (M0474) **Does this patient have at least one Stasis Ulcer that Cannot be Observed** due to the presence of a nonremovable dressing?

☒ 0 - No
☐ 1 - Yes

63. (M0476) **Status of Most Problematic (Observable) Stasis Ulcer:**

☐ 1 - Fully granulating
☒ 2 - Early/partial granulation
☐ 3 - Not healing
☐ NA - No observable stasis ulcer

64. (M0482) Does this patient have a **Surgical Wound?**

☒ 0 - No [If No, go to *Cardio/Respiratory Status*]
☐ 1 - Yes

65. (M0484) **Current Number of (Observable) Surgical Wounds:** (If a wound is partially closed but has *more* than one opening, consider each opening as a separate wound.)

☐ 0 - Zero
☐ 1 - One
☐ 2 - Two
☐ 3 - Three
☐ 4 - Four or more

66. (M0486) Does this patient have at least one **Surgical Wound that Cannot be Observed** due to the presence of a nonremovable dressing?

☐ 0 - No
☐ 1 - Yes

USING THE OASIS-BI FORM *(continued)*

67. (M0488) Status of Most Problematic (Observable) Surgical Wound:

- ☐ 1 - Fully granulating
- ☐ 2 - Early/partial granulation
- ☐ 3 - Not healing
- ☐ NA - No observable surgical wound

CARDIO/RESPIRATORY STATUS

Temperature *99*   Respirations *18*

Blood pressure
  Lying *132/80* Sitting *130/78* Standing *130/76*

Pulse
  Apical rate *72*   Radial rate *72*
  Rhythm *Regular*   Quality _____

Cardiovascular

N/A Palpitations	*N/A* Chest pains
S Claudication	*N/A* Murmurs
S Fatigues easily	*O* Edema
N/A BP problems	*N/A* Cyanosis
N/A Dyspnea on exertion	*N/A* Varicosities

  N/A Paroxysmal nocturnal dyspnea
  N/A Orthopnea (# of pillows)
  N/A Cardiac problems (specify)_____
  N/A Pacemaker _____
              (Date of last battery change)
  Other (specify) _____
  Comments _____
  _____
  _____
  _____

Respiratory
  History of

N/A Asthma	*N/A* Pleurisy
N/A TB	*N/A* Pneumonia
S Bronchitis	*N/A* Emphysema

  Other (specify) _____
  Present condition
  S Cough (describe) *Dry*
  O Breath sounds (describe) *Clear*
  N/A Sputum (character and amount) _____
  Other (specify) _____

68. (M0490) When is the patient dyspneic or noticeably Short of Breath?

- ☒ 0 - Never, patient is not short of breath
- ☐ 1 - When walking more than 20 feet, climbing stairs
- ☐ 2 - With moderate exertion (while dressing, using commode or bedpan, walking distances less than 20 feet)
- ☐ 3 - With minimal exertion (while eating, talking, or performing other ADLs) or with agitation
- ☐ 4 - At rest (during day or night)

69. (M0500) Respiratory Treatments utilized at home: (Mark all that apply.)

- ☐ 1 - Oxygen (intermittent or continuous)
- ☐ 2 - Ventilator (continually or at night)
- ☐ 3 - Continuous positive airway pressure
- ☒ 4 - None of the above

Comments _____
_____
_____
_____
_____

ELIMINATION STATUS

Genitourinary Tract

N/A Frequency	*N/A* Prostate disorder
N/A Pain	*N/A* Dysmenorrhea
N/A Hematuria	*N/A* Lesions
N/A Vaginal discharge/bleeding	*N/A* Hx hysterectomy
S Nocturia	*N/A* Gravida/Para
N/A Urgency	*N/A* Contraception

  N/A Date last PAP _____
  Other (specify) _____

70. (M0510) Has this patient been treated for a Urinary Tract Infection in the past 14 days?

- ☒ 0 - No
- ☐ 1 - Yes
- ☐ NA - Patient on prophylactic treatment
- ☐ UK - Unknown

(continued)

USING THE OASIS-B1 FORM *(continued)*

71. **(M0520) Urinary Incontinence or Urinary Catheter Presence:**

☒ 0 - No incontinence or catheter (includes anuria or ostomy for urinary drainage) [If No, go to *M0540*]

☐ 1 - Patient is incontinent

☐ 2 - Patient requires a urinary catheter (external, indwelling, intermittent, suprapubic) [Go to *M0540*]

72. **(M0530) When does Urinary Incontinence occur?**

☐ 0 - Timed-voiding defers incontinence

☐ 1 - During the night only

☐ 2 - During the day and night

Comments (appliances and care, bladder programs, cather type, frequency of irrigation and change) _____

_____

_____

_____

_____

Gastrointestinal Tract

N/A Indigestion   *N/A* Rectal bleeding

N/A Nausea/vomiting   *N/A* Hemorrhoids

N/A Ulcers   *N/A* Gallbladder problems

N/A Pain   *N/A* Jaundice

N/A Diarrhea/constipation *N/A* Tenderness

N/A Hernias (where)_____

Other (specify) _____

73. **(M0540) Bowel Incontinence Frequency:**

☒ 0 - Very rarely or never has bowel incontinence

☐ 1 - Less than once weekly

☐ 2 - One to three times weekly

☐ 3 - Four to six times weekly

☐ 4 - On a daily basis

☐ 5 - More often than once daily

☐ NA - Patient has ostomy for bowel elimination

☐ UK - Unknown

74. **(M0550) Ostomy for Bowel Elimination:** Does this patient have an ostomy for bowel elimination that (within the last 14 days):
a) was related to an inpatient facility stay, *or*
b) necessitated a change in medical or treatment regimen?

☒ 0 - Patient does *not* have an ostomy for bowel elimination.

☐ 1 - Patient's ostomy was *not* related to an inpatient stay and did *not* necessitate change in medical or treatment regimen.

☐ 2 - The ostomy *was* related to an inpatient stay or *did* necessitate change in medical or treatment regimen.

Comments (bowel function, stool color, bowel program, GI series, abd. girth) _____

_____

_____

_____

Nutritional status

N/A Weight loss/gain last 3 mos. (Give amount_____)

N/A Over/under weight   *N/A* Change in appetite

Diet *20% protein, 30% fat*

Other (specify) _____

Meals prepared by *Wife*

Comments _____

_____

_____

_____

Breasts (For both male and female)

N/A Lumps   *N/A* Tenderness

N/A Discharge   *N/A* Pain

Other (specify) _____

Comments _____

_____

_____

_____

USING THE OASIS-BI FORM *(continued)*

NEURO/EMOTIONAL/BEHAVIORAL STATUS

N/A Hx of previous psych. illness

Other (specify) _____

75. **(M0560) Cognitive Functioning:** (Patient's current level of alertness, orientation, comprehension, concentration, and immediate memory for simple commands.)

☐ 0 - Alert/oriented, able to focus and shift attention, comprehends and recalls task directions independently.

☒ 1 - Requires prompting (cuing, repetition, reminders) only under stressful or unfamiliar conditions.

☐ 2 - Requires assistance and some direction in specific situations (on all tasks involving shifting of attention), or consistently requires low stimulus environment due to distractibility.

☐ 3 - Requires considerable assistance in routine situations. Is not alert and oriented or is unable to shift attention and recall directions more than half the time.

☐ 4 - Totally dependent due to disturbances, such as constant disorientation, coma, persistent vegetative state, or delirium.

76. **(M0570) When Confused** (Reported or Observed):

☒ 0 - Never

☐ 1 - In new or complex situations only

☐ 2 - On awakening or at night only

☐ 3 - During the day and evening, but not constantly

☐ 4 - Constantly

☐ NA - Patient nonresponsive

77. **(M0580) When Anxious** (Reported or Observed):

☐ 0 - None of the time

☐ 1 - Less often than daily

☒ 2 - Daily, but not constantly

☐ 3 - All of the time

☐ NA - Patient nonresponsive

78. **(M0590) Depressive Feelings Reported or Observed in Patient:** (Mark all that apply.)

☐ 1 - Depressed mood (feeling sad, tearful)

☐ 2 - Sense of failure or self reproach

☒ 3 - Hopelessness

☐ 4 - Recurrent thoughts of death

☐ 5 - Thoughts of suicide

☐ 6 - None of the above feelings observed or reported

79. **(M0600) Patient Behaviors (Reported or Observed):** (Mark all that apply.)

☐ 1 - Indecisiveness, lack of concentration

☐ 2 - Diminished interest in most activities

☐ 3 - Sleep disturbances

☐ 4 - Recent change in appetite or weight

☐ 5 - Agitation

☐ 6 - A suicide attempt

☒ 7 - None of the above behaviors observed or reported

80. **(M0610) Behaviors Demonstrated *at Least Once a Week*** (Reported or Observed): (Mark all that apply.)

☐ 1 - Memory deficit: failure to recognize familiar persons/places, inability to recall events of past 24 hours, significant memory loss so that supervision is required

☐ 2 - Impaired decision-making: failure to perform usual ADLs or IADLs, inability to appropriately stop activities, jeopardizes safety through actions

☐ 3 - Verbal disruption: yelling, threatening, excessive profanity, sexual references

☐ 4 - Physical aggression: aggressive or combative to self and others (hits self, throws objects, punches, dangerous maneuvers with wheelchair or other objects)

☐ 5 - Disruptive, infantile, or socially inappropriate behavior (**excludes** verbal actions)

☐ 6 - Delusional, hallucinatory, or paranoid behavior

☒ 7 - None of the above behaviors demonstrated

USING THE OASIS-B1 FORM *(continued)*

81. (M0620) **Frequency of Behavior Problems (Reported or Observed)** (wandering episodes, self abuse, verbal disruption, physical aggression):

☒ 0 - Never
☐ 1 - Less than once a month
☐ 2 - Once a month
☐ 3 - Several times each month
☐ 4 - Several times a week
☐ 5 - At least daily

82. (M0630) Is this patient receiving **Psychiatric Nursing Services** at home provided by a qualified psychiatric nurse?

☒ 0 - No
☐ 1 - Yes
Comments _____

_____

_____

Endocrine and hematopoietic

_S_ Diabetes   _N/A_ Polydipsia
_N/A_ Polyuria   _N/A_ Thyroid problem
_N/A_ Excessive bleeding or bruising
_S_ Intolerance to heat and cold

Fractionals
Usual results _____
Frequency checked _____
Other (specify) _____
Comments _____

_____

_____

_____

ADL/IADLs

For M0640-M0800, complete the "Current" column for all patients. For these same items, complete the "Prior" column only at start of care and at resumption of care; mark the level that corresponds to the patient's condition 14 days prior to start of care date (M0030) or resumption of care date (M0032). In all cases, record what the patient is *able to do.*

83 (M0640) **Grooming:** Ability to tend to personal hygiene needs (washing face and hands, hair care, shaving or make up, teeth or denture care, fingernail care).

Prior   Current

☒   ☐   0 - Able to groom self unaided, with or without the use of assistive devices or adapted methods.

☐   ☒   1 - Grooming utensils must be placed within reach before able to complete grooming activities.

☐   ☐   2 - Someone must assist the patient to groom self.

☐   ☐   3 - Patient depends entirely upon someone else for grooming needs.

☐   ☐   UK - Unknown

84. (M0650) **Ability to Dress *Upper* Body** (with or without dressing aids), including undergarments, pullovers, front-opening shirts and blouses, managing zippers, buttons, and snaps:

Prior   Current

☒   ☐   0 - Able to get clothes out of closets and drawers, put them on and remove them from the upper body without assistance.

☐   ☒   1 - Able to dress upper body without assistance if clothing is laid out or handed to the patient.

☐   ☐   2 - Someone must help the patient put on upper body clothing.

☐   ☐   3 - Patient depends entirely upon another person to dress the upper body.

☐   UK - Unknown

USING THE OASIS-BI FORM *(continued)*

85. (M0660) Ability to Dress *Lower* Body (with or without dressing aids), including undergarments, slacks, socks or nylons, shoes:

Prior Current

[X]   [ ]   0 - Able to obtain, put on, and remove clothing and shoes without assistance.

[ ]   [ ]   1 - Able to dress lower body without assistance if clothing and shoes are laid out or handed to the patient.

[ ]   [X]   2 - Someone must help the patient put on undergarments, slacks, socks or nylons, and shoes.

[ ]   [ ]   3 - Patient depends entirely upon another person to dress lower body.

[ ]   UK - Unknown

86. (M0670) Bathing: Ability to wash entire body. *Excludes grooming (washing face and hands only).*

Prior Current

[ ]   [ ]   0 - Able to bathe self in s*hower or tub* independently.

[X]   [ ]   1 - With the use of devices, is able to bathe self in shower or tub independently.

[ ]   [ ]   2 - Able to bathe in shower or tub with the assistance of another person:
    (a) for intermittent supervision or encouragement or reminders, *OR*
    (b) to get in and out of the shower or tub, *OR*
    (c) for washing difficult to reach areas.

[ ]   [X]   3 - Participates in bathing self in shower or tub, *but* requires presence of another person throughout the bath for assistance or supervision.

[ ]   [ ]   4 - *Unable* to use the shower or tub and is bathed in *bed or bedside chair.*

[ ]   [ ]   5 - Unable to effectively participate in bathing and is totally bathed by another person.

[ ]   UK - Unknown

87. (M0680) Toileting: Ability to get to and from the toilet or bedside commode.

Prior Current

[X]   [ ]   0 - Able to get to and from the toilet independently with or without a device.

[ ]   [X]   1 - When reminded, assisted, or supervised by another person, able to get to and from the toilet.

[ ]   [ ]   2 - *Unable* to get to and from the toilet but is able to use a bedside commode (with or without assistance).

[ ]   [ ]   3 - *Unable* to get to and from the toilet or bedside commode but is able to use a bedpan/urinal independently.

[ ]   [ ]   4 - Is totally dependent in toileting.

[ ]   UK - Unknown

88. (M0690) Transferring: Ability to move from bed to chair, on and off toilet or commode, into and out of tub or shower, and ability to turn and position self in bed if patient is bedfast.

Prior Current

[ ]   [ ]   0 - Able to independently transfer.

[X]   [X]   1 - Transfers with minimal human assistance or with use of an assistive device.

[ ]   [ ]   2 - *Unable* to transfer self but is able to bear weight and pivot during the transfer process.

[ ]   [ ]   3 - Unable to transfer self and is *unable* to bear weight or pivot when transferred by another person.

[ ]   [ ]   4 - Bedfast, unable to transfer but is able to turn and position self in bed.

[ ]   [ ]   5 - Bedfast, unable to transfer and is *unable* to turn and position self.

[ ]   UK - Unknown

(continued)

USING THE OASIS-B1 FORM *(continued)*

89. (M0700) Ambulation/Locomotion: Ability to *safely* walk, once in a standing position, or use a wheelchair, once in a seated position, on a variety of surfaces.

Prior   Current

☒ ☐ 0 - Able to independently walk on even and uneven surfaces and climb stairs with or without railings (needs no human assistance or assistive device).

☐ ☒ 1 - Requires use of a device (cane, walker) to walk alone or requires human supervision or assistance to negotiate stairs, steps, or uneven surfaces.

☐ ☐ 2 - Able to walk only with the supervision or assistance of another person at all times.

☐ ☐ 3 - Chairfast, *unable* to ambulate but is able to wheel self independently.

☐ ☐ 4 - Chairfast, unable to ambulate and is *unable* to wheel self.

☐ ☐ 5 - Bedfast, unable to ambulate or be up in a chair.

☐ UK - Unknown

90. (M0710) Feeding or Eating: Ability to feed self meals and snacks. **Note: This** refers only to the process of *eating, chewing,* and *swallowing, not preparing* the food to be eaten.

Prior   Current

☒ ☒ 0 - Able to independently feed self.

☐ ☐ 1 - Able to feed self independently but requires:
(a) meal setup; *OR*
(b) intermittent assistance or supervision from another person; *OR*
(c) a liquid, pureed or ground meat diet.

☐ ☐ 2 - *Unable* to feed self and must be assisted or supervised throughout the meal/snack.

☐ ☐ 3 - Able to take in nutrients orally *and* receives supplemental nutrients through a nasogastric tube or gastrostomy.

☐ ☐ 4 - *Unable* to take in nutrients orally and is fed nutrients through a nasogastric tube or gastrostomy.

☐ ☐ 5 - Unable to take in nutrients orally or by tube feeding.

☐ UK - Unknown

91. (M0720) Planning and Preparing Light Meals (cereal, sandwich) or reheat delivered meals:

Prior   Current

☒ ☐ 0 - (a) Able to independently plan and prepare all light meals for self or reheat delivered meals; OR
(b) Is physically, cognitively, and mentally able to prepare light meals on a regular basis but has not routinely performed light meal preparation in the past (prior to this home care admission).

☐ ☒ 1 - *Unable* to prepare light meals on a regular basis due to physical, cognitive, or mental limitations.

☐ ☐ 2 - Unable to prepare any light meals or reheat any delivered meals.

☐ UK - Unknown

92. (M0730) Transportation: Physical and mental ability to *safely* use a car, taxi, or public transportation (bus, train, subway).

Prior   Current

☐ ☐ 0 - Able to independently drive a regular or adapted car; OR uses a regular or handicap-accessible public bus.

☒ ☒ 1 - Able to ride in a car only when driven by another person; OR able to use a bus or handicap van only when assisted or accompanied by another person.

☐ ☐ 2 - Unable to ride in a car, taxi, bus, or van, and requires transportation by ambulance.

☐ UK - Unknown

USING THE OASIS-BI FORM *(continued)*

93. (M0740) Laundry: Ability to do own laundry — to carry laundry to and from washing machine, to use washer and dryer, to wash small items by hand.

Prior   Current

☐   ☐   0 - (a) Able to independently take care of all laundry tasks; *OR*
    (b) Physically, cognitively, and mentally able to do laundry and access facilities, but has not routinely performed laundry tasks in the past (prior to this home care admission).

☒   ☐   1 - Able to do only light laundry, such as minor hand wash or light washer loads. Due to physical, cognitive, or mental limitations, needs assistance with heavy laundry such as carrying large loads of laundry.

☐   ☒   2 - *Unable* to do any laundry due to physical limitation or needs continual supervision and assistance due to cognitive or mental limitation.

☐   UK - Unknown

94. (M0750) Housekeeping: Ability to safely and effectively perform light housekeeping and heavier cleaning tasks.

Prior   Current

☐   ☐   0 - (a) Able to independently perform all housekeeping tasks; *OR*
    (b) Physically, cognitively, and mentally able to perform *all* housekeeping tasks but has not routinely participated in housekeeping tasks in the past (prior to this home care admission).

☐   ☐   1 - Able to perform only *light* housekeeping (dusting, wiping kitchen counters) tasks independently.

☐   ☐   2 - Able to perform housekeeping tasks with intermittent assistance or supervision from another person.

☐   ☐   3 - *Unable* to consistently perform any housekeeping tasks unless assisted by another person throughout the process.

☒   ☒   4 - Unable to effectively participate in any housekeeping tasks.

☐   UK - Unknown

95. (M0760) Shopping: Ability to plan for, select, and purchase items in a store and to carry them home or arrange delivery.

Prior   Current

☐   ☐   0 - (a) Able to plan for shopping needs and independently perform shopping tasks, including carrying packages; *OR*
    (b) Physically, cognitively, and mentally able to take care of shopping, but has not done shopping in the past (prior to this home care admission).

☐   ☐   1 - Able to go shopping, but needs some assistance:
    (a) By self is able to do only light shopping and carry small packages, but needs someone to do occasional major shopping; *OR*
    (b) *Unable* to go shopping alone, but can go with someone to assist.

☒   ☒   2 - *Unable* to go shopping, but is able to identify items needed, place orders, and arrange home delivery.

☐   ☐   3 - Needs someone to do all shopping and errands.

☐   UK - Unknown

96. (M0770) Ability to Use Telephone: Ability to answer the phone, dial numbers, and *effectively* use the telephone to communicate.

Prior   Current

☒   ☒   0 - Able to dial numbers and answer calls appropriately and as desired.

☐   ☐   1 - Able to use a specially adapted telephone (large numbers on the dial, teletype phone for the deaf) and call essential numbers.

☐   ☐   2 - Able to answer the telephone and carry on a normal conversation but has difficulty with placing calls.

☐   ☐   3 - Able to answer the telephone only some of the time or is able to carry on only a limited conversation.

☐   ☐   4 - *Unable* to answer the telephone at all but can listen if assisted with equipment.

☐   ☐   5 - Totally unable to use the telephone.

☐   ☐   NA - Patient does not have a telephone.

☐   UK - Unknown

(continued)

USING THE OASIS-B1 FORM *(continued)*

MEDICATIONS

97. (M0780) Management of Oral Medications: *Patient's ability* to prepare and take all prescribed oral medications reliably and safely, including administration of the correct dosage at the appropriate times/intervals. *Excludes* injectable and I.V. medications. (NOTE: This refers to ability, not compliance or willingness.)

Prior   Current

[X]   [X]   0 - Able to independently take the correct oral medication(s) and proper dosage(s) at the correct times.

☐   ☐   1 - Able to take medication(s) at the correct times if:
(a) individual dosages are prepared in advance by another person; *OR*
(b) given daily reminders; *OR*
(c) someone develops a drug diary or chart.

☐   ☐   2 - *Unable* to take medication unless administered by someone else.

☐   ☐   NA - No oral medications prescribed.

☐   UK - Unknown

98. (M0790) Management of Inhalant/Mist Medications: *Patient's ability* to prepare and take all prescribed inhalant/mist medications (nebulizers, metered-dose devices) reliably and safely, including administration of the correct dosage at the appropriate times/intervals. *Excludes* all other forms of medication (oral tablets, injectable and I.V. medications).

Prior   Current

☐   ☐   0 - Able to independently take the correct medication and proper dosage at the correct times.

☐   ☐   1 - Able to take medication at the correct times if:
(a) individual dosages are prepared in advance by another person, *OR*
(b) given daily reminders.

☐   ☐   2 - *Unable* to take medication unless administered by someone else.

[X]   [X]   NA - No inhalant/mist medications prescribed.

☐   UK - Unknown

99. (M0800) Management of Injectable Medications: *Patient's ability* to prepare and take all prescribed injectable medications reliably and safely, including administration of correct dosage at the appropriate times/intervals. *Excludes* I.V. medications.

Prior   Current

[X]   [X]   0 - Able to independently take the correct medication and proper dosage at the correct times.

☐   ☐   1 - Able to take injectable medication at correct times if:
(a) individual syringes are prepared in advance by another person, OR
(b) given daily reminders.

☐   ☐   2 - Unable to take injectable medications unless administered by someone else.

☐   ☐   NA - No injectable medications prescribed.

☐   UK - Unknown

EQUIPMENT MANAGEMENT

100. (M0810) Patient Management of Equipment (includes *only* oxygen, I.V./infusion therapy, enteral/parenteral nutrition equipment or supplies): *Patient's ability* to set up/monitor/change equipment reliably and safely, add appropriate fluids or medication, clean/store/dispose of equipment or supplies using proper technique. (NOTE: This refers to ability, not compliance or willingness.)

☐   0 - Patient manages all tasks related to equipment completely independently.

☐   1 - If someone else sets up equipment (fills portable oxygen tank, provides patient with prepared solutions), patient is able to manage all other aspects of equipment.

☐   2 - Patient requires considerable assistance from another person to manage equipment, but independently completes portions of the task.

☐   3 - Patient is only able to monitor equipment (liter flow, fluid in bag) and must call someone else to manage the equipment.

☐   4 - Patient is completely dependent on someone else to manage all equipment.

[X]   NA - No equipment of this type used in care [If NA, go to *M0825*]

USING THE OASIS-BI FORM *(continued)*

101. **(M0820) Caregiver Management of Equipment (includes** *only* **oxygen, I.V./infusion equipment, enteral/parenteral nutrition, ventilator therapy equipment or supplies):** *Caregiver's ability* to set up/monitor/change equipment reliably and safely, add appropriate fluids or medication, clean/store/dispose of equipment or supplies using proper technique. **(NOTE: This refers to ability, not compliance or willingness.)**

☐ 0 - Caregiver manages all tasks related to equipment completely independently.

☐ 1 - If someone else sets up equipment, caregiver is able to manage all other aspects.

☐ 2 - Caregiver requires considerable assistance from another person to manage equipment, but independently completes significant portions of task.

☐ 3 - Caregiver is only able to complete small portions of task (administer nebulizer treatment, clean/store/dispose of equipment or supplies).

☐ 4 - Caregiver is completely dependent on someone else to manage all equipment.

☐ NA - No caregiver

☐ UK - Unknown

THERAPY NEED

102. **(M0825) Therapy Need:** Does the care plan of the Medicare payment period for which this assessment will define a case mix group indicate a need for therapy (physical, occupational, or speech therapy) that meets the threshold for a Medicare high-therapy case mix group?

☐ 0 - No

☐ 1 - Yes

☐ NA - Not applicable

EQUIPMENT AND SUPPLIES

Equipment needs (check appropriate box)

Has	Needs	
☐	☐	Oxygen/Respiratory Equip.
☐	☐	Wheelchair
☐	☐	Hospital Bed
☒	☐	Other (specify) *walker*

Supplies needed and comments regarding equipment needs

Financial problems/needs

SAFETY

Safety measures recommended to protect patient from injury

NA

Emergency plans

Wife will call 911 for emergency care if needed

CONCLUSIONS

Conclusions/impressions and skilled interventions performed this visit

Wound care performed per care plan. Initiated teaching regarding wound care, signs & symptoms of wound infection, and emergency measures.

Date of assessment *7/2/05*

Signature of Assessor *Holly Dougherty, RN, BSN*

HOME CARE, INTERDISCIPLINARY COMMUNICATION IN

Communication between members of the home health care team is essential when caring for a patient at home. Ideally, the team works together toward similar goals to help the patient reach the expected outcomes. Agencies accomplish interdisciplinary communication in various ways. During patient care conferences, the team discusses the patient's care plan and any changes needed in treatment. Between these conferences, team members may communicate with one another through voice mail systems. However, the most important form of interdisciplinary communication is the agency's interdisciplinary communication form. Surveyors place a great deal of emphasis on this form, which shows when, why, and by whom a care plan was changed. It clearly defines deviations from the original care plan. Because the information documented on this form becomes part of the legal chart, follow the guidelines for accurate documentation.

ESSENTIAL DOCUMENTATION

When completing an interdisciplinary communication form, be sure to fill in the following:
- patient's name and identification number
- date and time
- your name and title
- name and title of the person to whom you're giving or from whom you're receiving the information
- subject matter discussed (for example, abnormal laboratory results)
- changes to the care plan as a result of this communication
- name of team members notified of the change in the care plan
- outcome of the conversation and any agreements made
- actions you took
- your signature and title.

When you speak to another member of the home health care team by phone or voice mail message, the same basic information should be documented.

See *Interdisciplinary communication form* for sample documentation.

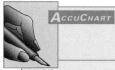

INTERDISCIPLINARY COMMUNICATION FORM

Changes concerning the patient or changes to the care plan can be documented on the interdisciplinary communication form.

INTERDISCIPLINARY COMMUNICATION FORM

Date	Time	Discipline	Change in status	Staff Signature
		RN		
		PT		
		OT		
		MSW		
9/21/05		RD	*Pt. has lost 5 lb. Increase dietary intake and add Ensure shakes 3X/day*	*Sue Smith, RD*
		HCA		

HOME CARE, PATIENT-TEACHING CERTIFICATION IN

Patient and caregiver teaching are integral parts of almost every care plan. The most common goal is for the patient to have increased knowledge of his disease or treatment, and a standardized tool helps achieve that goal in an organized manner. Teaching checklists and certifications help to ensure that information is provided to the patient in a timely manner and in such a way that the patient's and caregiver's level of understanding can be easily evaluated. It also aids interdisciplinary communication. Patient-teaching guides vary by facility, but the main content of the forms is the same.

ESSENTIAL DOCUMENTATION

The patient-teaching certification is a checklist that indicates that the instruction took place. Most forms begin with the type of therapy or specific disease that will be taught. Then the patient's comprehension level, motivational level, potential barriers to learning, knowledge of his disease or treatment, and skills are assessed. The patient's anticipated outcomes are determined and documented, and the nurse tailors the care plan and teaching plan to the individual needs of the patient or caregiver.

If your agency doesn't possess a specific patient or caregiver teaching tool, document this information in your progress note. Be sure to include all the above information, and remember to document clearly on subsequent notes the patient's or caregiver's verbal and nonverbal communication regarding the procedures or instructions, their knowledge, and level of understanding.

Refer to *Patient-teaching certification* for an example of a completed form.

AccuChart

PATIENT-TEACHING CERTIFICATION

The model patient-teaching form below shows what was taught to a home care patient with an I.V. line in place. This type of form will help you document your teaching sessions clearly and completely.

PATIENT-TEACHING
CHECKLIST/CERTIFICATION
OF INSTRUCTION

Patient name *Terry Elliott*
Caretaker *wife*
Type of Therapy *wound care*
Date *07/02/05*

CONTENT (Check all that apply; fill in blanks as indicated.)

1. ☑ Reason for Therapy
   Open wound
2. Drug/Solution
   ☐ Dose
   ☐ Schedule
   ☐ Label Accuracy
   ☐ Storage
   ☐ Container Integrity
3. Aseptic Technique
   ☑ Hand Washing
   ☐ Prepping Caps/Connections
   ☐ Tubing/Cap/Needle
   ☐ Needleless Adaptor Changes
4. Access Device Maintenance
   Type/Name _____

   ☐ Device/Site Inspection
   ☐ Site Care/Dressing Changes
   ☐ Catheter Clamping
   ☐ Maintaining Patency
   ☐ Saline Flushing
   ☐ Heparin Locking
   ☐ Feeding Tube Declogging
   ☐ Self-Insertion of Device
5. Drug Preparation
   ☐ Premixed Containers
   ☐ Compounding
   ☐ Patient Additives
   ☐ Piggyback Lipids
6. Method of Administration
   ☐ Gravity
   ☐ Pump (name)_____

   ☐ Continuous ☐ Intermittent
   ☐ Cycle/Taper

7. Administration Technique
   ☐ Pump Rate/Calibration
   ☐ Priming Tubing
   ☐ Filter
   ☐ Filling Syringe
   ☐ Loading Pump
   ☐ Access Device Hookup/
     Disconnect
8. Potential Complications/Adverse
   Effects
   ☐ Patient Drug Information Sheet
     Reviewed
   ☐ Pump Alarms/Troubleshooting
   ☐ Phlebitis/Infiltration
   ☐ Clotting/Dislodgment
   ☑ Infection
   ☐ Air Embolus
   ☐ Breakage/Cracking
   ☐ Electrolyte Imbalance
   ☐ Fluid Balance
   ☐ Glucose Intolerance
   ☐ Aspiration
   ☐ Nausea/vomiting/diarrhea/
     cramping
   ☐ Other: _____
   _____
9. Self-Monitoring
   ☐ Weight
   ☑ Temperature
   ☐ P ☐ BP
   ☐ Urine S & A
   ☐ Fingersticks
   ☐ Other: _____
   _____

10. Supply Handling/Disposal
    ☐ Disposal of Sharps/Supplies
    ☐ Opioids
    ☐ Cleaning Pump
    ☐ Changing Batteries
    ☐ Blood/Fluid Precautions
    ☐ Chemo/Spill Precautions
11. Information Given to Patient Re:
    ☐ Pharmacy Counseling
    ☑ Advance Directives
    ☐ Inventory Checks_____

    ☐ Deliveries _____

    ☑ 24-Hour On-Call Staff_____

    ☐ Reimbursement _____

    ☐ Service Complaints _____
12. Safety/Disaster Plan
    ☐ Backup Pump Batteries _____

    ☐ Emergency Room Use _____

    ☐ Electrical _____

    ☐ Disaster _____

    ☐ Other: _____
13. Written Instructions
    ☐ Yes ☐ No
    If No, Why_____
    _____
    _____

(continued)

PATIENT-TEACHING CERTIFICATION *(continued)*

Patient and/or caregiver demonstrates and/or verbalizes competency to perform home infusion therapy.

COMMENTS: *Pt. and wife instucted in signs and symptoms of wound infection with good understanding. Pt. and wife able to demonstrate adequate hand-washing technique and he'll check his temperature each evening and record result. Pt. appears motivated to take measures to improve his health. Because of pt.'s fatigue, information needs to be reviewed more than once.*

Theory/Skill Reviewed/Return Demonstration Completed:

Jane Smith, RN   *07/02/05*

Signature of RN Educator   Date

CONTENT (Check all that apply; fill in blanks as indicated.)

I agree that I have been instructed as described above and understand that the above functions will be performed in the home by myself and/or caregiver, outside a hospital or medically supervised environment.

John Dougherty   *01/02/05*

Patient/Caregiver Signature   Date

HOME CARE CERTIFICATION AND CARE PLAN

After you have made your initial visit to your patient and completed the Outcome and Assessment Information Set (OASIS), you must develop a comprehensive care plan. You'll need to prepare your care plan in cooperation with the patient and his caregivers. Remember that they may be providing much of the patient's care. Adjust your interventions, patient goals, and teaching accordingly.

Some agencies use a home health certification and care plan form, which is required for Medicare reimbursement, as their official care plan for Medicare patients. This form is also called Form 485. Other agencies use a multidisciplinary, integrated care plan. (See *The home care plan as legal evidence.*)

THE HOME CARE PLAN AS
LEGAL EVIDENCE

Your home care plan provides the most direct legal evidence of your nursing judgment. If you outline a care plan and then deviate from it without documenting a good reason for doing so, a court may decide that you strayed from a reasonable standard of care. Be sure to update your care plan routinely so it accurately reflects your clinical judgment about the care your patient requires to meet his changing needs.

ESSENTIAL DOCUMENTATION

The forms used for a care plan and the information necessary to complete the forms may vary from agency to agency. Record your patient's demographic information and diagnoses. Document drug information, nutritional requirements, use of durable medical equipment and supplies, safety measures, functional limitations, activities, mental status, prognosis, orders for discipline, and treatment (specify amount, frequency, and duration). Document the patient's goals, rehabilitation potential, and discharge plans.

Also, include information about the home environment, needed resources, and the emotional states and attitudes of the patient, family, and caregiver. Document physical changes needed in the patient's home for him to receive proper care. Note how you helped the family find the resources to implement the changes. Describe the primary caregiver, including whether he lives with the patient, their relationship, his age and physical ability, and his willingness to help the patient. Show in your documentation how you made the most of the patient's strengths and resources. Strengths include support systems, good health habits, coping behaviors, a safe and healthful environment, and financial security. Resources include the doctor, pharmacy, other health team members, and medical equipment.

If the patient is housebound, make sure you document that fact and the reasons behind it. (Remember that Medicare requires patients to be housebound to qualify for reimbursement of skilled services at home.)

Sign the care plan and include the date the verbal order was obtained to start care. The doctor must also sign the care plan.

Keep the patient's care plan updated. Note changes in the patient's condition or the care you think he needs. Document that you reported

AccuChart

HOME HEALTH CERTIFICATION AND CARE PLAN

Known as Form 485, the form below includes space for assessing functional abilities and documenting the care plan. This information is required for Medicare reimbursement.

1. Patient's HI Claim No. *000491675 5*	2. Start of Care Date *07/02/05*	3. Certification Period From: *07/02/05* To: *09/02/05*
4. Medical Record No. *541234*		5. Provider No. *0472*

6. Patient's Name and Address *Terry Elliot* *11 Second Street* *Hometown, PA 10981*	7. Provider's Name, Address, and Telephone Number *Very Good Home Care* *Health Rd* *Hometown, PA 10981*

8. Date of Birth *07/08/26*	9. Sex ☑ M ☐ F

10. Medications: Dose/Frequency/Route (N)ew (C)hanged
Humulin N 24units subQ every am (c)
Tylenol 325 mg-1000 mg q 4h prn pain
Darvocet N 100 one tab q 4h prn pain PO (N)
Mom 30 ml at bedtime prn P.O.

11. IDC-9-CM *891.0*	Principal Diagnosis *Open Wound Foot*	Date *07/01/05*
12. ICD-9-CM *86.28*	Surgical Procedure *Debridement Wound*	Date *07/01/05*
13. ICD-9-CM *250.03* *443.89*	Other Pertinent Diagnoses *Type 2 DM uncontrolled* *Perpiheral Vascular Disease*	Date *04/01/05* *04/01/05*

14. DME and Supplies *Walker Wound care Supplies*	15. Safety Measures *Correct use of supportive devices*

16. Nutritional requirements *20% protein 30% fat*	17. Allergies: *NKA*

18. a. Functional Limitations

1 ☑ Amputation	4 ☐ Hearing	8 ☐ Speech	B ☐ Other
2 ☐ Bowel/Bladder	5 ☐ Paralysis	9 ☐ Legally Blind	
(Incontinence)	6 ☑ Endurance	A ☐ Dyspnea with Minimal	
3 ☐ Contracture	7 ☑ Ambulation	Exertion	

18. b. Activities Permitted

1 ☐ Complete Bedrest	5 ☐ Exercises Prescribed	9 ☐ Cane	D ☐ Other (Specify)
2 ☐ Bedrest BRP	6 ☑ Partial Weight Bearing	A ☐ Wheelchair	
3 ☐ Up as Tolerated	7 ☑ Independent At Home	B ☑ Walker	
4 ☑ Transfer Bed/Chair	8 ☐ Crutches	C ☐ No Restrictions	

19. Mental Status

1 ☑ Oriented	3 ☑ Forgetful	5 ☐ Disoriented	7 ☐ Agitated
2 ☐ Comatose	4 ☐ Depressed	6 ☐ Lethargic	8 ☐ Other

20. Prognosis:

1 ☐ Poor	3 ☐ Fair	5 ☐ Excellent
2 ☑ Guarded	4 ☐ Good	

HOME HEALTH CERTIFICATION
AND CARE PLAN *(continued)*

21. Orders for Discipline and Treatments (Specify Amount/Frequency/Duration)

SN: Observe/assess: Cardiopulmonary, respiratory, musculoskeletal, gastrointestinal, and circulatory systems function. Assess: nutritional intake and dietary compliance related to wound healing; skin integrity and peripheral pulses; diabetic home management; and home safety. Instruct pt./caregiver in: diabetic management; signs/symptoms of wound infection; wound care; home safety; and emergency measures. SN to provide: wound care, until pt. is independent: daily wound care to ⓛ ankle area = clean area with saline and apply wet to dry saline dressing. SN visits: 5-7/wk X 3 wks; 2-4/wk X 3 wks; 1-3/wk X 3 wks
SN: GOALS: wound healing without infection or further complications, compliance with diabetic home management. Rehab potential to achieve goals: fair. Discharge plan: to family/self when care is independent.

23. Nurse's Signature and Date of Verbal SOC Where Applicable	25. Date HHA Received Signed POT
Jane Smith, RN 07/02/05	07/12/05

24. Physician's Name and Address	26. I certify/recertify that this patient is confined to his/her home and needs intermittent skilled nursing care, physical therapy and/or speech therapy or continues to need occupational therapy. The patient is under my care, and I have authorized the services on this care plan and will periodically review the plan.
Dr. Kyle Stevens *Dr's Medical Center* *Hometown, PA 10981*	

27. Attending Physician's Signature and Date Signed	28. Anyone who misrepresents, falsifies, or conceals essential information required for payment of Federal funds may be subject to fine, imprisonment, or civil penalty under applicable Federal laws.
KyLE Stevens, M.D. 01/01/05	

FORM HCFA-485-(C-4) (0-94) (Print Aligned)   PROVIDER

these changes to the doctor. Medicare, Medicaid, and certain third-party payers won't reimburse skilled services not reported to the doctor.

For sample documentation, see *Home health certification and care plan.*

HOME CARE DISCHARGE SUMMARY

When the patient is ready for discharge, either because he has met the goals set at admission or because he's no longer eligible for home care, you'll need to prepare a discharge summary for the doctor's approval to discharge, notifying reimbursers that services have been terminated, and

AccuChart

THE HOME CARE DISCHARGE SUMMARY

DISCHARGE SUMMARY

CODE _01_

Admission Date _07/02/05_
Discharge Date _09/30/05_

Name: _Terry Elliot_
Medical Record No.: _541234_

Address: _11 Second St., Hometown, PA 10981_ Phone No.: _881-555-2937_

Primary Diagnosis: _Open wound – Ⓛ foot_

Physician: _Dr. Kyle Stevens_   Date of Birth: _07/08/26_

Services Provided:
- ☑ Nursing
- ☐ Aide
- ☐ Other
- ☐ Occupational Therapy
- ☐ Physical Therapy
- ☐ Speech Therapy
- ☐ Social Work

Reason for Discharge:
- ☑ Condition Improved
- ☐ Self/Family Choice
- ☐ Moved Out of Area
- ☐ Referred to Another Agency
- ☐ Died at Home
- ☐ Died in Hospital
- ☐ Referred to Hospital
- ☐ Placed in Long-Term Institution
- ☐ Referred, Not Admitted
- ☐ Other

Physician Notified of Closure: ☑ Yes ☐ No   Date: _09/30/05_
Family Notified: ☑ Yes ☐ No   Date: _09/30/05_

Able to verbalize knowledge of the etiology, signs and symptoms, and sequelae/complications of health problem(s).
Patient: ☐ Yes ☑ Partially ☐ No
Family/Caregiver: ☑ Yes ☐ Partially ☐ No

Able to demonstrate knowledge and skills related to the treatment and management of health problem(s).
Patient: ☐ Yes ☑ Partially ☐ No
Family/Caregiver: ☐ Yes ☑ Partially ☐ No

Patient Status:
The patient's condition is: ☐ Stable ☐ Unstable ☑ Improving ☐ Declining ☐ Other

ADL STATUS: ☑ Improving ☐ Unchanged ☐ Declining

	Dependent	Partially Independent	Independent
Bathing			✓
Dressing			✓
Toileting			✓
Transferring			✓
Feeding			✓
Ambulation		✓	
Activity Tolerance	(poor)	(fair)	(good)

Functional Outcomes:	From	To
Knowledge	poor	fair
Skill	fair	good
Psychosocial	poor	fair
Health Status	poor	fair

SUPPORT SYSTEMS: ☑ Family ☐ Caregiver ☐ Friends
- ☐ Community Resources
- ☐ Support systems inadequate
- ☐ Other
- ☑ Patient uses support systems appropriately
- ☐ Patient uses support systems ineffectively

COMMENTS: _____

officially closing the case. The summary is completed on your last visit to the patient. Use the form provided by your agency for recording your discharge summary. This form may be multidisciplinary.

ESSENTIAL DOCUMENTATION

Depending on the form used, information included on a discharge summary may vary. Document your patient's demographic information, admission and discharge dates, the types of services provided, and the reason for discharge. Record the ability of the patient and caregiver to verbalize an understanding of the disease process, signs and symptoms, and complications, and to demonstrate the skills necessary to treat and manage the disease. The ability of the patient to perform activities of daily living and to use support systems should also be recorded. In addition to the patient's clinical condition at discharge, also describe his psychological condition. Provide outcomes attained and recommendations for further care.

Refer to *The home care discharge summary* for an example of documentation.

HOME CARE PROGRESS NOTES

In the home setting, as in the acute care setting, progress notes document the patient's condition and significant events that occur while he's under your care. You'll need to write a progress note each time you see a patient, describing his current condition and any skilled services provided during the visit. A skilled service must always be documented in order for the visit to be billable to Medicare. Your notes should also reflect the patient's progress toward his goals. Many agencies have the patient sign the progress note to prove that the service was provided on the date and time documented.

Complete your progress note within 24 hours of providing care and file it in the medical record within 7 days. Remember that Medicare certification reviews can occur without notice, and charts can be audited at any time.

AccuChart

DOCUMENTING ON A HOME CARE PROGRESS NOTE

Progress notes describe—in chronological order—patient problems and needs, nursing observations, reassessments, and interventions. A sample appears below.

☐ Phone Report   ☐ Coordination note   ☑ Clinical note continuation

Patient Name *Terry Elliot*   **ID#** *541234*   **Date** *08/10/05*

T=101°F   P=100   RR=28   BP=160/94. Pt. unaware of fever but complaining of increased pain at wound site. (Rates pain as 3 on a scale of 0 to 10, with 10 being worst pain imaginable.) Darvocet is controlling pain but pt. taking it q4hr while awake. Wound of Ⓛ ankle = 4 cm X 4.5 cm X 1 cm deep. Open area pink with increased amounts of thick, tan drainage. Wound is foul smelling. Dr. Jone's office contacted and pt. to start on cephalexin P.O. SN to increase visits for BID wound care. Pt. denies other complaints. Glucometer FBS = 160 this am. Lungs with diminished breath sounds at bases. Appetite good, bowels regular - had BM today. Began instruction to pt. on cephalexin dose, schedule, and adverse effects. Pt. appears quite anxious about wound condition. Explanation of signs, symptoms, and treatment of wound infection reinforced. Pt. able to repeat explanations. Support offered. SN to return for pm wound care today and pt. should have begun antibiotic therapy by then. ————————————————————Jane Smith, RN

Service by (Signature) Title

ESSENTIAL DOCUMENTATION

Complete a progress note each time you see the patient. If a patient receives more than one skilled nursing visit a day, you must complete a separate note for each visit.

Make sure your progress note provides a chronological accounting of at least the following:

- any changes in the patient's condition
- skilled nursing interventions performed related to the care plan
- the patient's responses to services provided
- the patient's vital signs
- what you taught the patient and caregiver, including a list of written instructional materials and brochures you gave them.

Refer to *Documenting on a home care progress note* for an example of progress note documentation.

HOME CARE RECERTIFICATION

To ensure continued home care services for patients who need them, you'll have to prove that the patient still requires it. Medicare and many managed care plans certify an initial 60-day period during which your agency can receive reimbursement for the patient's home care. When that period is over, the insurer may certify an additional 60-day period based on your written demonstration, and the doctor's agreement, that the patient needs continued care. The second 60-day period and every one after that are called recertification periods.

Your documentation requesting recertification must clearly support the patient's need for continued care within the insurer's guidelines. A clinical summary of care must be compiled and sent to the patient's doctor and then to the insurer. For Medicare, you'll also need to prepare a new certification and care plan form (Form 485) for the recertification period. (See *Home care certification and care plan,* pages 192 and 193.) You must return the form to your agency and Medicare before the current certification period expires. Make sure it includes all updated data as amended by verbal order since the start of care. You aren't required to submit Medicare's Medical Update and Patient Information form (Form 486) for recertification unless Medicare requests it.

ESSENTIAL DOCUMENTATION

When preparing a new certification and care plan for recertification, make sure the primary diagnosis reflects the patient's current needs, not the original reason for home care. For example, if your patient's primary diagnosis was heart failure but he developed a pressure ulcer that requires skilled visits to perform wound care, you'll need to change the original primary diagnosis to "open wound." Heart failure may be listed as a secondary diagnosis. (See "Home care certification and care plan," page 190, for full documentation guidelines.)

After you've completed Form 485, review the new orders with the patient's doctor and sign the "verbal order for start of care" line. This signature serves as a valid verbal order to continue home care services until the doctor signs the original document.

The clinical summary that you include with the new certification and care plan form must contain a summary of all disciplines represented on

ACCUCHART

MEDICAL UPDATE
AND PATIENT INFORMATION

When requested by Medicare, you'll have to complete Form 486, shown below. This form provides Medicare with information to support the need for skilled nursing care.

Department of Health and Human Services
Care Financing Administration

Form Approved
OMB No. 0938-0357

MEDICAL UPDATE AND PATIENT INFORMATION

1. Patient's HI Claim No. *000491675*	2. SOC Date *07/02/05*	3. Certification Period From: *09/02/05*　　To: *11/02/05*

4. Medical Record No. *541234*	5. Provider No. *0472*

6. Patient's Name and Address *Terry Elliot, 11 Second St., Hometown, PA*	7. Provider's Name *Very Good Home Care*

8. Medicare Coverered: ☑ Y ☐ N	9. Date Physician Last Saw Patient: *08/01/05*

10. Date Last Contacted Physician: *08/02/05*

11. Is the Patient Receiving Care in an 1861 (J)(1) Skilled Nursing Facility or Equivalent?
　☐ Y　☑ N　☐ Do Not Know

12. ☐ Certification	☑ Recertification	☐ Modified

13. Dates of Last Inpatient Stay: Admission *N/A* 　　Discharge *N/A*	14. Type of Facility: *N/A*

15. Updated information: New Orders/Treatments/Clinical Facts/Summary from Each Discipline

SN: 08/02/05: Dr. Jones contacted to report temp = 101° F orally, increased amt. thick, tan, foul smelling drainage. Pt. started on cephalexin 500 mg BID po X 10 days, increase wound care to BID and increase SN visits for wound care to 12–14 X 3 wks.
PT: 08/01/05: Verbal order received to increase pt. to ambulation with straight cane. Continue strengthening home exercise program.
SN: 08/08/05: Decrease wound care to daily. Decrease SN visits to 5–7 X 7 wks.

16. Functional Limitations (Expand From 485 and Level of ADL) Reason Homebound/Prior Functional Status
FL: Ambulation, endurance, open, draining wound. RH: Unable to ambulate more than 15 ft. before becoming exhausted. PFS: Independent ambulation.

17. Supplementary Care Plan on File from Physician Other than Referring Physician: ☐ Y ☑ N
(If Yes, Please Specify Giving Goals/Rehab. Potential/Discharge Plan)

18. Unusual Home/Social Environment

19. Indicate Any Time When the Home Health Agency Made a Visit and Patient was Not Home and Reason Why if Ascertainable 　*N/A*	20. Specify Any Known Medical and/or Non-Medical Reason the Patient Regularly Leaves Home and Frequency of Occurrence *Doctor's office visits as needed.*

21. Nurse or Therapist Completing or Reviewing Form *Jane Smith, RN*	Date (Mo., Day, Yr.) *08/02/05*

HCFA-486 (C3) (02-94) (Print Aligned)　　　　　　　　PROVIDER

the patient's care team, including the home health nursing assistant, along with updated treatments and goals and the frequency and duration of visits. Also, include what has already been accomplished in addition to realistic goals for continued treatment. (See *Medical update and patient information.*)

HOME CARE REFERRAL

Before you begin caring for a patient in his home, your agency will receive information about that patient on a referral, or intake, form. Either you or someone in your agency will use this form to make sure the patient is eligible for home care, and that the agency can provide the services he needs, before taking the new case.

To meet Medicare's criteria for home care reimbursement, the patient will need to meet the following conditions:

- Patient must be confined to his home.
- Patient must need skilled services.
- Patient must need skilled services on an intermittent basis.
- The care must be reasonable and medically necessary.
- Patient must be under the care of a doctor.

ESSENTIAL DOCUMENTATION

Document your patient's demographic information, including the name and telephone number of the doctor and primary caregiver, and insurance information. Record orders and services required, specifying the amount, frequency, and duration. Note the patient's functional limitations and activities permitted. List drug orders and allergy information. Record advance directive information. Include your patient's medical and psychosocial histories, cultural and religious considerations, environmental assessment, vital signs, and physical assessment findings. Date and sign your entry.

See *Referral for home care,* pages 200 and 201, for sample documentation.

AccuChart

REFERRAL FOR HOME CARE

Also called the intake form, this form is used to document a new patient's needs when you begin your evaluation. Use the form below as a guide.

ELECTION BENEFIT PERIOD   ① 2 3 4

Date of Referral: *07/01/05*   Branch _____   Chart#: *0001234*   H _____
Info Taken By: *Jane Smith, RN*   Admit Date: *07/02/05*
Patient's Name: *Terry Elliot*
Address: *11 Second St.*
City: *Hometown*   State: *PA*   Zip: *10981*
Phone: *881-555-2937*   Date of Birth: *07/08/26*
Primary Caregiver Name & #: *Susan Elliot*   *881-555-2937*
Insurance Name: *Medicare*   Ins.#: *123-45-6789A*
Is this a managed care policy (HMO): *No*
Primary Dx: (Code *891.00*) *Open wound Foot/Complications (Onset)*   Date: *07/11/05*
        (Code *250.72*) *Type 2 DM Uncontrolled*   *(Exac.)*   Date: *07/11/05*
        (Code *443.89*) *Periph Vascular Disease*   *(Exac.)*   Date: *07/11/05*
Procedures: (Code *86.28*) *Debridement Wound*   *(Onset)*   Date: *07/11/05*
Referral Source: *Doctor's office*   Phone: *881-555-6900*
Physician Name & Phone #: (UPIN *22222*)   *Dr. Kyle Stevens*
Phone: *881-555-6900*
Physician Address: *Dr's Medical Center, Hometown, PA 10981*
Hospital   *N/A*   Admit *N/A*   Discharge *N/A*
Functional Limitations: Pain Management,   *Pain, ambulation dysfunction*

ORDERS/SERVICES (specify amount, frequency, and duration):
SN: *5-7 visits/wk X 9 wks for assessment and wound care @ foot: Saline wet to dry drsg*
AI: *3-5 visits/wk X 9 wks for assistance with ADLs and personal care*
PT, OT, ST: *PT 1-3 visits/wk X 9 wks to assess mobility and safety, and develop home exercise*
    program.
MSW: *1-2 visits X 1 mo. for financial assessment and long-term planning*
Spiritual Coordinator: *N/A*   Counselor: *N/A*
Volunteer: *N/A*
Other Services Provided: *N/A*
Goals: *Wound healing without complications.*
Equipment: *walker and dressing supplies*
Company & Phone #: *Best Med Equip. Co 881-260-1026*
Safety Measures: *Correct use of supportive devices*   Nutritional Req: *20% protein 30% fat*

FUNCTIONAL LIMITATIONS: (Circle Applicable)

①Amputation	5 Paralysis	9 Legally Blind
2 Bowel/Bladder	⑥Endurance	A Dyspnea With
3 Contracture	⑦Ambulation	Minimal Exer
4 Hearing	8 Speech	B Other

ACTIVITIES PERMITTED: (Circle Applicable)

1. Complete Bedrest	5. Partial Wgt Bearing	A. Wheelchair
2. Bedrest BRP	6. Independent at Home	ⒷWalker
3. Up as Tolerated	7. Crutches	C. No Restriction
④Transfer Bed/Chair	8. Cane	D. Other — specify

REFERRAL FOR HOME CARE *(continued)*

Accessibility to   Bath Y (N)   Shower Y (N)   Bathroom (Y) N   Exit (Y) N

Mental Status: (Circle)   (Oriented)   Comatose   (Forgetful)   Depressed   Disoriented   Lethargic   Agitated   Other

Allergies: _NKA_

- Hospice Appropriate Meds   • Med company: _N/A_

MEDICATIONS: _Humulin N   24 units subQ every am_   _changed_

Tylenol   325-1000 mg q4hr prn pain P.O.   _unchanged_

Darvocet N 100   one tab q4hr prn pain P.O.   _new_

MOM 30 ml at bedtime prn P.O.   _unchanged_

Living Will   Yes _____   No _X_   Obtained _____   Family to mail to office _____

Guardian, POA, or Responsible Person: _wife_

Address & Phone Number: _same_

Other Family Members: _N/A_

ETOH: _0_   Drug Use: _X_   Smoker _1-2 ppd X 25 yrs_

HISTORY: _Chronic peripheral vascular disease with periodic open wounds of feet and legs._
Seen by doctor in office 04/01/05 and new wound of ① foot debrided.

Social History (place of birth, education, jobs, retirement, etc.): _Korean War veteran retired   (X 18 yrs)_
construction worker

ADMISSION NOTES: VS: T _99°F orally_   AP _88_   RR _22_   BP _150/82_

Lungs: _diminished bilat. at bases_   Extremities: _® BKA, ① foot pale, DP and PT pulses +._

Wgt: _155 lb_   Recent wgt loss/gain of _denies_

Admission Narrative: _Pt. independent in Insulin administration and instructed in Insulin_
dosage change with good understanding. Wound of ① ankle-outer malleolar area = 4 cm
X 5 cm X 1 cm deep; open with beefy red appearance, wound edges pink, moderate
amount serosanguineous drainage present. Wound care performed by RN per care plan.
Pain controlled with Darvocet prn.

Psychosocial Issues _N/A_

Environmental Concerns _None_

Are there any cultural or spiritual customs or beliefs of which we should be aware before providing Hospice services? _____
_N/A_

Funeral Home: _N/A_   Contact made   YES _____   NO _____

DIRECTIONS: _1 block before intersection of Main St, on Second St._

Agency Representative

Signature: _Jane Smith, RN_   Date: _07/02/05_

HOME CARE TELEPHONE ORDERS

Typically, a doctor's order to change some aspect of home care for your patient will come to you by telephone. Either you or the doctor may initiate this conversation for various reasons. No matter who originated the contact or how it came about, it's your job to immediately read back and document any orders received. You'll need to use the appropriate verbal order form and send it to the doctor for a signature.

ᴀᴄᴄᴜCʜᴀʀᴛ

HOME CARE TELEPHONE ORDER FORM

Here's an example of a form used by one agency to fulfill the documentation requirements for telephone orders. The doctor must sign the order within 48 hours.

Facility name		Address	
Very Good Home Care		*Health Rd, Hometown, PA*	
Last name	**First name**	**Attending doctor**	**Patient ID #**
Elliot	*Terry*	*Dr. Kyle Stevens*	*123456789*

Date ordered	Date discontinued	ORDERS
07/10/05		*Start cephalexin 500 mg BID P.O.*
		Increase wound care to BID
		Increase SN visits to daily X 2 wks per
		Dr. Goodman's order. Read back and
		confirmed by Dr. Goodman.

Signature of nurse receiving order	Time	Signature of doctor	Date
Jane Smith, RN	*1400*	*M. Goodman, MD*	*07/11/05*

Keep a copy of your signed verbal order in the patient's record until the original copy with the doctor's signature is returned to the office. The original order must be placed in the patient's medical record within 10 days.

ᴇssᴇɴᴛɪᴀʟ ᴅᴏᴄᴜᴍᴇɴᴛᴀᴛɪᴏɴ

Make sure your verbal order form includes the patient's complete name and identification number. Record the complete name, title, and signature of the person who received the order and the complete name of the doctor who gave the order. Include a place for the doctor's signature. Document the complete contents of the order as it was given and that the order was read back and confirmed.

In addition to writing up the verbal order, document in the patient's record the reason it was initiated. Describe the circumstances that prompted your conversation with the patient's doctor as well as the doctor's reason for giving the order. Be sure to communicate the order to everyone on the patient's health care team who needs to know it.

See *Home care telephone order form* for sample documentation.

4/10/05	1400	Called Dr. Goodman to report increase in yellow drain-
		age from leg wound, no odor. Skin around wound red,
		warm, and tender. P 88, BP 138/74, oral T 100.6° F.
		Dr. Goodman gave telephone order to start cephalexin
		500 mg BID P.O., increase skilled nurse visits to daily
		X 14 days, and to call doctor in 2 weeks for follow-up
		orders. Orders read back and confirmed with Dr.
		Goodman and transcribed on telephone order sheet.
		Explained to pt. and caregiver the indications for
		antibiotic, frequency, dosage, and possible adverse
		effects. Also explained the need for more frequent
		wound care. Instructed them on signs and symptoms
		to report to doctor and home care agency, including
		increase in drainage, dressing saturation, odor from
		wound, and increase in temperature. Pt. and caregiver
		verbalized understanding of antibiotic, signs and
		symptoms to report, and more frequent wound care.
		—————————— Jane Smith, RN

HYPERGLYCEMIA

Defined as an elevated blood glucose level, hyperglycemia results from not enough insulin or the body's inability to effectively use insulin. Extremely high blood glucose levels can lead to ketoacidosis, a potentially life-threatening condition.

Diabetes mellitus is the most common cause of hyperglycemia, but it may also be attributable to Cushing's syndrome; stresses, such as trauma, infections, burns, and surgery; and drugs such as corticosteroids. Patients with diabetes may develop hyperglycemia as a result of not enough insulin, poor compliance with diet, and illness.

If your patient develops hyperglycemia, notify the doctor and anticipate orders for regular insulin therapy and fluid and electrolyte replacement. Your prompt interventions are necessary to prevent ketoacidosis and a potentially fatal outcome.

ESSENTIAL DOCUMENTATION

Caring for a patient with hyperglycemia requires frequent assessments and interventions. Document on a timely basis and avoid block charting.

Record the date and time of your entry. Record the patient's blood glucose level and your assessment findings, such as polyuria, polydipsia, polyphagia, glycosuria, ketonuria, blurry vision, flushed cheeks, dry skin and mucous membranes, poor skin turgor, weak and rapid pulse, hypotension, Kussmaul's respirations, acetone breath odor, weakness, fatigue, and altered level of consciousness. Document the name of the doctor notified, the time of notification, and the orders given. Record your interventions, such as subcutaneous or I.V. administration of regular insulin, frequent blood glucose monitoring, and I.V. fluid and electrolyte replacement. Include your patient's response to these interventions. Use the appropriate flow sheets to record intake and output, I.V. fluids, drugs, and frequent vital signs and blood glucose level. Document any patient education, such as proper nutrition, proper use of insulin, and disease management that you provide.

9/27/05	1800	Pt. states, "I vomited and feel weak and dizzy." Face
		flushed, skin and mucous membranes dry, skin tents
		when pinched, breath has acetone odor, BP 100/50, P 98
		and weak, RR 28 and deep, oral T 98.8° F, blood
		glucose 462 mg/dl by fingerstick. Dr. Kelly notified at
		1740 and orders given. I.V. infusion of 1000 ml NSS
		started in ℚ forearm with 22G catheter at 100 ml/hr.
		Regular insulin 15 units SubQ given in ℚ upper arm. Lab
		called to draw blood for electrolytes and blood glucose
		levels. Explained rationales for therapy to pt. See flow
		sheets for frequent documentation of VS, I/O, I.V.
		fluids, and blood glucose levels.—— Cass McGuigan, RN
	1815	Pt. states, "I'm feeling a little better. I don't feel
		light-headed any more." BP 118/54, P 94, RR 20, slight
		acetone odor still noted on breath. Voided 800 ml pale
		yellow urine, neg. ketones, +2 glucose. ——————
		————————————— Cass McGuigan, RN
	1830	BP 122/60, P 90 and strong, RR 18. Pt. denies nausea,
		vomiting, and dizziness. Lab called to report blood
		glucose of 375 mg/dl, potassium 3.0 mEq/L. Dr. Moore
		notified of results and ordered 20 mEq of KCL to be
		added to 1000 ml of NSS to infuse at 100 ml/hr. ——
		————————————— Cass McGuigan, RN

HYPEROSMOLAR HYPERGLYCEMIC NONKETOTIC SYNDROME

A complication of type 2 (non-insulin-dependent) diabetes mellitus, hyperosmolar hyperglycemic nonketotic syndrome (HHNS) is a condition marked by blood glucose levels as high as 1,000 mg/dl but without ketosis. Although the patient with HHNS produces enough insulin to prevent diabetic ketoacidosis, it isn't enough insulin to prevent dangerously high hyperglycemia, vast diuresis, and extracellular fluid losses. If left untreated, HHNS can lead to dehydration, seizures, coma, and death.

If your patient with type 2 diabetes mellitus develops hyperglycemia, call the doctor and anticipate orders for administering large amounts of I.V. fluids and, possibly, a transfer to intensive care.

ESSENTIAL DOCUMENTATION

Record the date and time of your entry. Record your patient's blood glucose level and your assessment findings, such as dry skin and mucous membranes, poor skin turgor, extreme polyuria, hypotension, tachycardia, seizures, aphasia, somnolence, and coma. Document the name of the doctor notified, the time of notification, and the orders given. Record your interventions, such as cardiac monitoring, seizure precautions, maintaining a patent airway, and I.V. fluid, insulin, and electrolyte administration. Document your patient's response to these interventions. Record your frequent cardiopulmonary, renal, and neurologic assessments. Use the appropriate flow sheets to record intake and output, I.V. fluids, drugs, frequent vital signs, and electrolyte and blood glucose levels.

9/15/05	1900	Blood glucose level by fingerstick 950 mg/dl at 1830.
		P 104, BP 88/64, RR 18, oral T 99.4° F. Pt. drowsy, but
		arousable, oriented to person but not place and time.
		Skin and mucous membranes dry, skin tents when
		pinched. Foley catheter drained 35 ml over last hour.
		Breath sounds clear. Placed on portable cardiac monitor
		showing sinus tachycardia. Side rails padded, bed in low
		position, airway taped to headboard of bed, suction
		equipment placed in room. Dr. Ramirez notified of
		assessment findings and elevated blood glucose level at
		1835. Came to see pt. at 1840 and orders given. O₂
		started at 2 L/min via NC. I.V. infusion of 1000 ml
		NSS in Ⓛ antecubital increased to 1 L/hr. Infusion of
		100 units regular insulin/100 ml of NSS started at 0.1
		units/kg/hr. Respiratory therapy called to obtain blood
		sample for ABG. Lab notified for stat CBC, BUN, creati-
		nine, electrolytes, and blood glucose levels. Pt. being
		transferred to ICU, report called to Rose D'Amato, RN.
		Nursing supervisor, Marie Stone, RN, notified. Called
		pt.'s husband and notified him of wife's condition and
		transfer to ICU. ———————— Tom Woods, RN

HYPERTENSIVE CRISIS

Hypertensive crisis is a medical emergency in which the patient's diastolic blood pressure suddenly rises above 120 mm Hg. Precipitating factors include abrupt discontinuation of antihypertensive drugs; increased salt consumption; increased production of renin, epinephrine, and norepinephrine; and added stress.

Your prompt recognition of hypertensive crisis and nursing interventions to lower blood pressure are vital for preventing stroke, blindness, renal failure, hypertensive encephalopathy, left-sided heart failure, pulmonary edema, and even death. Anticipate assisting with insertion of an arterial catheter for continuous blood pressure monitoring, administering I.V. antihypertensive drugs, and preparing your patient for transfer to intensive care.

ESSENTIAL DOCUMENTATION

Record the date and time of your entry. Record the patient's blood pressure and the findings of your assessment, including the patient's cardiopulmonary, neurologic, and renal systems, such as headache, nausea, vomiting, seizures, blurred vision, transient blindness, confusion, drowsiness, heart failure, pulmonary edema, chest pain, and oliguria. Document the measures you took to ensure a patent airway. Record the name of the doctor you notified, the time of notification, and orders given, such as continuous blood pressure and cardiac monitoring, I.V. antihypertensive drugs, blood work, supplemental oxygen, and seizure precautions. See "Arterial line insertion," page 25, for documenting the insertion of an arterial line in your patient. Document your patient's response to these interventions. Use the appropriate flow sheets to record intake and output, I.V. fluids, drugs, and frequent vital signs. Include patient education and emotional support given.

3/2/05	1500	Pt. arrived in ED with c/o headache, blurred vision, and
		vomiting. BP 220/120, P 104 bounding, RR 16 unlabored,
		oral T 97.4° F. Pt. states, "I stopped taking my blood
		pressure pills 2 days ago when I ran out." Drowsy, but
		oriented to place and person, knew year but not day of
		week or time of day. No c/o chest pain, neck veins not
		distended, lungs clear. Cardiac monitor shows sinus
		tachycardia, no arrhythmias noted. Dr. Kelly notified and
		in to see pt. at 1045, orders written. O₂ at 4 L/min.
		administered via NC. Dr. Kelly explained need for arterial
		line for BP monitoring. Pt. understands procedure and
		signed consent. Assisted Dr. Kelly with insertion of
		arterial line in ® radial artery using 20G 2½" arterial
		catheter, after a positive Allen's test. Catheter secured
		with 1 suture. 4" X 4" gauze pad with povidone-iodine
		ointment applied. ® hand and wrist secured to arm
		board. Transducer leveled and zeroed. Initial BP reading
		238/124, mean arterial pressure 162 mm Hg with pt.'s
		head at 30°. Readings accurate to cuff pressures. Line
		flushes easily. I.V. line inserted in ® forearm with 18G
		catheter. Nitroprusside sodium 50 mg in 250 ml D₅W
		started at 0.30 mcg/kg/min. See frequent vital signs flow
		sheet for frequent vital signs. Blood sent to lab for stat
		CBC, ABG, electrolytes, BUN, creatinine, blood glucose level.
		Stat ECG and portable CXR done, results pending. Foley
		catheter inserted, urine sent for UA. Side rails padded,
		bed in low position, airway taped to headboard of bed,
		suction equipment placed in room. All procedures
		explained to pt. and wife. Pt. resting comfortably in bed,
		with HOB at 30°. Pt. states he's no longer nauseated and
		headache "is much better". ———— Alan Walker, RN

HYPERTHERMIA-HYPOTHERMIA BLANKET

A blanket-sized aquathermia pad, the hyperthermia-hypothermia blanket raises, lowers, or maintains body temperature through conductive heat or cold transfer between the blanket and the patient. It can be operated manually or automatically.

The blanket is used most commonly to reduce high fever when more conservative measures, such as baths, ice packs, and antipyretics, are unsuccessful. Its other uses include maintaining normal temperature during surgery or shock; inducing hypothermia during surgery to decrease metabolic activity and thereby reduce oxygen requirements; reducing intracranial pressure; controlling bleeding and intractable pain in patients with amputations, burns, or cancer; and providing warmth in cases of severe hypothermia.

ESSENTIAL DOCUMENTATION

Record the date and time of your entry. Document that the procedure was explained to the patient and a signed informed consent form is in the chart if required by your facility. Record the patient's vital signs, neurologic signs, fluid intake and output, skin condition, and position change. Record vital signs and the findings of your neurologic assessment every 5 minutes until the desired body temperature is reached and then every 15 minutes until the temperature is stable, or as ordered. These frequent assessments may be documented on a frequent vital signs assessment sheet. (See "Vital signs, frequent," page 442.) Also, document the type of hyperthermia-hypothermia unit used and control settings (manual or automatic, and temperature settings). Note the duration of the procedure and the patient's tolerance of treatment. Describe any measures taken to prevent skin injury. Record signs of complications, such as shivering, marked changes in vital signs, increased intracranial pressure, respiratory distress or arrest, cardiac arrest, oliguria, and anuria; the name of the doctor notified; the time of notification; the orders given; your actions; and the patient's response.

1/19/06	1000	Need for hypothermia blanket explained to pt.'s wife by
		Dr. Albright. Wife signed consent form. Preprocedure VS:
		Rectal T 104.3° F, P 112 and regular, RR 28, BP 138/88.
		Automatic hypothermia blanket, set at 99° F, placed
		under pt. at 0945. Sheet placed between pt. and
		hypothermia blanket. Lanolin applied to back, buttocks,
		and undersides of legs, arms, and feet. Skin intact,
		flushed, warm to the touch. Rectal probe in place and
		secured with tape. Pt. drowsy, but easily arousable and
		oriented to place and person but not time, able to feel
		light touch in all extremities, moving all extremities on
		own, no c/o numbness or tingling, PEARL. See I/O and
		frequent vital signs flow sheets for hourly intake and
		output, and q5min. VS and neuro. assessments. No
		shivering noted, Foley catheter intact draining clear
		amber urine, no dyspnea.————— Jane Walters, RN

HYPOGLYCEMIA

Occurring when the blood glucose level drops below 60 mg/dl, hypoglycemia is a potentially fatal metabolic disorder. Hypoglycemia may occur as a complication of diabetes mellitus, but it may also occur as a result of adrenal insufficiency, myxedema, poor nutrition, hepatic disease, alcoholism, vigorous exercise, and certain drugs such as pentamidine. If you recognize signs and symptoms of hypoglycemia in your patient, obtain a blood glucose level, immediately notify the doctor, and administer a carbohydrate or glucagon, as ordered, to prevent irreversible brain damage and death.

ESSENTIAL DOCUMENTATION

Record the date and time of your entry. Record your patient's signs and symptoms of hypoglycemia, such as hunger, weakness, shakiness, paresthesia, nervousness, palpitations, tachycardia, diaphoresis, and pallor. With more severe hypoglycemia you may assess drowsiness, reduced level of consciousness, slurred speech, behavior changes, incoordination, seizures, and coma. Document the results of the blood glucose level determined by fingerstick. Note the name of the doctor notified, the time of notification, and the orders given. For a conscious patient, record the type, amount, and route of carbohydrate given and the patient's response. If your patient is unconscious, record whether I.V. carbohydrates or subcutaneous glucagon was administered. Again, record the amount given, the route, and the patient's response.

Record all repeat blood glucose determinations and the measurement method used. If repeat doses are necessary, write a separate note for each administration, including the patient's response. Avoid block charting. Document other nursing interventions that may be necessary, such as maintaining a patent airway and seizure precautions, and the patient's response. Use the appropriate flow sheets to record intake and output, I.V. fluids, drugs, and frequent vital signs and blood glucose levels. Document any patient education, such as signs and symptoms of hypoglycemia, treating hypoglycemic episodes, preventive measures to avoid hypoglycemia, and disease management.

7/19/05	1845	While performing p.m. care at 1840, noted pt. had slurred speech and shaky hands. When questioned, pt. stated, "I feel OK, just a little headache." Pt. stated she wasn't very hungry at dinner. P 108, RR 14, BP 110/60, oral T 97.4° F. Skin pale and diaphoretic. Denies paresthesia. Received glyburide 5 mg at 1700. Blood glucose level by fingerstick 62 mg/dl. Dr. Luu notified at 1845 and ordered 15 g of oral carbohydrate. Gave ½ cup of orange juice. ——————— Mary Kelly, RN
	1900	Blood glucose level 71 mg/dl by fingerstick. Speech remains slurred, skin pale and diaphoretic, denies paresthesia, still c/o headache. P 104, RR16, BP 118/70. Gave pt. an additional ½ cup orange juice. ————— Mary Kelly, RN
	1915	Blood glucose level by fingerstick 98 mg/dl. P 88, RR 16, BP 118/68. Speech clear, skin pink, sl. diaphoresis noted, reports headache gone. Pt. states, "I feel much better. I didn't know my blood sugar was so low." Explained relationship between oral hypoglycemic and timing of meals, reviewed s/s of hypoglycemia and its treatment. ——————————————— Mary Kelly, RN

HYPOTENSION

Defined as blood pressure below 90/60 mm Hg, hypotension reduces perfusion to the tissues and organs of the body. Severe hypotension is a medical emergency that may progress to shock and death.

Various disorders of the cardiopulmonary, neurologic, and metabolic systems may cause hypotension. It may also result from the use of certain drugs, stress, and position changes. Moreover, changes in heart rate, the pumping action of the heart, and fluid balance may result in hypotension.

Because hypotension can be fatal, your prompt recognition and interventions are necessary to save your patient's life. Notify the doctor immediately, insert an I.V. line to administer fluids, begin cardiac monitoring, and administer oxygen. Anticipate administering vasopressor drugs and hemodynamic monitoring. Follow Advanced Cardiac Life Support (ACLS) protocols, as necessary.

ESSENTIAL DOCUMENTATION

Record the date and time of your entry. Record your patient's blood pressure and other vital signs. Document your assessment findings, such as bradycardia, tachycardia, weak pulses, cool, clammy skin, oliguria, reduced bowel sounds, dizziness, syncope, reduced level of consciousness, and myocardial ischemia. Note the name of the doctor notified, the time of notification, and any orders given, such as continuous blood pressure and cardiac monitoring, obtaining a 12-lead ECG, administering supplemental oxygen, and inserting an I.V. line for fluids and vasopressor drugs. Describe other interventions, such as lowering the head of the bed, inserting an indwelling urinary catheter, and assisting with insertion of hemodynamic monitoring lines. Document adherence to ACLS protocols, using a code sheet to record interventions, if necessary. (See "Cardiopulmonary arrest and resuscitation," page 53). Use the appropriate flow sheets to record intake and output, I.V. fluids, drugs, and frequent vital signs. Record the patient's responses to these interventions. Include any emotional support and patient education.

8/1/05	1235	Pt. c/o dizziness at 1220. P 48, RR 18, BP 86/48, oral T 97.6° F. Peripheral pulses weak, skin cool and diaphoretic, normal bowel sounds, clear breath sounds, alert and oriented to time, place, and person, no c/o chest pain. Continuous cardiac monitoring via portable monitor shows failure of permanent pacemaker to capture. Rhythm strip mounted below. Dr. King called at 1225, came to see pt., and orders given. 12-lead ECG done and confirms failure to capture. Placed on O₂ 2L by NC. Intermittent infusion device started in ® forearm with 18G catheter. VS recorded q5min on frequent VS sheet. Stat portable CXR done at 1230. Explained pacemaker malfunction to pt. Assured her that she's being monitored and that a temporary pacemaker is available, if needed. Dr. King called pt.'s husband and told him of situation. ————————— Kathy Thompson, RN
Koller, Johanna ID# 543929		8/1/05 1235
	1240	Dr. King explained that CXR showed a lead fracture in pacemaker wire requiring replacement. Procedure explained by doctor and informed consent form signed. Pt. still c/o dizziness. P 46, R 20, BP 88/46. Preoperative teaching performed. Pt. states she remembers the procedure from last year when the pacemaker was inserted. Report called to Sally Lane, RN, in operating room. ——————————— Kathy Thompson, RN

HYPOVOLEMIA

When a patient is hypovolemic, reduced intravascular blood volume causes circulatory dysfunction and inadequate tissue perfusion. Without sufficient blood or fluid replacement, the patient develops hypovolemic shock, which can progress to irreversible cerebral and renal damage, cardiac arrest and, ultimately, death.

The most common cause of hypovolemic shock is acute blood loss. Other causes include severe burns, intestinal obstruction, peritonitis, acute pancreatitis, ascites, dehydration from excessive perspiration, severe diarrhea or protracted vomiting, diabetes insipidus, diuresis, and inadequate fluid intake.

When your patient is hypovolemic, assess for and maintain a patent airway, breathing, and circulation. Expect to administer blood or fluid replacement. Inotropic and vasopressor drugs may also be administered. Other nursing interventions focus on identifying and treating the underlying cause.

ESSENTIAL DOCUMENTATION

Record the date and time of your entry. Record your assessment findings, such as hypotension; tachycardia; rapid, shallow respirations; reduced urine output; cold, pale, clammy skin; weight loss; poor skin turgor; weak, diminished, or absent pulses; and reduced level of consciousness. Document the measures you took to ensure a patent airway, breathing, and circulation, and the patient's responses to your interventions. Record the name of the doctor you notified, the time of notification, the orders given, and your actions, such as continuous blood pressure and cardiac monitoring, I.V. inotropic and vasopressor drugs, I.V. blood and fluid replacement, blood work, supplemental oxygen, and assisting with insertion of hemodynamic monitoring lines. Chart the patient's response to these interventions. Refer to "Arterial line insertion," page 25, and "Hemodynamic monitoring," page 164, for instruction on documenting insertion of these lines in your patient. Use the appropriate flow sheets to record intake and output, I.V. fluids, drugs, and frequent vital signs. Include patient education and emotional support given.

10/17/05	1435	Pt. restless and confused to time and place. P 120 reg, BP
		88/58, RR 28 shallow, rectal T 96.8° F. Lungs clear, neck
		veins flat, skin cold and clammy, skin tents when pinched,
		peripheral pulses weak. Urine output last hour 25 ml via
		Foley catheter. Placed pt. flat in bed, on ℚ side. Notified
		Dr. Diegidio at 1410, came to see pt., and orders written.
		Continuous cardiac monitoring shows sinus tachycardia.
		Automated cuff placed for continuous BP monitoring. Dr.
		Diegidio explained need for hemodynamic monitoring to
		pt.'s husband who signed consent. Assisted Dr. Diegidio with
		insertion of 6-lumen catheter into ℝ subclavian vein.
		Pressures on insertion: CVP 2 mm Hg, PAD 4 mm Hg, PAWP
		3 mm Hg. Wedge tracing obtained with 1.5 ml balloon
		inflation. NSS 1000 ml at 125 ml/hr infusing in proximal
		infusion port. Using flush solution of 500 units heparin in
		500 ml NSS. Catheter sutured in place and site covered with
		transparent semipermeable dressing. Portable CXR confirmed
		line placement. Lab in to draw blood for CBC, electrolytes,
		BUN, creatinine, serum lactate, and coagulation studies at
		1420. ABG drawn by Thomas Reilly, RPT, at 1423. O₂ at
		4L via NC w/pulse oximetry of 95%. See flow sheets for
		frequent VS, I/O, and hemodynamic readings. All procedures
		explained to pt. and husband. Pt. lying comfortably in bed,
		oriented to time, place, and person. Given Tylenol 2 tabs
		p.o. at 1430 for mild discomfort at catheter insertion site.
		—————————— Andrew Miller, RN

HYPOXEMIA

Defined as a low concentration of oxygen in the arterial blood, hypoxemia occurs when the partial pressure of arterial oxygen (PaO_2) falls below 60 mm Hg. Hypoxemia causes poor tissue perfusion and may lead to respiratory failure. Hypoxemia may be caused by any condition that results in hypoventilation abnormalities (such as head trauma, stroke, or central nervous system depressant drugs), diffusion abnormalities (including pulmonary edema, pulmonary fibrosis, and emphysema), ventilation/perfusion mismatches (such as chronic obstructive pulmonary disease or restrictive lung disorders), and shunting of blood (such as pneumonia, atelectasis, acute respiratory distress syndrome, pulmonary edema, and pulmonary embolism).

If you suspect your patient is hypoxemic, notify the doctor immediately and anticipate interventions to prevent and treat respiratory failure.

ESSENTIAL DOCUMENTATION

Record the date and time of your entry. Record your patient's PaO_2 level and cardiopulmonary assessment findings, such as change in level of consciousness, tachycardia, increased blood pressure, tachypnea, dyspnea, mottled skin, cyanosis, and, in patients with severe hypoxemia, bradycardia and hypotension. Chart the name of the doctor notified, the time of notification, and any orders given. Record your interventions, such as measuring oxygen saturation by pulse oximetry, obtaining arterial blood gas values, providing supplemental oxygen, positioning the patient in a high Fowler's position, assisting with endotracheal intubation, monitoring mechanical ventilation, and providing continuous cardiac monitoring. Document the patient's responses to these interventions. Use the appropriate flow sheets to record intake and output, I.V. fluids, drugs, and frequent vital signs. Include any emotional support and patient education.

| 7/19/05 | 1400 | Pt. restless and confused, SOB, skin mottled. P 112, BP 148/78, RR 32 labored, rectal T 97.4° F. Dr. Bouchard notified and came to see pt. ABGs drawn by doctor and sent to lab. Pulse oximetry 86% on O₂ 3 L/min by NC. Placed on O₂ 100% via nonrebreather mask with pulse oximetry 92%. Pt. positioned in high Fowler's position. Continuous cardiac monitoring shows sinus tachycardia at 116, no arrhythmias noted. Radiology called for stat portable CXR. Doctor. notified wife of change in husband's status.————————— Donna Damico, RN |

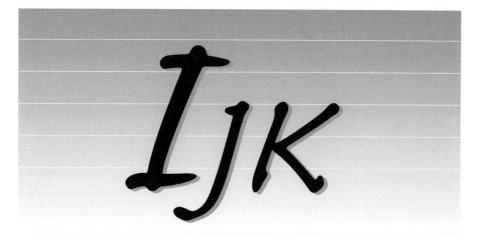

ILLEGAL ALTERATION OF A MEDICAL RECORD

As a general rule, the medical record is presumed to be accurate if there's no evidence of fraud or tampering. Tampering or illegal alteration of a medical record includes adding to someone else's note, destroying the patient's chart, not recording important details, recording false information, writing an incorrect date or time, adding to previous notes without marking the entry as being late, and rewriting notes. Evidence of tampering can cause the medical record to be ruled inadmissible as evidence in court.

LEGAL CASEBOOK

REWRITING RECORDS

In *Thor v. Boska (1974)*, a rewritten copy of a patient's record was suspected of being an altered record. This lawsuit involved a woman who had seen her doctor several times because of a breast lump. Each time, the doctor examined her and made a record of her visit. After 2 years, the woman sought a second opinion and learned that she had breast cancer. She sued her first doctor. Rather than producing his records in court, the doctor brought copies of the records and said he had copied the originals for legibility. The court reasoned that he was withholding evidence and held in favor of the plaintiff.

In a suspected case of notes written after litigation, the plaintiff's attorney retains handwriting experts to determine when portions were written. An alteration in the record can make a defensible case indefensible.

AccuChart

DOCUMENTING AN ALTERED MEDICAL RECORD ON THE INCIDENT REPORT

When you discover that a medical record has been altered, document your findings on an incident report.

INCIDENT REPORT		Name *Greta Manning*
DATE OF INCIDENT *11-14-05*	**TIME OF INCIDENT** *0400*	Address *7 Worth Way, Boston, MA* Phone *(617) 555-1122*

EXACT LOCATION OF INCIDENT (Bldg, Floor, Room No, Area)
4-Main, Rm. 447

Addressograph if patient _____

TYPE OF INCIDENT
(CHECK ONE ONLY) ☑ PATIENT ☐ EMPLOYEE ☐ VISITOR ☐ VOLUNTEER ☐ OTHER (specify)

DESCRIPTION OF THE INCIDENT (WHO, WHAT, WHEN, WHERE, HOW, WHY)
(Use back of form if necessary) *Called Dr. James at 0400 on 11/14/05 to report pt. had chest pain, radiating to jaw. Doctor said to give pt. Mylanta 30 ml X 1. 0430 called doctor to report continuing chest pain despite Mylanta 30 ml. X 1 dose. Doctor said to put nitroglycerin patch on now, rather than 6 a.m. When asked, doctor stated pt. didn't need nitro s.l. Tonight, 11/15/05, when I came in, found doctor's order timed for 0400, 11/14/05, for nitro 1/150 gr SL q5min X 3 for chest pain.*

If you suspect that another health care professional has made changes to a medical record, notify your nursing supervisor or risk manager immediately. Avoid the urge to correct the medical record. Moreover, don't change your notes if requested to do so by another colleague. Complete an incident report, according to your facility's policy, documenting the alterations that you noted in the medical record or the request by a colleague to change your notes. (See *Rewriting records,* page 215.)

ESSENTIAL DOCUMENTATION

Record the date and time that you complete the incident report. Write a factual account of what you observed in the medical record or your conversations with the colleague asking you to alter the record. Include the names and titles of persons you notified.

See *Documenting an altered medical record on the incident report* for how to report an altered medical record.

INAPPROPRIATE COMMENT IN THE MEDICAL RECORD

Negative language and inappropriate information don't belong in a medical record. Such comments are unprofessional and can also trigger diffi-

UNPROFESSIONAL DOCUMENTATION

Negative language and inappropriate information don't belong in a medical record and can be used against you in a lawsuit. For example, one elderly patient's family became upset after the patient developed pressure ulcers. They complained that the patient wasn't receiving adequate care. The patient later died of natural causes.

However, because the patient's family was dissatisfied with the care that the patient received, they sued. In the patient's chart, under prognosis, the doctor had written "PBBB." After learning that this stood for "pine box by bedside," the insurance company was only too happy to settle for a significant sum.

culties in legal cases. A lawyer may use negative or inappropriate comments to show that a patient received poor care. (See *Unprofessional documentation.*)

ESSENTIAL DOCUMENTATION

Your documentation in the medical record should contain descriptive, objective information: what you see, hear, feel, smell, measure, and count – not what you suppose, infer, conclude, or assume. Describe events or behaviors objectively and avoid labeling them with such expressions as "bizarre," "spaced out," or "obnoxious." (See *Charting objectively,* page 218.)

The following note is an example of a nurse using inappropriate words with negative connotations:

1/19/06	1400	Pt. was obnoxious when I went to give him his medi-
		cations and threw me out of his room. ————
		———————————————— Anne Curry, RN

The next note concerns the same situation, but is written objectively:

1/19/06	1400	Attempted to give pt. his medication, but he said, "I've
		had enough pills. Now leave me alone." Explained the
		importance of the medication and attempted to deter-
		mine why he wouldn't take it. Pt. refused to talk. Dr.
		Ellis notified that medication was refused. ————
		———————————————— Anne Curry, RN

CHARTING OBJECTIVELY

What you say and how you say it are of utmost importance in documentation. Keeping the patient's chart free from negative, inappropriate information—potential legal bombshells—can be quite a challenge when you're writing detailed narrative notes. Here are some guidelines to help you sidestep charting pitfalls and record an accurate account of your patient's care and status.

AVOID REPORTING STAFFING PROBLEMS

Even though staff shortages may affect patient care or contribute to an incident, you shouldn't refer to staffing problems in a patient's chart. Instead, discuss them in a forum that can help resolve the problem. In a confidential memo or an incident report, call the situation to the attention of the appropriate personnel such as your nurse-manager. Also review your hospital's policy and procedure manuals to determine how you're expected to handle this situation.

KEEP STAFF CONFLICTS AND RIVALRIES OUT OF THE RECORD

Entries about disputes with nursing colleagues (including characterization and criticism of care provided), questions about a doctor's treatment decisions, or reports of a colleague's rude or abusive behavior reflect personality clashes and don't belong in the medical record. They aren't legitimate concerns about patient care.

As with staffing problems, address concerns about a colleague's judgment or competence in the appropriate setting. After making sure that you have the facts, talk with your nurse-manager. Consult with the doctor directly if an order concerns you. Share your opinions, observations, or reservations about colleagues with your nurse-manager only; avoid mentioning them in a patient's chart.

If you discover personal accusations or charges of incompetence in a chart, discuss this with your supervisor.

STEER CLEAR OF WORDS ASSOCIATED WITH ERRORS

Terms such as by mistake, accidentally, somehow, unintentionally, miscalculated, and confusing can be interpreted as admissions of wrongdoing. Instead, let the facts speak for themselves—for example, "Pt. was given Demerol 100 mg I.M. at 1300 hours for abdominal pain. Doctor Jones was notified at 1305 and is on his way here. Pt.'s vital signs are BP 120/82, P 80, RR 20, T 98.4° F."

If the ordered drug dose was 50 mg, this entry will let other health care providers know that the patient was overmedicated.

AVOID BIAS

Don't use words that suggest a negative attitude toward the patient. For example, don't use unflattering or unprofessional adjectives, such as obstinate, drunk, obnoxious, bizarre, or abusive, to describe the patient's behavior. If a patient is difficult or uncooperative, document the behavior objectively. Negative words could cause a plaintiff's attorney to attack your professionalism with an argument such as this: "Look at how this nurse felt about my client—she called him 'rude, difficult, and uncooperative.' No wonder she didn't take good care of him; she didn't like him."

DON'T ASSUME

Always aim to record the facts about a situation, not your assumptions or conclusions. Record only what you see and hear. For example, don't record that a patient pulled out an I.V. line if you didn't witness him doing so. Do, however, describe your findings—for example, "Found pt., arm board, and bed linens covered with blood. I.V. line and venipuncture device were untaped and hanging free."

INCIDENT REPORT

An incident is an event that's inconsistent with the facility's ordinary routine, regardless of whether injury occurs. In most health care facilities, any injury to a patient requires an incident report (also known as an event report or occurrance report). Patient complaints, medication errors, and injuries to employees and visitors require incident reports as well. (See *Reporting an incident.*)

An incident report serves two main purposes:

▪ to inform hospital administration of the incident so that it can monitor patterns and trends, thereby helping to prevent future similar incidents (risk management)

▪ to alert the administration and the hospital's insurance company to the possibility of liability claims and the need for further investigation (claims management).

ESSENTIAL DOCUMENTATION

When filing an incident report, include only the following information:

▪ the exact time and place of the incident

▪ the names of the persons involved and any witnesses

LEGAL CASEBOOK

REPORTING AN INCIDENT

As a nurse, you have a duty to report any incident of which you have first-hand knowledge. Not only can failure to report an incident lead to your being fired, but it can also expose you to personal liability for malpractice—especially if your failure to report the incident causes injury to a patient.

When you do file an incident report, don't indicate in the patient's chart that an incident report has been completed. This destroys the confidential nature of the report and may result in a lawsuit.

An incident involving a patient should also be recorded in his medical record. If you don't document the incident, treatment, follow-up care, and patient's response, the plaintiff's attorney might think you're hiding something. If the case goes to court, the jury may be asked to determine if the patient received appropriate care after the incident.

Include in the incident report and progress note any statements made by the patient or his family concerning their role in the incident. For example, "Patient stated, 'The nurse told me to ask for help before I went to the bathroom, but I decided to go on my own.'" This kind of statement helps the defense attorney prove that the patient was entirely or partially at fault. If the jury finds that the patient was partially at fault, the concept of contributory negligence may be used to reduce or even eliminate the patient's recovery of damages.

TIPS FOR WRITING AN INCIDENT REPORT

When a malpractice lawsuit reached the courtroom in years past, the plaintiff's attorney wasn't allowed to see incident reports. Today, in many states, the plaintiff is legally entitled to a record of the incident if he requests it through the proper channels.

When writing an incident report, keep in mind the people who may read it and follow these guidelines.

WRITE OBJECTIVELY

Record the details of the incident in objective terms, describing exactly what you saw and heard. For example, unless you actually saw a patient fall, write: "Found patient lying on the floor." Then describe only the actions you took to provide care at the scene, such as helping the patient back into bed, assessing him for injuries, and calling the doctor.

AVOID OPINIONS

Don't commit your opinions to writing in the incident report. Rather, verbally share your suggestions or opinions on how an incident may

be avoided with your supervisor and risk manager.

ASSIGN NO BLAME

Don't admit to liability and don't blame or point your finger at colleagues or administrators. Steer clear of such statements as "Better staffing would have prevented this incident." State only what happened.

AVOID HEARSAY AND ASSUMPTIONS

Each staff member who knows about the incident should write a separate incident report. If one of your patients is injured in another department, the staff members in that department are responsible for documenting the details of the incident.

FILE THE REPORT PROPERLY

Don't file the incident report with the medical record. Send the report to the person designated to review it according to your facility's policy.

- factual information about what happened and the consequences to the person involved (supply enough information so administration can decide whether the matter needs further investigation)
- any relevant facts (such as your immediate actions in response to the incident; for example, notifying the patient's doctor).

After completing the incident report, sign and date it. (See *Tips for writing an incident report.*)

An incident must also be documented in the patient's medical record. Write a factual account of the incident, including the treatment, follow-up care, and the patient's response. Include in the progress note and in the incident report anything the patient or his family says about their role in the incident.

See *Completing an incident report* for how to document a patient incident.

AccuChart

COMPLETING AN INCIDENT REPORT

When you discover a reportable event, you must fill out an incident report. Forms vary but most include the following information.

INCIDENT REPORT

DATE OF INCIDENT	**TIME OF INCIDENT**
6-25-05	1300

EXACT LOCATION OF INCIDENT (Bldg, Floor, Room No, Area)
3B-Room 310

Name   Greta Manning
Address   7 Worth Way, Boston, MA
Phone   (617) 555-1122

Addressograph if patient _____

TYPE OF INCIDENT
(CHECK ONE ONLY)   ☑ PATIENT   ☐ EMPLOYEE   ☐ VISITOR   ☐ VOLUNTEER   ☐ OTHER (specify)

DESCRIPTION OF THE INCIDENT (WHO, WHAT, WHEN, WHERE, HOW, WHY)
(Use back of form if necessary)   Pt. found on floor next to bed. States she was trying to reach her slippers, which were under the bed, and lost her balance.

Patient fall incidents	**FLOOR CONDITIONS** ☐ OTHER _____ ☑ CLEAN & SMOOTH ☐ SLIPPERY (WET)	**FRAME OF BED** ☑ LOW ☐ HIGH	**NIGHT LIGHT** ☐ YES ☑ NO
	WERE BED RAILS PRESENT? ☐ NO ☑ 1 UP ☐ 2 UP ☐ 3 UP ☐ 4 UP	**OTHER RESTRAINTS** (TYPE AND EXTENT) N/A	
	AMBULATION PRIVILEGE ☑ UNLIMITED ☐ LIMITED WITH ASSISTANCE ☐ COMPLETE BEDREST ☐ OTHER		
	WERE OPIOIDS, ANALGESICS, HYPNOTICS, SEDATIVES, DIURETICS, ANTIHYPERTENSIVES, OR ANTICONVULSANTS GIVEN DURING LAST 4 HOURS? ☐ YES ☑ NO DRUG _____ AMOUNT _____ TIME _____		

Patient incidents	**PHYSICIAN NOTIFIED** Name of Physician J. Reynolds, MD	DATE 6/25/05	TIME 1310	COMPLETE IF APPLICABLE

Employee incidents	**DEPARTMENT**	**JOB TITLE**	**SOCIAL SECURITY #**
	MARITAL STATUS		

All incidents	**NOTIFIED** DATE TIME C. Smith, RN 6/25/05 1310	**LOCATION WHERE TREATMENT WAS RENDERED**

NAME, ADDRESS AND TELEPHONE NUMBERS OF WITNESS(ES) OR PERSONS FAMILIAR WITH INCIDENT - WITNESS OR NOT
Janet Adams   (617) 555-0912   1 Main St., Boston, MA

SIGNATURE OF PERSON PREPARING REPORT	**TITLE**	**DATE OF REPORT**
Connie Smith	RN	6/25/05

PHYSICIAN'S REPORT — To be completed for all cases involving injury or illness   (do not use abbreviations) (Use back if necessary)

DIAGNOSIS AND TREATMENT

DISPOSITION

PERSON NOTIFIED OTHER THAN HOSPITAL PERSONNEL   DATE   TIME
NAME AND ADDRESS

PHYSICIAN'S SIGNATURE   DATE

INCREASED INTRACRANIAL PRESSURE

The skull is a rigid compartment filled to capacity with three components: brain tissue, blood, and cerebrospinal fluid. Intracranial pressure (ICP) is the pressure exerted by these three components against the skull. When the volume of one or more of these components increases, the volume of the other two must decrease or ICP will rise. If increased ICP goes untreated, it can lead to brain herniation and death.

Causes of increased ICP include tumors, abscesses, hemorrhage, head injuries, brain surgery, infection, cerebral infarct, conditions that obstruct venous outflow, lead or arsenic poisoning, renal failure, hepatic failure, and Reye's syndrome.

If you suspect increased ICP in your patient, immediately notify the doctor and ensure adequate airway, breathing, and circulation. Anticipate endotracheal intubation and mechanical ventilation, monitor for changes in level of consciousness (LOC), prepare for ICP monitoring, and anticipate orders for osmotic diuretics.

ESSENTIAL DOCUMENTATION

Record the date and time of your entry. Record your patient's ICP if he has continuous ICP monitoring. Record your assessment findings, such as reduced LOC (for example, confused, restless, agitated, lethargic, or comatose), pupillary changes (including unequal size and sluggish or absent response to light), headache, seizures, focal neurologic signs, increased blood pressure, widened pulse pressure, bradycardia, decorticate or decerebrate posturing, and vomiting. Record the name of the doctor notified, the time of notification, and the orders given. Document your actions, such as maintaining a patent airway and ventilation, administering oxygen, administering osmotic diuretics, proper head positioning, and monitoring ICP. Use the appropriate flow sheets to record ICP readings, Glasgow Coma Scale scores, intake and output, I.V. fluids given, drugs administered, and frequent vital signs. Monitor your patient frequently, as ordered, and time and record each assessment. Chart all patient education and emotional support provided.

12/28/05	1300	Pt. fell 10' and hit head at 0900. Now c/o headache,
		pupils equal with sluggish response on right. P 66,
		BP 146/50, RR 12. Rectal T 97.2° F. No evidence of
		seizures, hand grasp on ® sl. weaker than Ⓛ, opens
		eyes to verbal command, localizes and pushes away
		painful stimulus, oriented to name but not time and
		place. Glasgow Coma score 10. Dr. Harper notified at
		1250 and came to examine pt., orders given. O₂ at
		2 L/min via NC started. HOB elevated and maintained
		at 15-degree angle, head maintained in straight align-
		ment. Lights low, noise level to a minimum. Doctor
		Harper will contact pt.'s wife to discuss ICP monitor-
		ing and obtain consent for insertion of ICP monitor.
		See flow sheets for frequent VS, I/O, and Glasgow
		Coma scores. Reorienting pt. to time and place. Ex-
		plaining all procedures to pt. ——— Erin O'Leary, RN

INFECTION CONTROL

Meticulous record keeping is an important contributor to effective infection control. Various federal agencies require documentation of infections so that the data can be assessed and used to help prevent and control future infections. In addition, the data you record help your health care facility meet national and local accreditation standards.

Typically, you must report to your facility's infection control department any culture result that shows a positive infection and any surgery, drug, elevated temperature, X-ray finding, or specific treatment related to infection.

ESSENTIAL DOCUMENTATION

Record the date and time of your entry. Document to whom you reported the signs and symptoms of suspected infection, instructions received, and treatments initiated. Record that you have followed standard precautions against direct contact with blood and body fluids. Record that you have taught the patient and his family about these precautions. Record the dates and times of your interventions in the patient's chart and on the Kardex. Document any breach in an isolation technique, and file an incident report should this occur.

Note the name of the doctor that you notified of the results of any culture and sensitivity studies, and record the time of notification. If the doctor prescribes a drug to treat the infection, record this as well along with the patient's response. Transcribe any new or modified drug orders to the patient's medication Kardex. Also, inform the infection control practitioner. Record the patient's response to this drug.

11/28/05	1300	Standard precautions maintained. P 96, BP 132/82, rectal T 102.3° F. Large amount of purulent yellow-green, foul-smelling drainage from incision soaked through 6 4" X 4" gauze pads in 2 hr. Dr. Levin notified. Ordered Tylenol 650 mg P.O. q 4hr prn for temp greater than 101° F, given at 1250. Repeat C&S obtained and sent to lab. Wound cleaned w/NSS and covered with 4 sterile 4" X 4" pads using sterile technique. Reinforced standard precautions to pt. and wife. ———— Lynne Kasoff, RN

INFORMATION FROM OTHER DEPARTMENTS

Because health care involves teamwork, all interdepartmental and interdisciplinary communication about the patient must be documented. When receiving critical laboratory test results, be sure to read the results back to verify them.

ESSENTIAL DOCUMENTATION

When you speak with another department, either to give them information or to receive information, record the date, time, name of the person you spoke with, and the results. If you need to notify the doctor of any results, document your notification, including the doctor's name and the time that he was notified.

1/4/06	1400	Lab technician Donald Boyle called floor to report pt.'s random blood glucose of 486 mg/dl. Dr. Somers notified. Stat blood glucose ordered. Pt. placed on bed rest and being monitored q 15 min until results available. P 98 strong, BP 98/68, RR 24, oral T 98.2° F. Alert and oriented to time, place, and person. No acetone odor on breath. Skin warm and dry. ———— ———————————————————— Peggy Irwin, RN

INFORMED CONSENT, INABILITY TO GIVE

Informed consent relies on an individual's capacity or ability to make decisions at a particular time under specific circumstances. To make medical decisions, a person must possess not only the capacity, but also the competence to make such decisions.

If you have reason to believe that a patient is incompetent to participate in giving consent because of a medical condition or sedation, you have an obligation to bring it to the doctor's attention immediately. Should you learn that the doctor has discussed consent issues with the patient at a time when the patient was heavily sedated or medicated, you need to bring your concerns to the doctor's attention. If the doctor isn't available, discuss your concerns with your supervisor.

Along with discussing the matter with the doctor and your supervisor, you must assess your patient's understanding of the information provided by the practitioner. If the patient can't provide consent, follow facility policy on contacting legal guardians or family members for consent before the procedure. (See *When a patient can't give consent.*)

LEGAL CASEBOOK

WHEN A PATIENT CAN'T GIVE CONSENT

If you believe your patient is incompetent to participate in giving consent because of medication or sedation and you do nothing, and the patient undergoes the procedure without giving proper consent, you might find yourself as a co-defendant in a battery lawsuit. Patient's lawyers, judges, and juries will look closely at the medication records to see when, in relation to the signing of the consent form, the patient was last medicated and the patient's response to the medication as documented in the record. You could be held jointly responsible for the patient undergoing a procedure that he didn't consent to if:

- you took part in the battery by assisting with the treatment
- you knew it was taking place and you didn't try to stop it.

If the doctor fails to provide adequate information for consent because of the patient's medicated status, the patient may sue the doctor for lack of informed consent due to temporary incapacitation. The courts might hold you responsible if, knowing the doctor hasn't provided adequate information to a patient, you fail to try to stop the procedure until proper consent can be obtained.

ESSENTIAL DOCUMENTATION

Document conversations with the patient, including his mental status and understanding of the procedure, complications, and expected outcomes. Record that your patient is confused or medicated, you can't provide the information the patient needs, the patient doesn't understand the procedure, or you assessed that the patient wasn't competent to provide consent when speaking with the doctor because of medication or sedation. Record the names of the doctor and nursing supervisor that you notified, and note the time of notification.

07/19/05	0700	Pt. given morphine 4 mg I.V. push at 0630 for chest pain. Dr. James in to see pt. at 0645 to explain cardiac cath procedure and obtain informed consent. Pt. keeps asking, "Where am I? What is happening?" Dr. James explained that she was in CCU with chest pain and was scheduled for a cardiac catheterization this a.m. Pt. keeps asking, "What is this test and why do I need it?" Cardiac cath. canceled for this a.m. Doctor will come back to see pt. later today. ———————— Mary Higgins, RN

INFORMED CONSENT IN EMERGENCY SITUATION

A patient must sign a consent form before most treatments and procedures. Informed consent means that the patient understands the proposed therapy, alternative therapies, the risks, and the hazards of not undergoing any treatment at all.

However, in specific circumstances, emergency treatment (to save a patient's life or to prevent loss of organ, limb, or a function) may be done without first obtaining consent. If the patient is unconscious or a minor who can't give consent, emergency treatment may be performed without first obtaining consent. The presumption is that the patient would have consented if he had been able unless there's a reason to believe otherwise. For example, to sustain the life of unconscious patients in the emergency department, intubation has been held to be appropriate even if no one is available to consent to the procedure.

Courts will uphold emergency medical treatment as long as reasonable effort was made to obtain consent and no alternative treatments were available to save life or limb.

ESSENTIAL DOCUMENTATION

Record the date and time of your entry. Document the emergency and the reason your patient can't give informed consent such as being unconsciousness. Describe efforts to reach family members to obtain consent. List the names, addresses, telephone numbers, and relationships of the people you or the doctor attempted to reach. Record that no alternative treatment was available to save life or limb.

| 8/19/05 | 1000 | Pt. arrived in ED at 0940 via ambulance following MVC. Pt. not responding to verbal commands, opens eyes and pushes at stimulus in response to pain, making no verbal responses. Pt. has bruising across upper chest, labored breathing, skin pale and cool, normal S_1 and S_2 heart sounds, diminished breath sounds throughout Ⓛ lung, normal breath sounds Ⓡ lung, no tracheal deviation. P 112, BP 88/52, RR 26. Dr. Mallory called at 0945 and come to see pt. I.V. line inserted in Ⓡ antecubital with 20G catheter. 1000 ml NSS infusing at 125 ml/hr. 100% oxygen given via nonrebreather mask. Stat CXR ordered to confirm pneumothorax. Pt. identified by driver's license and credit cards as Michael Brown of 123 Maple St., Valley View. Doctor Mallory called house to speak with family about need for immediate chest tube and treatment, no answer, left message on machine. Business card of Michelle Brown found in wallet. Company receptionist confirms she is wife of Michael Brown, but she's out of the office and won't return until this afternoon. Left message at 0945 for wife to call doctor. ———————— Sandy Becker, RN |
| | 1015 | Tracheal deviation to Ⓛ side, difficulty breathing, cyanosis of lips, and mucous membranes, distended neck veins, absent breath sounds in Ⓡ lung, muffled heart sounds. P 120, BP 88/58, RR 32. Neurologic status unchanged. See neuro flow sheet. Dr. Mallory called pt.'s home and wife's place of business but was unable to speak with her. Again, left messages. Because of pt.'s deteriorating condition, pt.'s inability to give consent, and inability to reach wife, Dr. Mallory has ordered chest tube to be inserted on Ⓡ side to relieve tension pneumothorax. ——— Sandy Becker, RN |

INFORMED CONSENT, LACK OF UNDERSTANDING OF

Informed consent means that your patient has consented to a procedure after receiving a full explanation of it, its risks and complications, and the risk if the procedure isn't performed at this time. As a patient advocate, it's your responsibility to help ensure that the patient is truly making an informed choice. If you determine that the patient didn't understand the informed consent discussion with the doctor, treatment shouldn't proceed. Notify the doctor that the patient can't give informed consent without further information from the doctor. If the informed consent has already been signed, notify the doctor that the patient's decision wasn't an informed one. After the doctor clarifies the procedure or treatment, ask the patient to explain in her own words what she was just told. Also, ask the patient questions to determine whether she fully understands the intent and implications.

ESSENTIAL DOCUMENTATION

Document the date and time of your discussion with the patient. Record the conversation in which you determined that the patient didn't fully understand the procedure or treatment. Use the patient's own words, placing them in quotations. Note whether the patient signed the consent form. Record the name of the doctor notified, the time of notification, what you told the doctor, and his response. Document any further explanations by the doctor and the patient's response. Record whether the patient could explain the procedure and her ability to answer your questions.

7/6/05	0945	While performing morning care, pt. asked, "Will I have
		periods after my tubal ligation?" and "How will I know
		if I am pregnant?" Tubal ligation is scheduled for
		tomorrow morning and signed consent is in chart.
		Notified Dr. Newcomb at 0915 that, because pt. is asking
		questions about getting pregnant, she doesn't under-
		stand the full implications of the procedure and that
		her consent wasn't informed. Dr. Newcomb came to see
		pt. and husband at 0930 and explained the procedure
		and consequences of tubal ligation. When asked to
		repeat back what the doctor said, pt. replied, "I under-
		stand now. I'll still get periods. This surgery will pre-
		vent eggs from reaching my uterus so they won't be
		able to be fertilized by sperm. I won't be able to have
		any more children. But, that's OK since we don't want
		any more. Four is enough." ———— Fran Cervone, RN

INFORMED CONSENT WHEN PATIENT IS A MINOR

Informed consent involves ensuring that the patient or someone acting on his behalf has enough information to know the risks and consequences of

WHEN A MINOR CAN GIVE CONSENT

The ability of a minor to give consent varies with the condition being treated, the age of the minor, and the state where the condition is being treated. Because privacy issues are involved, the nurse must understand the specific circumstances in which a minor can give consent and when to contact the parent or legal guardian.

A teenage mother must give consent before her baby can receive treatment but in general isn't permitted to determine the course of her own health care. Under federal law, adolescents can be tested and treated for human immunodeficiency virus without parental involvement. However, parental consent is required to set an adolescent's fractured arm in most cases.

Every state will allow an emancipated minor to consent to his own medical care and treatment. State definitions of emancipation vary, but it's generally recognized that to be emancipated, the individual must be a minor by state definition and must have obtained a legal declaration of freedom from the custody, care, and control of his parents.

Most states will allow teenagers to consent to treatment in cases involving pregnancy and sexually transmitted diseases.

An unemancipated minor in his mid- to late teens, who shows signs of intellectual and emotional maturity, is considered a "mature minor" and, in some cases, is allowed to exercise some of the rights regarding health care that are generally reserved for adults.

a treatment, procedure, drug, or surgery. When the patient is a minor, it's essential that the doctor give a full explanation of care to the parent or designated adult responsible for signing the consent. (See *When a minor can give consent.*) Ethically, there's certainly a duty to inform a minor of the procedure and risks regardless of whether he can consent to care. Wherever and whenever possible, children should at least be given the opportunity to participate in the decision making for their care. Parents ultimately have the responsibility for making health care decisions, but children benefit greatly by involvement in their care and treatment. Generally, when controversies arise and a court hearing ensues, the older the minor is, the more likely his wishes will be followed.

ESSENTIAL DOCUMENTATION

Record the date and time that the patient or health care proxy gave consent. Describe the involvement of the child, where possible. Include information on other persons present. Record any questions or comments that the child, parents, or significant others had. Witness the signature of the responsible adult per facility policy. Ask the responsible adult to restate the purpose of the procedure, medication, or surgery in his own words.

Record his responses. Also, ask the child to do the same, and chart the response. You may ask the child to draw a picture for you and place that in the chart. Describe any teaching done with the adults and child.

11/12/05	1420	Consent obtained by Dr. Mason for Scott Jones' tonsillectomy from Mr. and Mrs. Jones, parents of Scott, at 1400 at the preop clinic appt. Parents were able to state the purpose of the surgery and the risks involved. Asked Scott to draw a picture of what was going to happen, and he drew a picture of the oper-ating room with the doctor "pulling out" his tonsils. When asked how he felt about having the surgery he said, "I keep missing swim practice. I'll be glad to be able to go all the time." ——————————— Richard Lyons, RN

INTAKE AND OUTPUT

Many patients require 24-hour intake and output monitoring. They include surgical patients, patients on I.V. therapy, patients with fluid and electrolyte imbalances, and patients with burns, hemorrhage, or edema.

For easy reference, list the volumes of specific containers. Infusion devices make documenting enteral and I.V. intake more accurate. However, keeping track of intake that isn't premeasured – for example, food such as gelatin that's normally fluid at room temperature – requires the cooperation of the patient, family members (who may bring the patient snacks and soft drinks or help him to eat at the health care facility), and other caregivers. Therefore, you must make sure that everyone understands how to record or report all foods and fluids that the patient consumes orally.

Don't forget to count I.V. piggyback infusions, drugs given by I.V. push, patient-controlled analgesics, and any irrigation solutions that aren't withdrawn. You'll also need to know whether the patient receives any fluids orally or I.V. while he's off your unit.

Recording fluid output accurately requires the cooperation of the patient and staff members in any other departments your patient goes to. If he's ambulatory, remind him to use a urinal or a commode.

The amount of fluid lost through the GI tract is normally 100 ml or less daily. However, if the patient's stools become excessive or watery, they must be counted as output. Vomiting, drainage from suction devices and wound drains, and bleeding are other measurable sources of fluid

ACCUCHART

INTAKE AND OUTPUT

As the sample shows, you can monitor your patient's fluid balance by using an intake and output record.

Name: _Josephine Klein_
Medical record #: _49731_
Admission date: _2/13/05_

INTAKE AND OUTPUT RECORD

	Oral	Tube feeding	Instilled	I.V. and IVPB	TPN	Total	Urine	Emesis Tubes	NG	Other	Total
Date 2/15/05											
0700–1500	250	320	H₂O 50	1100		1720	1355				1355
1500–2300	200	320	H₂O 50	1100		1670	1200				1200
2300–0700		320	H₂O 50	1100		1470	1500				1500
24hr total	450	960	H₂O 150	3300		4860	4055				4055
Date											
24hr total											
Date											
24hr total											
Date											
24hr total											

The INTAKE columns are Oral, Tube feeding, Instilled, I.V. and IVPB, TPN, Total. The OUTPUT columns are Urine, Emesis Tubes, NG, Other, Total.

Key: IVPB = I.V. piggyback   TPN = total parenteral nutrition   NG = nasogastric

Standard measures

Styrofoam cup	240 ml	Water (large)	600 ml	Milk (large)	600 ml	Ice cream,	120 ml
Juice	120 ml	Water pitcher	750 ml	Coffee	240 ml	sherbet, or gelatin	
Water (small)	120 ml	Milk (small)	120 ml	Soup	180 ml		

loss. If the patient is incontinent, document this as well as tube drainage and irrigation volumes.

Make sure your patient's name is on the intake and output record. Record the date and time of your shift on the appropriate line. Record the total intake and output for each category of fluid for your shift, then total these categories and provide a shift total for intake and output. At the end of 24 hours, a daily total is calculated, usually by the night nurse. Make sure all nurses use the same units of measurement. In most cases, this will be milliliters.

See *Intake and output,* page 231, for an example of proper documentation.

INTESTINAL OBSTRUCTION

An intestinal obstruction is a partial or complete blockage of the lumen in the small or large bowel. A small-bowel obstruction is far more common and usually more serious. A complete obstruction can cause death within hours from shock and vascular collapse. Intestinal obstructions are most likely to occur from adhesions caused by previous abdominal surgery, external hernias, volvulus, Crohn's disease, radiation enteritis, intestinal wall hematomas (after trauma or anticoagulant therapy), and neoplasms.

When your patient has an intestinal obstruction, assess and treat him for peritonitis and shock, which are life-threatening conditions. Anticipate administering I.V. fluids, electrolytes, blood, and antibiotics. Assist with insertion of a nasogastric or intestinal tube for decompression of the bowel. Prepare your patient for surgery, if necessary.

ESSENTIAL DOCUMENTATION

Record the date and time of your entry. Record the results of your GI assessment, such as colicky pain, abdominal tenderness, rebound tenderness, nausea, vomiting, constipation, liquid stools, borborygmi or absent bowel sounds, and abdominal distention. Also, record the results of your cardiopulmonary, renal, and neurologic assessments. Document the name of the doctor notified, the time of notification, the orders given, your actions, and the patient's response. Use the appropriate flow sheets to record intake and output, I.V. fluids given, drugs administered, and frequent vital signs. A critical care flow sheet may also be used. Record the type of decompression tube inserted; the name of the doctor inserting the tube; the suction type and amount; the color, amount, and consistency of drainage; and mouth and nose care provided. Note the patient's tolerance of the procedure. Document the patient's level of pain on a scale of 0 to 10, with 10 being the worst pain imaginable, your interventions, and the patient's response. Record all drugs given on the medication Kardex and document the patient's response in your note. Include patient education and emotional support given.

9/19/05	1810	Pt. c/o nausea and cramping abdominal pain. Vomited
		150 ml green liquid. States he hasn't had BM X 5 days. P
		112, BP 128/72, RR 28, oral T 99.0° F. Abdominal exam
		shows rebound tenderness, distention, and high-pitched
		hyperactive bowel sounds. Pt. is alert and oriented to
		time, place, and person. Normal heart sounds. Breath
		sounds clear. Skin pale, cool, peripheral pulses palpable.
		Voiding approx. 400 ml q4hr. Notified Dr. Brunell at
		1745 of pt.'s condition. Orders given. Pt. NPO. Explained
		NPO to pt. and wife, answered their questions, and
		explained treatments being done. Stat abdominal X-ray
		done at 1755. Lab in to draw blood for electrolytes,
		BUN, creatinine, CBC w/diff. at 1800. I.V. infusion
		started in ® forearm with 18G catheter. 1000 ml of
		D₅NSS w/KCL 20 mEq/L infusing at 75 ml/hr. Dr.
		Brunell in at 1805 to explain possible bowel obstruction
		to pt. and wife. Told them that depending on the
		results of X-ray, pt. may need decompression tube, and
		explained to them the reasons for this treatment. See
		I.V., I/O, and VS flow sheets. ——— Mary Wagner, RN

INTRA-AORTIC BALLOON COUNTERPULSATION CARE

The patient receiving intra-aortic balloon counterpulsation (IABC) therapy requires continuous monitoring and care to ensure proper IABC function, patient comfort, and early detection and treatment of complications. Refer to "Intra-aortic balloon insertion," pages 235 and 236, for a discussion of common uses of IABC therapy.

ESSENTIAL DOCUMENTATION

Record the patient's arm and foot pulses, sensation and movement, color, and temperature every 15 minutes for 1 hour, then reassess the arms every 2 hours and the legs every hour while the balloon is in place.

Document hourly intake and output. Monitor and record bowel sounds, abdominal distention, tenderness, and elimination patterns every 4 hours. Record vital signs, pulmonary artery pressure, and pulmonary artery wedge pressure frequently, as ordered. Monitor and record laboratory values, such as arterial blood gases, BUN, creatinine, complete blood count with differential, partial thromboplastin time, and electrolytes. Place a waveform strip in the chart to document balloon function. Check the insertion site for redness, swelling, bleeding, hematoma, and drainage, and record all site care according to facility policy. Record the name of the doctor notified of any changes in the patient's condition or complications, the time of notification, the orders given, your actions, and the patient's response. Use the appropriate flow sheets to record intake and output, I.V. fluids given, drugs administered, and frequent hemodynamic measurements and vital signs. A critical care flow sheet may also be used to document frequent assessments. Include any teaching and emotional support given. Record routine checks of equipment, problems, and troubleshooting.

9/24/05	0900	Monitor shows normal inflation-deflation timing and
		augmentation, NSR, no arrhythmias noted. Radial pulses
		strong, hands pink and warm, able to move fingers and
		feel light touch bilaterally. Pedal pulse palpable and
		strong, feet warm to touch, able to move toes and
		ankles and feel light touch bilaterally. + bowel sounds in
		all 4 quadrants, medium-sized BM this a.m. No abdom-
		inal tenderness or distention. P 94, BP 122/72, RR 18,
		oral T 98.8° F, PAP 15/5, PAWP 4. Normal heart sounds.
		Breath sounds clear. Blood drawn and sent to lab at
		0845 for BUN, creatinine, CBC w/diff., PT/PTT. Results
		pending. ABC insertion site without redness, warmth,
		bleeding, hematoma, or drainage. See critical care flow
		sheet for I/O, I.V. fluids, frequent assessments. Re-
		minded pt. to keep affected leg straight, HOB not more
		than 30 degrees, and to call for help to move in bed.
		Call bell placed within reach. ———— Darcy Stone, RN

Mr. Goodrich   9/24/05
ID#: 445591   0900

INTRA-AORTIC BALLOON INSERTION

Providing temporary support for the heart's left ventricle, intra-aortic balloon counterpulsation (IABC) mechanically displaces blood within the aorta by means of an intra-aortic balloon (IAB) attached to an external pump console. The IAB is inserted through the common femoral artery and positioned with its tip just distal to the left subclavian artery. It monitors myocardial perfusion and the effects of drugs on myocardial function and perfusion. IABC improves two key aspects of myocardial physiology: It increases the supply of oxygen-rich blood to the myocardium, and it decreases myocardial oxygen demand.

IABC is indicated for patients with low-cardiac output disorders or cardiac instability, including refractory angina, ventricular arrhythmias associated with ischemia, and pump failure caused by cardiogenic shock, intraoperative myocardial infarction (MI), or low cardiac output after bypass surgery. IABC is also indicated for patients with low cardiac output secondary to acute mechanical defects after MI, such as ventricular septal defect, papillary muscle rupture, or left ventricular aneurysm.

ESSENTIAL DOCUMENTATION

Record the date and time of IAB insertion. Note that the patient or family understands the procedure and that a signed consent form is in the chart. Before insertion, document vital signs as well as the pulses, sensation, movement, color, and temperature of all extremities. If a sedative was ordered, chart it on the medication Kardex. Record the name of the doctor performing the procedure, other assistants, and the leg used. Describe the patient's tolerance of the procedure. After IAB insertion, document that a chest X-ray was done to confirm placement. Record the patient's arm and foot pulses, sensation and movement, color, and temperature every 15 minutes for 1 hour, then reassess the arms every 2 hours and the legs every hour while the balloon is in place.

9/23/05	1300	Pt. and wife verbalize understanding of IAB procedure, signed consent form is in chart. P 98, BP 102/68, RR 18, oral T 98.4° F. Dorsalis pedis, posterior tibial, and radial pulses palpable bilaterally. Pt. able to feel light touch and move all extremities bilaterally. Hands pink and warm, feet pink and cool to touch bilaterally. Transported to cardiac cath lab via stretcher for IAB insertion. ——————————————— Barry Moore, RN
	1400	Returned from cath lab. P 92, BP 114/88, RR 16, oral T 98.6° F. IAB inserted into ® femoral artery. Hands warm to touch, skin pink, radial arteries strong, able to feel light touch and move hands and fingers bilaterally. Feet cool, dorsalis pedis and posterior tibial pulses palpable, able to move ® leg, foot, and toes without difficulty, moving Ⓛ foot and toes without problem. + bowel sounds active in all 4 quadrants, no abdominal tenderness or distention. Monitor shows normal waveform, strip mounted below. No bleeding, hematoma, drainage, redness, or swelling at insertion site. Reminded pt. to keep ® leg straight and to call nurse with complaints of pain in leg, numbness or tingling. Call bell placed within reach. No c/o discomfort at insertion site. ——————————————— Barry Moore, RN
		Mr. Goodrich 9/23/05 ID#:445591 1300

INTRA-AORTIC BALLOON REMOVAL

The intra-aortic balloon may be removed when the patient's hemodynamic status remains stable after the frequency of balloon augmentation is decreased. The control system should be turned off and the connective tubing disconnected from the catheter to ensure balloon deflation. After the balloon and introducer sheath are removed, pressure is applied manually, then by pressure dressing, sandbag, or both. Provide wound care according to your facility's policy.

ESSENTIAL DOCUMENTATION

Record the time and date of balloon removal. Chart the name of the doctor removing the balloon. Indicate how pressure is applied and for how long. Record the patient's pedal pulses and the color, temperature, and sensation of the affected limb. Describe the type of dressing applied. Record any bleeding and hematoma formation. Document your frequent assessments of the insertion site and circulation to the affected leg according to your facility's policy. Include any patient education.

9/26/05	1015	IAB in ® groin removed by Dr. Johnson. Pressure applied for 30 minutes by Dr. Johnson followed by application of a pressure dressing. Pt. instructed to keep ® leg straight. ® foot warm and pink, strong dorsalis pedis and posterior tibial pulses, able to feel light touch. No bleeding or hematoma noted at ® groin site. ———————————————— Pat Schuler, RN

INTRACEREBRAL HEMORRHAGE

The rupture of a cerebral vessel causes bleeding into the brain tissue, resulting in intracerebral hemorrhage. This type of hemorrhage usually causes extensive loss of function and has a very slow recovery period and poor prognosis. The effects of the hemorrhage depend on the site and extent of the bleeding. Intracerebral hemorrhage may occur in patients with hypertension or atherosclerosis. Other causes include aneurysm, arteriovenous malformation, tumors, trauma, or bleeding disorders.

If you suspect an intracerebral hemorrhage or stroke in your patient, ensure a patent airway, breathing, and circulation (ABC). Perform a neurologic examination and alert the doctor of your findings.

ESSENTIAL DOCUMENTATION

Record the date and time of your entry. Evaluate the patient's ABC, and document your findings, actions taken, and the patient's response. Record your neurologic assessment (such as reduced level of consciousness, confused, restless, agitated, lethargic, or comatose), pupillary changes (including unequal size and sluggish or absent response to light), headache, seizures, focal neurologic signs, increased blood pressure, widened pulse pressure, bradycardia, decorticate or decerebrate posturing, and vomiting. Document the name of the doctor notified, the time of notification, and the orders given. Record your actions, such as drug and fluid administration, assisting with intracranial pressure monitoring insertion, administering oxygen, assisting intubation, and maintaining mechanical ventilation. Chart your patient's responses to these interventions. Record any patient and family education and support given.

Assess your patient frequently and record the specific time and results of your assessments. Use the appropriate flow sheets to record intake and output, I.V. fluids given, drugs administered, and frequent hemodynamic measurements and vital signs. A critical care flow sheet may also be used to document frequent assessments. A neurologic flow sheet, such as the Glasgow Coma Scale or the National Institutes of Health Stroke Scale, may be used to record your frequent neurologic assessments.

2/1/05	0810	Pt. found in bed at 0735 unresponsive to verbal stimuli
		but grimaces and opens eyes with painful stimuli. PERRL.
		Moving ® side of body but not Ⓛ. Airway is patent, with
		unlabored breathing. BP 100/60, P 72 and regular, RR 16,
		rectal T 98° F. Breath sounds clear, normal heart sounds.
		Skin cool, dry. Peripheral pulses palpable. Dr. Martinez
		notified at 0740 and orders given. Administering O₂ at
		2 L/min by NC. I.V. infusion started in ® forearm with
		18G catheter. NSS infusing at 30 ml/hr. #16 Fr. Foley
		catheter inserted. MRI scheduled for 0900. Dr. Martinez
		in to see pt. at 0750. Dr. called wife, Patricia Newman,
		to notify her of change in pt.'s condition. Wife consented
		to MRI. Glasgow Coma score of 7. See Glasgow Coma
		Scale, I.V., I/O, and VS flow sheets for frequent assess-
		ments. ———————————————— Juanita Perez, RN

INTRACRANIAL PRESSURE MONITORING

Intracranial pressure (ICP) monitoring measures pressure exerted by the brain, blood, and cerebrospinal fluid (CSF). Indications for monitoring ICP include head trauma with bleeding or edema, overproduction or insufficient absorption of CSF, cerebral hemorrhage, and space-occupying brain lesions. ICP monitoring can detect elevated ICP early, before clinical danger signs develop. Your prompt interventions can then help avert or diminish neurologic damage caused by cerebral hypoxia and shifts of brain mass. The procedure is always performed by a neurosurgeon in the operating room, emergency department, or critical care unit.

ESSENTIAL DOCUMENTATION

Document that the procedure has been explained to the patient or his family and that the patient or a responsible family member has signed the consent form. Record the time and date of the insertion procedure, the name of the doctor performing the procedure, and the patient's response.

Note the insertion site and the type of monitoring system used. Record ICP digital readings and waveforms and cerebral perfusion pressure hourly in your notes, on a flow sheet, or directly on readout strips, depending on your facility's policy. Document any factors that may affect ICP (for example, drug administration, stressful procedures, or sleep).

Record routine and neurologic vital signs hourly (including temperature, pulse, respirations, blood pressure, level of consciousness, pupillary activity, and orientation to time, place, person, and date), and describe the patient's clinical status. Note the amount, character, and frequency of any CSF drainage (for example, "between 1800 and 1900, 15 ml of blood-tinged CSF"). Also, record the ICP reading in response to drainage. Describe the insertion site and any site care and dressing changes performed. Describe any patient and family education and support given.

4/29/05	1100	ICP insertion and monitoring procedures explained to
		pt.'s wife by Dr. Norton. Wife verbalized understanding
		of procedure and signed consent form. Subarachnoid
		bolt placed by Dr. Norton on ℗ side of skull behind
		hairline. Initial ICP 16 mm Hg, MAP 110 mm Hg, monitor
		strip mounted below. Site clean, no drainage or redness,
		covered with sterile dressing. See flow sheets for hourly
		ICP, VS, neuro, checks. BP 154/88, P 98 and regular, RR
		24 and regular, rectal T 99.4° F. Opens eyes and moves
		℗ extremities to painful stimuli, makes incomprehensible
		sounds. PERRLA. No purposeful movement on ℗ side.
		Breath sounds clear, normal heart sounds, peripheral
		pulses palpable. Skin pale, cool. Foley catheter drained
		100 ml of clear amber urine last hr.
		———————————— Mary Steward, RN

Mr. Paul   1100
4/29/05   ID#: 563421

I.V. CATHETER INSERTION

Peripheral I.V. line insertion involves the selection of a venipuncture device and an insertion site, application of a tourniquet, preparation of the site, and venipuncture. Selection of a venipuncture device and site depends on the type of solution to be used; frequency and duration of infusion; patency and location of accessible veins; the patient's age, size, and condition; and, when possible, the patient's preference.

I.V. catheters are inserted to administer medications, blood, or blood products, or to correct fluid and electrolyte imbalances.

ESSENTIAL DOCUMENTATION

In your note or on the appropriate I.V. sheets, record the date and time of the venipuncture; the type, gauge, and length of the needle or catheter; and the anatomic location of the insertion site. Also, document the number of attempts at venipuncture (if you made more than one), the type and flow rate of the I.V. solution, the name and amount of medication in the solution (if any), and any adverse reactions and actions taken to correct them. If the I.V. site was changed, document the reason for the change. Document patient teaching and evidence of patient understanding.

10/3/05	1100	20G 1½" catheter inserted in ® forearm without
		difficulty on the first attempt. Site dressed with trans-
		parent dressing and tape. I.V. infusion of 1000 ml D₅W
		started at 100 ml/hr. I.V. infusing without difficulty. Pt.
		instructed to notify nurse if the site becomes swollen
		or painful, or catheter becomes dislodged or leaks. No
		c/o pain after insertion. ————— David Stevens, RN

I.V. CATHETER REMOVAL

A peripheral I.V. line is removed on completion of therapy, for cannula site changes, and for suspected infection or infiltration.

ESSENTIAL DOCUMENTATION

After removing an I.V. line, document the date and time of removal. Describe the condition of the site. If drainage was present at the puncture site, document that you sent the tip of the device and a sample of the drainage to the laboratory for culture, according to your facility's policy. Record any site care given and the type of dressing applied. Include any patient instructions.

10/15/05	1000	I.V. catheter removed from ® forearm vein. Pressure
		held for 2 min. until bleeding stopped. Site clean and
		dry, no redness, drainage, warmth, or pain noted. Dry
		sterile dressing applied to site. Pt. instructed to call
		nurse if bleeding, swelling, redness, or pain occurs at the
		removal site. ————————— Jane Newport, RN

I.V. SITE CARE

Proper I.V. site care is the single most important intervention for prevention of infection and other complications. Typically, I.V. dressings are changed every 48 hours or whenever the dressing becomes wet, soiled, or nonocclusive. The site should be assessed every 2 hours if a transparent semipermeable dressing is used or with every dressing change otherwise. Check your facility's policy for frequency of I.V. dressing changes and the type of site care to be performed.

ESSENTIAL DOCUMENTATION

In your notes or on the appropriate I.V. sheets, record the date and time of the dressing change. Chart the condition of the insertion site, noting whether there are signs of infection (redness and pain), infiltration (coolness, blanching, and edema), or thrombophlebitis (redness, firmness, pain along the path of the vein, and edema). If complications are present, note the name of the doctor notified, the time of notification, the orders given, your interventions, and the patient's response. Record site care given and the type of dressing applied. Document patient education.

12/3/05	0910	Transparent I.V. dressing wet and curling at edges.
		Dressing removed. Skin cleaned with alcohol, air dried. No
		redness, blanching, warmth, coolness, edema, drainage, or
		induration noted. No c/o pain at site. New trans-
		parent dressing applied and secured with tape. Pt. told
		to report any pain at site. ———— Gina Antenucci, RN

I.V. SITE CHANGE

Routine maintenance of an I.V. site and rotation of the site help prevent complications, such as thrombophlebitis and infection. The I.V. site is changed every 48 to 72 hours, according to your facility's policy. An I.V. site that shows signs of infection, infiltration, or thrombophlebitis should be changed immediately.

ESSENTIAL DOCUMENTATION

In your note or on the appropriate I.V. sheets, record the date and time that the I.V. line was removed. Note whether the site change is routine or due to a complication. Describe the condition of the site. Record any site care given and the type of dressing applied.

Document the new I.V. insertion site. Record the type, gauge, and length of the needle or catheter. Chart the number of attempts at venipuncture, if you made more than one. Include the type and flow rate of the I.V. solution, the name and amount of medication in the solution (if any), and any adverse effects as well as actions taken to correct them. Describe any patient education.

9/2/05	0900	I.V. line in place for 72 hours and removed from ® forearm according to facility policy. Site without redness, warmth, swelling, or pain. 2" x 2" gauze dressing applied. I.V. infusion restarted in ⓛ forearm using 20G 1½" catheter on first attempt. Site dressed with transparent dressing. I.V. infusion of 500 ml of NSS at 50 ml/hr without difficulty. Pt. instructed to call nurse immediately for any pain at I.V. site. ———————————— Leigh Adams, RN

I.V. SITE INFILTRATION

Infiltration of an I.V. site occurs when an I.V. solution enters the surrounding tissue as a result of a punctured vein or leakage around a venipuncture site. If vesicant drugs or fluids infiltrate, severe local tissue damage may result. Because infiltration can occur without pain or in unresponsive patients, the I.V. site must be monitored frequently.

Document your assessments of the I.V. site and the site care you provide. Such documentation is important in the prevention and early detection of infiltration and other complications. Many malpractice cases are brought annually because of the severe nerve and tissue damage from infiltrated I.V. sites that nurses failed to monitor. In some cases, amputations have been necessary because of the nerve and tissue damage.

ESSENTIAL DOCUMENTATION

Record the date and time of your entry. Record signs and symptoms of infiltration at the I.V. site, such as swelling, burning, discomfort, or pain; tight feeling; decreased skin temperature; and blanching. Chart your assessment of circulation to the affected and unaffected limbs, such as skin color, capillary refill, pulses, and circumference. Document your actions such as stopping the infusion. Estimate the amount of fluid infiltrated. Record the name of the doctor notified, the time of notification, the orders given (such as vesicant antidotes, limb elevation, and ice or warm soaks), your actions, and the patient's response. Restart the infusion and note the new location above the infiltration or in the unaffected limb. Record any emotional support and patient education.

10/31/05	1900	I.V. site in ® forearm swollen and cool at 1820. Pt.
		c/o of some discomfort at the site. Hands warm with
		capillary refill less than 3 seconds, strong radial pulses
		bilaterally. ® forearm circumference 9½", Ⓛ forearm
		circumference 9". I.V. line removed and sterile gauze
		dressing applied. Approx. 30 ml of NSS infiltrated.
		Dr. Horning notified at 1830, and orders given that
		I.V. therapy may be discontinued. ® arm elevated on 2
		pillows and ice applied in wrapped towel for 20 min.
		After ice application, skin cool, intact. No c/o burning
		or numbness. Explained importance of keeping arm
		elevated and to call nurse immediately for any pain,
		burning, numbness in ® forearm. — Betsy Rothman, RN

I.V. THERAPY, CONTINUOUS

More than 89% of hospitalized patients receive some form of I.V. therapy. Whether providing fluid or electrolyte replacement, total parenteral nutrition, drugs, or blood products, you'll need to carefully document all

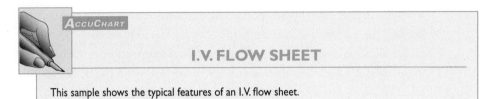

I.V. FLOW SHEET

This sample shows the typical features of an I.V. flow sheet.

INTRAVENOUS CARE RECORD

INTRAVENOUS CARE COMMENT CODES C = CAP F = FILTER T= TUBING D = DRESSING								
START DATE/ TIME	INITIALS	I.V. VOLUME & SOLUTION	ADDITIVES	FLOW RATE	SITE	STOP DATE/ TIME	TUBING CHANGE	COMMENTS/ASSESSMENT OF SITE
6/30/05 1100	DS	1000 cc D₅W	20 mEq KCL	100/hr	RFA	6/30/05 2100	T	
6/30/05 2100	JM	1000 cc D₅W	20 mEq KCL	100/hr	RFA	7/1/05 0700		
7/1/05 0700	DS	1000 cc D₅W	20 mEq KCL	100/hr	LFA	7/2/05	TD	

facets of I.V. therapy — including administration and any subsequent complications of I.V. therapy.

Keep in mind that an accurate description of your care provides a clear record of treatments and drugs received by your patient. This record provides legal protection for you and your employer and furnishes health care insurers with the data they need to approve and provide reimbursement for equipment and supplies.

Depending on your facility's policy, you'll document I.V. therapy on a special I.V. therapy sheet, nursing flow sheet, or in another format.

ESSENTIAL DOCUMENTATION

On each shift, document the type, amount, and flow rate of I.V. fluid, along with the condition of the I.V. site. Chart each time you flush the I.V. line, and identify any drug used to flush the line. Any change in routine care should be documented, along with follow-up assessments. Record any patient teaching that you perform with the patient and his family.

See *I.V. flow sheet* for documentation of routine care during continuous I.V. administration.

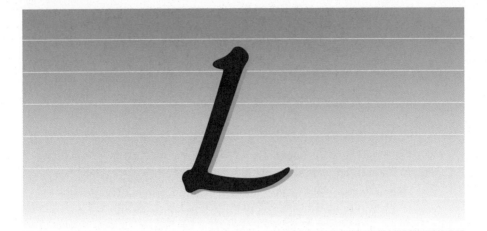

LANGUAGE DIFFICULTIES

Entering a health care facility or using a health care service can be a daunting experience for a person who doesn't speak English. Nurses and other health care workers face similar obstacles to communication. A patient may be unable to communicate his questions, concerns, needs, and fears, and the nurse may be unable to perform a health history, ask about symptoms, or provide education. In fact, every part of the nurse-patient relationship may be compromised.

When a patient doesn't speak English, you'll need to find an interpreter. Interpreters may be found among staff members or family members. Telephone interpretation services are also available. Make sure that the patient trusts and approves of the family member. Be aware that the patient may not want to discuss his problems in front of family members and that family translators may be protective of the patient and may not relay all information. In some cultures, it may not be appropriate for a translator to discuss certain matters with members of the opposite sex. Failure to have a reliable translator can result in lack of informed consent and subsequent claims of false imprisonment, battery, or assault.

ESSENTIAL DOCUMENTATION

Document the primary language spoken by the patient. Include the names, addresses, and telephone numbers of family interpreters approved by the patient. Place in the patient's chart a list of staff members approved by your facility to act as interpreters. When a translator is used for an event, such as patient education, discharge instructions, or informed consent, record the name of the translator on the appropriate form or in your note. Describe alternative forms of communication used, such as a picture board or flash cards.

11/31/05	1310	Pt. only speaks Taiwanese. Her daughter, Miss Hung, translated during the process of informed consent and signed the consent form. A set of flash cards was developed with which Mrs. Hung will indicate her need for such items as pain medication or toileting. Miss Hung agreed to meet with the staff every a.m. between 0800 and 0900 to describe the day's events and activities to the pt. and to translate questions the pt. may have. — ———————————————— Debbie Hancy, RN

LAST WILL AND TESTAMENT, PATIENT REQUEST FOR WITNESS OF

A patient, especially one who believes he's dying, may ask you to witness a last will and testament. In many states, a nurse can witness a patient's signature on a will. However, you don't have a legal or ethical responsibility to act as a witness. Check your facility's policy or ask your facility's legal consultant before you witness a will. (See *Witnessing a will,* page 248.)

If a patient asks you to be a witness when he draws his will, notify the doctor and your supervisor before you act as a witness. Don't give any legal advice or offer assistance in wording the document. Don't comment on the nature of the patient's choices. Document your actions in your nurse's note.

ESSENTIAL DOCUMENTATION

When you witness a written will, document that it was signed and witnessed, who signed and witnessed it, who was present, what was done with it after signing, and what the patient's condition was at the time. Document the name of the doctor, facility attorney, or any other person (such as the nursing supervisor) who was notified, and note the time of notification. Record instructions that were given and your actions. Record that

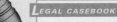

WITNESSING A WILL

In many states, your signature on a will certifies that:
- you witnessed the signing of the will
- you heard the maker of the will declare it to be his will
- all witnesses and the maker of the will were actually present during the signing.

By attesting to the last two facts, you help ensure the authenticity of the will and the signatures. However, your signature doesn't certify that the maker of the will is competent.

Before you sign any document, read at least enough of it to make sure it's the type of document the maker represents it to be. Usually you won't have to read all the text and, legally, that isn't necessary for your signature to be valid. You should, however, always examine the document's title and first page and give careful attention to what's written immediately above the place for your signature.

you heard the maker of the will declare it to be his will and that all witnesses and the maker of the will were actually present during the signing.

| 12/17/05 | 1300 | Pt. asked me to witness his will. Dr. Pershing; Edward Ewing, hospital attorney; and Nancy Strom, RN, nursing supervisor, were contacted at 1245. Mr. Ewing; Ms. Strom; pt.'s daughter, Mrs. Pope; pt.; and I were present at the signing. The document was entitled "My last will and testament." Pt. signed the will. It was witnessed by the above people and me. Will was placed with pt.'s personal belongings in his closet after signing. At pt.'s request, a copy was given to Mrs. Pope. At the signing, pt. was alert and oriented to time, place, and person. Pt. is also aware of his poor prognosis and has had many discussions with me about "putting my affairs in order before I die." ——————— Sally Ball, RN |
| | | |

LATE DOCUMENTATION ENTRY

Late documentation entries are appropriate in several situations:
- if the chart was unavailable when it was needed – for example, when the patient was away from the unit (for X-rays or physical therapy)
- if you need to add important information after completing your notes
- if you forgot to write notes on a particular chart.

LEGAL CASEBOOK

AVOIDING LATE ENTRIES

If the court uncovers alterations in a patient's chart during the course of a trial, suspicions may be aroused. The court may logically infer that additional alterations were made. In such situations, the value of the entire medical record may be brought into question.

That's what happened to the nurse involved in one case. She failed to chart her observations of a patient for 7 hours after a surgery, during which time the patient died. The patient's family later sued the hospital, charging the nurse with malpractice. The nurse insisted that she had observed the patient but, because her particular unit was understaffed and overpopulated, she wasn't able to record her observations. She explained that the assistant director of nursing later instructed her about the hospital's policy on charting late additions. The nurse subsequently added her observations to the patient's medical record.

However, the court wasn't convinced that the nurse had indeed observed the patient during the postoperative period. Suspicious of the altered record, it ruled that the nurse's failure to chart her observations at the proper time supported the plaintiff's claim that she had made no such observations.

Keep in mind, however, that a late or altered chart entry can arouse suspicions and can be a significant problem in the event of a malpractice lawsuit. (See *Avoiding late entries*.)

ESSENTIAL DOCUMENTATION

If you must make a late entry or alter an entry, find out if your facility has a protocol for doing so (many do). If not, the best approach is to add the entry to the first available line, and label it "late entry" to indicate that it's out of sequence. Then record the date and time of the entry and, in the body of the entry, record the date and time it should have been made.

| 12/14/05 | 0900
Late entry | (Chart not available 12/13/05 at 1500; pt. was in radiology) On 12/13/05 at 1300, pt. stated she felt faint when getting OOB on 12/13/05 at 1200 and she fell to the floor. Pt. states she didn't hurt herself at the time and didn't think she had to tell anyone about this until her husband encouraged her to report it. ℞ wrist bruised and slightly swollen. Pt. c/o some tenderness. Dr. Muir notified at 1310 and came to see pt. at 1320 on 12/13/05. X-ray of wrist ordered. —————————————— Elaine Kasmer, RN |

LATEX HYPERSENSITIVITY

Latex, derived from the sap of the rubber tree, is used throughout the health care industry. The increased use of latex may be related to the increased hypersensitivity reactions experienced by health care workers and patients, ranging from local dermatitis to anaphylactic reaction.

If your patient has latex hypersensitivity, use only nonlatex products. Be prepared to treat life-threatening hypersensitivity with antihistamines, epinephrine, corticosteroids, I.V. fluids, oxygen, intubation, and mechanical ventilation, if necessary. Alert the pharmacy and other departments that the patient has a latex allergy so that latex-free materials can be provided. Place a band on the patient's wrist and on the medical record to identify the hypersensitivity to latex.

ESSENTIAL DOCUMENTATION

Record the date and time of your entry. On admission, record all allergies, including reactions to latex. Document signs and symptoms that you observe or that the patient reports to you, such as red skin, itching, itchy or runny eyes and nose, coughing, hives, wheezing, bronchospasm, or laryngeal edema. Include information about diagnostic testing the patient may undergo to confirm latex hypersensitivity. Record that other departments have been notified of the patient's latex allergy and that identification of this allergy has been placed on the patient's wrist and on the front of the medical record. Describe measures taken to prevent latex exposure. Be sure to chart your patient teaching about latex reactions.

3/31/05	1120	Pt. reports that she has a latex allergy and has devel-
		oped red skin and itching with past exposures to latex.
		Latex allergy wristband placed on pt.'s Ⓛ wrist. Latex
		precautions stickers placed on pt.'s medical record,
		MAR, nursing Kardex, and door to pt.'s room. Pharmacy,
		dietary, lab, and other departments notified of latex
		allergy by automated record-keeping system. Supply cart
		with latex-free products kept by pt.'s room. Pt. very
		knowledgeable about her latex allergy and was able to
		describe s/s of reactions, products to avoid, and how to
		respond to a reaction with autoinjectable epinephrine,
		if necessary. Pt. already sent away for an ID bracelet to
		identify her latex allergy, but she hasn't yet received it.
		—————————————————— Kate Wilson, RN

LEVEL OF CONSCIOUSNESS, CHANGES IN

A patient's level of consciousness (LOC) provides information about his respiratory, cardiovascular, and neurologic status. The Glasgow Coma Scale (see below) provides a standard reference for assessing or monitoring the LOC of a patient with a suspected or confirmed brain injury. This scale measures three responses to stimuli—eye opening response, motor

AccuChart

USING THE GLASGOW COMA SCALE

The Glasgow Coma Scale is a standard reference that is used to assess or monitor level of consciousness in a patient with a suspected or confirmed brain injury. This scale measures three responses to stimuli—eye opening response, motor response, and verbal response—and assigns a number to each of the possible responses within these categories.

The lowest possible score is 3; the highest is 15. A score of 7 or lower indicates coma. This scale is commonly used in the emergency department, at the scene of an accident, and for the evaluation of a hospitalized patient.

GLASGOW COMA SCALE

Characteristic	Response	Score
Eye opening response	▪ Spontaneous	4
	▪ To verbal command	③
	▪ To pain	2
	▪ No response	1
Best motor response	▪ Obeys commands	⑥
	▪ To painful stimulus:	
	– Localizes pain; pushes stimulus away	5
	– Flexes and withdraws	4
	– Abnormal flexion	3
	– Extension	2
	– No response	1
Best verbal response (arouse patient with painful stimulus, if necessary)	▪ Oriented and converses	5
	▪ Disoriented and converses	④
	▪ Uses inappropriate words	3
	▪ Makes incomprehensible sounds	2
	▪ No response	1
	Total:	/3

response, and verbal response – and assigns a number to each of the possible responses within these categories. The lowest possible score is 3; the highest is 15. A score of 7 or lower indicates a coma.

ESSENTIAL DOCUMENTATION

Record the date and time of your assessment. Depending on your facility's Glasgow Coma Scale flow sheet, you'll either circle the number that describes your patient's response to stimuli or you'll write in the number of the corresponding response. Then record the total of these three responses.

See *Using the Glasgow Coma Scale,* page 251, for an example of how to document your patient's LOC.

LUMBAR PUNCTURE

Lumbar puncture involves the insertion of a sterile needle into the subarachnoid space of the spinal canal, usually between the third and fourth lumbar vertebrae. This process is used to detect increased intracranial pressure (ICP) or the presence of blood in cerebrospinal fluid (CSF), obtain CSF specimens for laboratory analysis, and inject dyes or gases for contrast in radiologic studies. It's also used to administer drugs (including anesthetics) and to relieve ICP by removing CSF. This procedure should be used with caution in patients with increased ICP because the rapid reduction in pressure that follows the withdrawal of CSF can cause tonsillar herniation and medullary compression.

ESSENTIAL DOCUMENTATION

Document that the patient understands the procedure and has signed a consent form. Record your patient teaching about what to expect before, during, and after the procedure. Record the date of the procedure as well as the initiation and completion times. Document adverse reactions, such as changes in level of consciousness or vital signs or dizziness. Chart that you reported these responses to the doctor and note his response, your actions, and the patient's response. Record the number of test tube specimens of CSF that were collected and the time they were transported to the laboratory. Describe the color, consistency, and other characteristics of the collected specimens. Document the patient's tolerance of the procedure. After the procedure, document your interventions, such as keeping the patient flat in bed for 6 to 12 hours, encouraging fluid intake, assessing for headache, and checking the puncture site for leakage of CSF. Record the patient's responses to these interventions.

10/8/05	0900	Lumbar puncture explained to pt. by Dr. Wells. Pt. verbalized
		understanding of the procedure and signed consent form.
		Explained what to expect before, during, and after the
		procedure and answered his questions. Pt. positioned on ⓛ
		side for lumbar puncture. Pt. draped and prepped by Dr.
		Wells. Specimen obtained by dr. on first attempt. One test
		tube obtained and sent to lab. Specimen clear and straw
		colored. Preprocedure, 0815, P 88, BP 126/82, RR 18, oral T
		98.2° F. During procedure, 0830, P 92, BP 128/80, RR 18.
		After procedure, 0845, P 86, BP 132/82, RR 20, oral T
		98.0° F. Pt. maintained in supine position as instructed. I.V.
		of NSS infusing at 100 ml/hr in ® forearm. Puncture site
		dressed by Dr. Wells. Site clear, dry, and intact. No leakage.
		Pt. has no c/o of headache or dizziness. Pt. reports no pain
		after procedure. Pt. lying flat in bed without difficulty. Pt.
		drank 240 ml ginger ale. ———— Jeanette Kane, RN

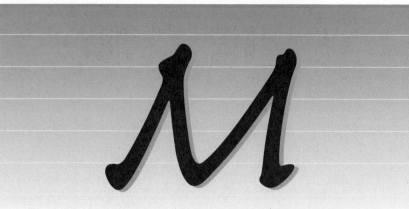

MECHANICAL VENTILATION

A mechanical ventilator moves air in and out of a patient's lungs. Although the equipment ventilates a patient, it doesn't ensure adequate gas exchange. Mechanical ventilation may use either positive or negative pressure to ventilate a patient.

Positive-pressure ventilators exert a positive pressure on the airway, which causes inspiration while increasing tidal volume. The inspiratory cycles of these ventilators may vary in volume, pressure, or time. A high-frequency ventilator uses high respiratory rates and low tidal volume to maintain alveolar ventilation.

Negative-pressure ventilators create negative pressure, which pulls the thorax outward and allows air to flow into the lungs. Examples of such ventilators are the iron lung, the cuirass (chest shell), and the body wrap. Negative-pressure ventilators are used mainly to treat neuromuscular disorders, such as Guillain-Barré syndrome, myasthenia gravis, and poliomyelitis.

Other indications for ventilator use include central nervous system disorders, such as cerebral hemorrhage and spinal cord transsection, acute respiratory distress syndrome, pulmonary edema, chronic obstructive pulmonary disease, flail chest, and acute hypoventilation.

ESSENTIAL DOCUMENTATION

Document the date and time that mechanical ventilation began. Note the type of ventilator used as well as its settings, such as ventilatory mode, tidal volume, rate, fraction of inspired oxygen, positive end-expiratory pressure, and peak inspiratory flow. Record the size of the endotracheal (ET) tube, centimeter mark of the ET tube, and cuff pressure. Describe the patient's subjective and objective responses to mechanical ventilation, including vital signs, breath sounds, use of accessory muscles, comfort level, and physical appearance.

Throughout mechanical ventilation, list any complications and subsequent interventions. Record pertinent laboratory data, including arterial blood gas (ABG) analyses and oxygen saturation findings. Also, record tracheal suctioning and the character of secretions.

If the patient is receiving pressure-support ventilation or is using a T-piece or tracheostomy collar, note the duration of spontaneous breathing and the patient's ability to maintain the weaning schedule. If the patient is receiving intermittent mandatory ventilation, with or without pressure-support ventilation, record the control breath rate, time of each breath reduction, and rate of spontaneous respirations.

Record adjustments made in ventilator settings as a result of ABG levels, and document adjustments of ventilator components, such as draining condensate into a collection trap and changing, cleaning, or discarding the tubing. Also, record teaching efforts and emotional support given.

3/16/05	1015	Pt. on Servo ventilator set at TV 750, F$_{IO_2}$ 45%, 5 cm
		PEEP, Assist-control mode of 12. RR 20 and nonlabored;
		no SOB noted. #8 ETT in Ⓡ corner of mouth taped
		securely at 22-cm mark. Suctioned via ETT for large
		amt. of thick white secretions. Pulse oximetry reading
		98%. Ⓛ lung clear. Ⓡ lung with basilar crackles and expir-
		atory wheezes. Dr. Short notified at 1000; no treatment
		at this time. Explained all procedures including suctioning
		to pt. Pt. nodded head "yes" when asked if he understood
		explanations.————————— Janice Del Vecchio, RN

MEDICATION ERROR

Medication errors are the most common, and potentially the most dangerous, nursing errors. Mistakes in dosage, patient identification, or drug selection by nurses have led to vision loss, brain damage, cardiac arrest, and death. (See *Lawsuits and medication errors,* page 256.)

LAWSUITS AND MEDICATION ERRORS

Unfortunately, lawsuits involving nurses' drug errors are common. The court determines liability based on the standards of care required of nurses who administer drugs. In many instances, if the nurse had known more about the proper dosage, administration route, or procedure connected with a drug's use, she might have avoided the mistake.

In *Norton v. Argonaut Insurance Co. (1962)*, an infant died after a nurse administered injectable digoxin at a dosage level appropriate for elixir of Lanoxin, an oral drug. The nurse was unaware that digoxin was available in an oral form. The nurse questioned two doctors who weren't treating the infant about the order but failed to mention to them that the order was written for elixir of Lanoxin. She also failed to clarify the order with the doctor who wrote it.

The nurse, the doctor who ordered the drug, and the hospital were found liable.

A medication event report or incident report should be completed when a medication error is discovered. The nurse who discovers the medication error is responsible for completing the medication event report or incident report and for communicating the error to the patient's doctor and the nursing supervisor.

ESSENTIAL DOCUMENTATION

In your nurse's note, describe the situation objectively and include the name of the doctor notified, the time of notification, and the doctor's response. Let the facts speak for themselves. Avoid the use of such terms as "by mistake," "somehow," "unintentionally," "miscalculated," and "confusing," which can be interpreted as admissions of wrongdoing.

Document the medication error on an incident report or medication event report. (See *Medication event quality review form*.)

10/8/05	1315	Pt. was given Demerol 100 mg I.M. at 1300 for abdominal
		pain. Dr. Miller was notified at 1305 and is on his way to
		see pt. P 80, BP 120/82, RR 20, oral T 98.4° F. Alert and
		oriented to time, place, and person. — Aleisha Adams, RN

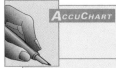

MEDICATION EVENT QUALITY REVIEW FORM

When a medication error occurs, most facilities require the nurse to complete a medication event report. The information is used to investigate the incident and develop an action plan to avoid future incidents.

QUALITY REVIEW FORM

Confidential — This is a peer review document and may be protected by applicable law. ***Not for distribution.***

Patient information

Event data

Date and time of event: __10/8/05__ __1300__   Date and time reported: __10/8/05__ __1315__

Primary event type (check one only):
- ☐ Wrong drug
- ☐ Wrong dose
- ☐ Omitted dose
- ☐ Wrong route
- ☑ Wrong time
- ☐ Wrong patient
- ☐ Other _____

For wrong dose or omitted doses,
\# doses involved: _____

Event severity (check only one):
- ☐ 0 - potential error only
- ☐ 1 - error occurred, no harm to the patient
- ☑ 2 - error occurred, increased monitoring only
- ☐ 3 - error occurred, change in VS, additional labs, no permanent harm
- ☐ 4 - error occurred, required additional treatment, increased LOS
- ☐ 5 - error occurred, permanent harm to patient
- ☐ 6 - error resulted in patient's death

Contributing causes of event

Order related (check all that apply):
Type of order: ☐ Written   ☐ Oral   ☐ Telephone
- ☐ Order incomplete:
  - ☐ Not dated
  - ☐ No frequency
  - ☐ Not timed
  - ☐ No route
  - ☐ No dose
  - ☐ No drug parameters indicated
  - ☐ No signature
  - ☐ Signature illegible
- ☐ Order illegible
- ☐ Unacceptable abbreviation used: _____
- ☐ Decimal misplaced
- ☐ Inappropriate use of leading or trailing zeros
- ☐ Order not flagged correctly
- ☐ Order written on wrong patient's chart
- ☐ Inappropriate drug selection
- ☐ Inappropriate route selection
- ☐ Patient drug allergies not identified or documented
- ☐ Drug not renewed
- ☐ Drug not discontinued
- ☐ Drug not reordered postop
- ☐ Nonformulary request

Transcription related (check all that apply):
- ☐ Order not faxed
- ☐ Order not transcribed
- ☐ Pharmacy clarification of order not transcribed
- ☐ Incomplete order not clarified
- ☐ Order not completely signed off
- ☐ Incorrect transcription onto:
  - ☐ MAR
  - ☐ Recopied MAR

- ☐ Transcription illegible on:
  - ☐ MAR
  - ☐ Recopied MAR
- ☐ Incomplete allergy documentation
- ☐ Allergies not transcribed onto:
  - ☐ Order sheets ☐ MAR   ☐ Recopied MAR
- ☐ Unacceptable abbreviations

Patient related (check all that apply):
- ☐ Took own meds
- ☐ Altered infusion rate
- ☐ Loss of venous access
- ☐ Medication refused

Dispensing related (check all that apply):
- ☐ Drug incompatibility
- ☐ Outdated product dispensed
- ☐ Patient allergies not identified
- ☐ Incorrect product chosen
- ☐ Product incorrectly labeled
- ☐ Product not delivered to nursing unit
- ☐ Delay in delivery due to:
  - ☐ Nonformulary request   ☐ Illegible order
  - ☐ Out of stock   ☐ Illegible fax
  - ☐ Further investigation required
  - ☐ Pneumatic tube problem ☐ Other: _____
- ☐ Product incorrectly prepared in:
  - ☐ Pharmacy   ☐ Nursing unit   ☐ Other: _____
- ☐ Miscalculation
- ☐ No physician order

(continued)

MEDICATION EVENT QUALITY
REVIEW FORM (continued)

☐ Incomplete physician order not clarified
☐ Unacceptable abbreviation used: _____
☐ Computer entry errors (pharmacy only):
   ☐ Duplicate   ☐ Wrong patient   ☐ Wrong drug
   ☐ Missed order   ☐ Other _____
☐ Pharmacy clarification of order not documented

Administration related (check all that apply):
☐ Incorrect drug storage method
☐ Patient allergies not correctly checked against:
   ☐ Allergy band   ☐ MAR
☐ Patient allergy band not intact
☐ Patient not correctly identified
☐ No physician order
☐ Drug incompatibility
☐ Available product incorrectly prepared
☐ Miscalculation

☐ Incorrectly labeled
☐ Medication or I.V. not checked with MAR, order, I.V. record
☑ Time of last p.r.n. medication administration not checked
☐ Patient not observed taking medication
☐ Med. or I.V. not charted at time of administration
☐ Med. or I.V. not charted correctly
☐ Incorrect I.V. line used
☐ Incorrect setting on infusion pump
☐ Lock-out on infusion pump not used
☐ Outdated product given
☐ Forgotten or overlooked
☐ Product not available
☐ Extra or duplicated dose
☐ Monitoring, insufficient or not done

Event analysis

(Include additional information, such as staffing patterns, activity level, patient outcome, action plan, and conclusion)
Susan Jones, RN, had administered and documented giving p.r.n. Demerol 100 mg I.M. to the pt. at 1215. I did not review the p.r.n. MAR and administered the dose again at 1300. Pt. monitored q 15 min. for 2 hours. No adverse effects. Pt. alert and oriented to time, place, and person. Dr. Miller notified at 1305 and came to see pt. _____

Completed by: _Aleisha Adams, RN_ _____   Date completed: _10/8/05_

MISCONDUCT

The American Nurses Association's Code for Nurses outlines the nurse's obligation to report acts of negligence and incompetence by other health care providers. It states that "the nurse acts to safeguard the patient and public when health care and safety are affected by incompetent, unethical, or illegal practice by any person."

Usually, there are institutional channels through which you can report the misconduct of another nurse or nursing assistant without fear of reprisal. In many cases, a nurse-manager and the human resources department assume joint responsibility for investigating allegations of misconduct.

If you suspect misconduct, write an official memo to your supervisor. Avoid focusing on personalities. Personal accusations detract from the disclosure and may invite a lawsuit for libel or slander. Have other professionals verify the information, if possible. This will lend objectivity to the information and may shield you from retaliation.

ESSENTIAL DOCUMENTATION

Record your disclosures carefully. Write a clear, objective summary of the relevant facts. Be specific. Record the dates and times that the incidents occurred or when they were discovered. Explain why the information is significant and what needs to be done. If the misconduct involved a patient, record the consequences to the patient, the results of your patient assessment, the name of the doctor notified, the time of notification, the orders given, your actions, and the patient's response. You may need to file an incident report when misconduct involves a patient.

To: Mary Stone, RN
    Nursing Supervisor
From: Jan Finnegan, RN
Date: 5/31/05
Time: 1400
At 1330, observed Kathy Kane, RN, prepare Demerol 25 mg I.M. injection for the
patient, Robert Slone. When Ms. Kane entered the room, the patient stated, "It's
about time." Ms. Kane responded, "Oh, I think you can wait longer," and she left the
patient's room. She then squirted the medication into the trash container on the
medication cart. Ms. Kane stated to me, "If he's gonna complain about how long it
took me to get it to him, he must not need the medication." I entered Mr. Slone's
room and found him grimacing and clutching his abdomen. When asked, Mr. Slone
stated his pain was 7 on a scale of 0 to 10, with 10 being the worst pain imaginable.
I then told Ms. Kane I was giving Mr. Slone his pain medication. Demerol 25 mg
I.M. given in ® lateral thigh region at 1340. Assisted Mr. Slone into comfortable
position and showed him how to splint his incision with a pillow. Medication
documented on the MAR. Incident report filed, and nursing supervisor Mary Stone
contacted at 1345. —————————————————————————— Jan Finnegan, RN

MISSING PATIENT

If a patient leaves your unit without your knowledge, immediately look for him on the unit and notify your nursing supervisor, security, and the patient's doctor and family. Notify the police if there's a possibility that the patient may hurt himself or others, especially if he has left the facility with any medical devices. The legal consequences of a patient leaving the facility without medical permission can be particularly severe if the patient is confused or mentally incompetent, especially if he's injured or dies of exposure as a result of his absence.

ESSENTIAL DOCUMENTATION

Document the time that you discovered the patient missing, your attempts to find him, and the people you notified, including his doctor, the nursing supervisor, security, and his family. Include any other pertinent information. Your facility's policy may require you to complete an incident report.

9/7/05	1900	Pt. not in room at 1845 for meds. Checked pt.'s bath-
		room, day room, and all conference rooms and offices
		on nursing unit. Pt. last seen at 1800 in his room
		eating dinner. Contacted Mary Collins, RN, nurse-
		supervisor, and security officer Bill Newman at 1850.
		Called pt.'s home at 1855 and spoke with wife who said
		pt. wasn't at home. Dr. Thomas notified at 1900 that
		pt. was missing. —————————— Stacey Miller, RN

MISUSE OF EQUIPMENT

At times, a patient may manipulate equipment or misuse supplies (for example, pressing keys on a pump or monitor, detaching tubing, or playing with switches) without understanding the consequences. If your patient misuses equipment, explain that such misuse can harm him. Tell him to call for the nurse if he feels the equipment isn't working properly, is causing him discomfort, or if he has other concerns. Notify the patient's doctor of any misuse.

ESSENTIAL DOCUMENTATION

Record the date and time that your patient misused the equipment. Describe the patient's actions and record what he tells you, using his own words in quotes. Record how you corrected the problem.

Document your assessment of the patient's condition. Chart the name of the doctor notified, the time of notification, the orders given, your actions, and the patient's response. Include any patient teaching performed.

2/6/05	0930	I.V. of 1000 ml D₅W hung at 0915 infusing at rate of 60
		ml/hr via infusion pump. ——— Kate Comerford, RN
	1015	Assessed I.V. infusion; 840 ml left in bag. Pt. stated,
		"I flicked the switch because I didn't see anything
		happening. Then I pressed the green button and the
		arrow." I.V. pump reset to 60 ml/hr. P 80, BP 110/82,
		RR 18, oral T 98.4° F. Breath sounds clear; normal heart
		sounds; no peripheral edema. Instructed pt. not to
		touch the pump or I.V. line. I.V. pump placed on lock
		setting. Told him to call the nurse if he feels they
		aren't working properly. Pt. verbalized understanding
		and agreed not to touch equipment. Dr. Huang notified
		at 1030. No new orders. ——— Kate Comerford, RN

MIXED VENOUS OXYGEN SATURATION MONITORING

This procedure uses a fiber-optic thermodilution pulmonary artery catheter to continuously monitor oxygen delivery to tissues and oxygen consumption by tissues. Monitoring of mixed venous oxygen saturation ($S\bar{v}O_2$) allows rapid detection of impaired oxygen delivery, such as that from decreased cardiac output, hemoglobin level, or arterial oxygen saturation. It also helps evaluate a patient's response to drug therapy, endotracheal tube suctioning, ventilator setting changes, positive end-expiratory pressure (PEEP), and fraction of inspired oxygen. The $S\bar{v}O_2$ level usually ranges from 60% to 80%; the normal value is 75%.

ESSENTIAL DOCUMENTATION

Record the $S\bar{v}O_2$ value on a flowchart and attach a tracing as ordered. Note significant changes in the patient's status and the results of any interventions. For comparison, note the $S\bar{v}O_2$ value as measured by the fiber-optic catheter whenever a blood sample is obtained for laboratory analysis of $S\bar{v}O_2$.

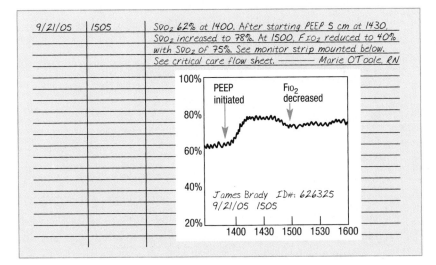

9/21/05	1505	SvO_2 62% at 1400. After starting PEEP 5 cm at 1430,
		SvO_2 increased to 78%. At 1500, F_{IO_2} reduced to 40%
		with SvO_2 of 75%. See monitor strip mounted below.
		See critical care flow sheet. ——— Marie O'Toole, RN

MULTIPLE TRAUMA

The patient with multiple trauma has injuries to more than one body system caused by such situations as vehicular accident, violence, a fall, or a burn. His injuries may involve penetrating wounds, blunt trauma, or both. Your patient's chances of survival are improved when health care workers follow a systematic team approach of assessment, resuscitation, and treatment. You'll need to document your assessments, your interventions, and the patient's response. Moreover, you'll need to document emotional care given to the patient and his family.

ESSENTIAL DOCUMENTATION

Immediately upon arrival at the health care facility, the patient will undergo a primary survey of airway, breathing, and circulation with resuscitation and treatment of life-threatening problems. Documentation at this point in the patient's care must reflect:
- date and time that the patient is admitted to the facility
- assessment of airway, breathing, and circulation (including hemorrhage) and resuscitation and emergency treatment, such as cardiopulmonary resuscitation, intubation, mechanical ventilation, oxygen therapy, fluid or blood replacement, and direct pressure to bleeding
- level of responsiveness.

When the primary survey is complete, document a more thorough secondary survey, including:
- cause and physical evidence of trauma
- vital signs
- head-to-toe assessment
- history
- diagnostic tests.

Record treatments provided, such as insertion of a nasogastric, urinary, or chest tube; neck and spine stabilization; drug therapy; splinting fractures; and wound care. Include patient and family teaching and emotional support provided.

Continue to document ongoing frequent assessments and treatments until the patient's condition has stabilized. A critical care or trauma flow sheet may be used.

8/15/05	1330	18 y.o. male brought to ED after being struck by a car
		at 1245 while riding his bike. Pt. was wearing a helmet.
		Parents are present. Pt. is awake, alert, and oriented to
		person and place but not time. Pt. has trauma to face,
		airway is open, no stridor, RR 18 and nonlabored,
		Administering O₂ 2 L/min by NC. Cervical spine main-
		tained in alignment. P 104, BP 90/62. Monitor shows
		sinus tachycardia, no arrhythmias. Bruising over abdomen.
		Pt. splinting abdomen and c/o abdominal pain. Is
		nauseated but no vomiting. #16 Fr Foley catheter placed;
		no blood in urine. I.V. line started in Ⓡ antecubital vein
		with 18G catheter. 1000 ml of lactated Ringer's infusing
		at 100 ml/hr. X-rays of neck, spine, and pelvis done at
		1315; results pending. Moving upper extremities
		spontaneously and without pain. Moving Ⓛ leg on own,
		without pain, Ⓡ thigh has bruising and deformity, c/o of
		Ⓡ thigh pain. Radial pulses palpable. Dorsalis pedis and
		posterior tibial pulses palpable and weak. Able to feel
		light touch to both legs. Dr. Moore discussing need for
		exploratory abdominal surgery and reduction of Ⓡ thigh
		fracture with parents. See I.V., I/O, and VS flow sheets
		for frequent assessments. Explaining all procedures to
		pt., allowing parents to be with pt. —— Carrie Burke, RN

MYOCARDIAL INFARCTION, ACUTE

A myocardial infarction (MI) is an occlusion of a coronary artery that leads to oxygen deprivation, myocardial ischemia and, eventually, necrosis. The extent of functional impairment depends on the size and location of the infarct, the condition of the uninvolved myocardium, the potential for collateral circulation, and the effectiveness of compensatory mechanisms.

Mortality is high when treatment for MI is delayed; however, prognosis improves if vigorous treatment begins immediately. Therefore, prompt recognition of MI and nursing interventions to relieve chest pain, stabilize heart rhythm, reduce cardiac workload, and revascularize the coronary artery are essential to preserving myocardial tissue and preventing complications, including death. Expect to assist with thrombolytic therapy, administer oxygen, assist with the insertion of hemodynamic monitoring catheters, and prepare your patient for invasive procedures to improve coronary circulation. Also, anticipate administering drugs to relieve pain, inhibit platelet aggregation, treat arrhythmias, reduce myocardial oxygen demands, increase myocardial oxygen supply, and improve the patient's chance of survival.

ESSENTIAL DOCUMENTATION

Record the date and time of your entry. Describe your patient's chest pain and other symptoms of MI, using his own words whenever possible. Record your assessment findings, such as feelings of impending doom, anxiety, restlessness, fatigue, nausea, vomiting, dyspnea, tachypnea, cool extremities, weak peripheral pulses, diaphoresis, third or fourth heart sounds, a new murmur, pericardial friction rub, low-grade fever, hypotension or hypertension, bradycardia or tachycardia, and crackles on lung auscultation.

Document the name of the doctor that you notified, the time of notification, and the orders given, such as transfer to the coronary care unit, continuous cardiac monitoring, supplemental oxygen, 12-lead ECG, I.V. therapy, cardiac enzymes (including troponin and myoglobin), nitroglycerin (sublingual or via an I.V. line), thrombolytic therapy, aspirin, morphine, bed rest, antiarrhythmics, beta-adrenergic blockers, angiotensin-converting enzyme inhibitors, and heparin.

Document your actions and your patient's response to these therapies. Use the appropriate flow sheets to record intake and output, hemodynamic parameters, I.V. fluids given, drugs administered, and frequent vital signs. Record what you teach the patient, such as details about the disease process, treatments, drugs, signs and symptoms to report, exercise, sexual activity, proper nutrition, smoking cessation, support groups, and cardiac rehabilitation programs. Include emotional support given to the patient and his family.

| 12/30/05 | 2310 | Pt. c/o severe crushing midsternal chest pain with radiation to Ⓛ arm at 2240. Pt. pointed to center of chest and stated, "I feel like I have an elephant on my chest." Rates pain at 9 on a scale of 0 to 10, w/ 10 being the worst pain imaginable. Pt. is restless in bed and diaphoretic, c/o nausea. P 84 and regular, BP 128/82, RR 24, oral T 98.8° F. Extremities cool, pedal pulses weak, normal heart sounds, breath sounds clear. Dr. Boone notified of pt.'s chest pain and physical findings at 2245 and came to see pt. and orders given. O₂ started at 2 L by NC. 12-lead ECG obtained; showed ST-segment elevation in anterior leads. Pt. placed on portable cardiac monitor. I.V. line started in Ⓛ forearm with 18 G catheter with NSS at 30 ml/hr. Stat cardiac enzymes, troponin, myoglobin, and electrolytes sent to lab at 2255. Nitroglycerin 1/150 gr given SL, 5 minutes apart X 3 with no relief. Explaining all procedures to pt., who verbalizes understanding. Assuring him that he's being monitored closely and will be transferred to CCU for closer monitoring and treatment. Dr. Boone called wife and notified her of husband's chest pain and transfer. Report called to CCU at 2255 and given to Laurie Feldman, RN. ———— Patricia Silver, RN |

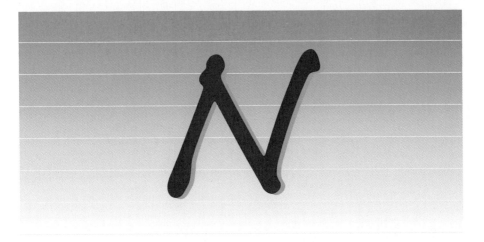

NASOGASTRIC TUBE CARE

Providing effective nasogastric (NG) tube care requires meticulous monitoring of the patient and the equipment. Monitoring the patient involves checking drainage from the NG tube and assessing the patient's GI function. Monitoring the equipment involves verifying correct tube placement and irrigating the tube to ensure patency to prevent mucosal damage.

Specific care measures vary only slightly for the most commonly used NG tubes: the single-lumen Levin tube and the double-lumen Salem sump tube.

ESSENTIAL DOCUMENTATION

Record the date and time that care was provided. Regularly record tube placement confirmation (usually every 4 to 8 hours). Record fluids you instill in the NG tube and any NG output. This may be recorded on an intake and output flow sheet. Describe the NG drainage, noting its color, consistency, and odor. Track the irrigation schedule, and note the actual time of each irrigation. Describe the condition of the patient's skin, mouth, and nares as well as care provided. Record tape changes and skin care you provide. Chart your assessment of bowel sounds. Note instructions and explanations that you give the patient.

11/30/05	1100	NG tube placement verified by aspirating 10 ml of clear
		and colorless fluid with mucus shreds and pH test strip
		result of 5. NG tube drained 100 ml of clear and
		colorless fluid with mucus shreds over 4 hr. Active bowel
		sounds in all 4 quadrants. Skin around mouth and nose
		intact. Helped pt. brush his teeth and rinse mouth,
		petroleum jelly applied to lips, water-soluble lubricants
		applied to nares. Tape secure around nose and not
		moved at this time. Explained importance of good oral
		hygiene to pt. ———————————— Clarissa Stone, RN

NASOGASTRIC TUBE INSERTION

Usually inserted to decompress the stomach, a nasogastric (NG) tube can prevent vomiting after major surgery. An NG tube is typically in place for 48 to 72 hours after surgery, by which time peristalsis usually resumes. However, the NG tube may remain in place for shorter or longer periods, depending on its use.

The NG tube has other diagnostic and therapeutic applications, especially in assessing and treating upper GI bleeding, collecting gastric contents for analysis, performing gastric lavage, aspirating gastric secretions, and administering drugs and nutrients.

Insertion of an NG tube demands close observation of the patient and verification of proper tube placement.

ESSENTIAL DOCUMENTATION

Record the type and size of the NG tube inserted; the date, time, and route of insertion; and confirmation of proper placement. Describe the type and amount of suction, if applicable; the drainage characteristics, such as amount, color (for example, green, brown, or brown-flecked), character, consistency, and odor; and the patient's tolerance of the insertion procedure.

Include in your note signs and symptoms signaling complications, such as nausea, vomiting, and abdominal distention. Document subsequent irrigation procedures and continuing problems after irrigations.

4/22/05	1700	Procedure explained to pt. by Dr. Thomas. #12 Fr. NG
		tube inserted via Ⓛ nostril by Dr. Thomas. Placement
		verified by aspiration of green stomach contents and
		pH test strip result of 5. Tube attached to low inter-
		mittent suction as ordered. Tube taped in place to
		nose. Drainage pale green, Hematest negative. Irrigated
		with 30 ml NSS per order. Hypoactive bowel sounds in
		all 4 quadrants. Pt. resting comfortably in bed. No c/o
		nausea or pain. ———————— Carol Allen, RN

NASOGASTRIC TUBE REMOVAL

A nasogastric (NG) tube typically remains in place for 48 to 72 hours after surgery and is removed when peristalsis resumes. Depending on its use, it may remain in place for shorter or longer periods.

ESSENTIAL DOCUMENTATION

Record the date and time that the NG tube is removed. Chart that you have explained the procedure to the patient. Describe the color, consistency, and amount of gastric drainage. Note the patient's tolerance of the procedure.

4/24/05	0900	Explained the procedure of NG tube removal to pt.
		Active bowel sounds heard in all 4 quadrants. Drained
		25 ml of pale green odorless drainage over last 2 hr.
		Tolerating ice chips without nausea, vomiting, discom-
		fort, or abdominal distention. NG tube removed without
		difficulty. Pt. taking small sips of water without c/o
		nausea. Pt. stated, "Taking the tube out wasn't as bad as
		I thought." ———————— Carol Allen, RN

NEGLIGENT COLLEAGUE, SUSPICION OF

The nurse practice act in each state emphasizes that a nurse's primary duty is to protect patients from harm. Nurses are required by the American Nurses Association to report a colleague's unsafe practice. A nurse who reports a negligent colleague is legally protected by the doctrine of qualified privilege. This doctrine protects the nurse against being charged with libel (written defamation of character) or slander (oral defamation of character) so that the patient's physical and mental well-being can remain her primary concern. When addressing a colleague's negligence, notify your nursing supervisor. In some cases, you may also be required to notify the facility's high-level administrators and the board of directors.

ESSENTIAL DOCUMENTATION

Most facilities require you to complete an incident report in the case of suspected negligence. In the report, use objective wording, describing only the specific incident about which you're concerned. Include statements provided by witnesses, the names and titles of people you interviewed about the incident, and the names of those notified regarding the occurrence. Describe actions taken to prevent further patient injury. Notify the patient's doctor that you're filing an incident report, and submit the report to the nursing supervisor. In your nurse's note, don't record that you have filed an incident report, but do indicate your interventions to minimize harm to the patient.

11/21/05	1500	Found pt., who is quadriplegic, lying face down in his pillow
		at 1440. Pt. was cyanotic when turned over and reposi-
		tioned for comfort. P 102, BP 102/62, RR 34, axillary temp
		97.2° F. O₂ sat. 88% by pulse oximetry. Placed on 2 L O₂ by
		NC. After 5 minutes, O₂ sat. 96%. Dr. Santini notified at
		1450, gave order to discontinue O₂ if O₂ sat. remains
		greater than 95% for next hour. Pt. also noted to have
		dried feces covering a large area of buttocks. Pt. bathed,
		cleaned; skin care regimen applied to reddened sacrum.
		1455, pt. resting comfortably in bed. Skin pink and warm.
		P 84, BP 112/64, RR 18 and unlabored. O₂ sat. 96%, O₂
		discontinued. ———————————— Pam Davis, RN

NONCOMPLIANCE, PATIENT

Occasionally, a patient does something – or fails to do something – that may contribute to an injury or explain why he hasn't responded to nursing and medical care.

ESSENTIAL DOCUMENTATION

Record the date and time of your entry. Document noncompliant patient behaviors and their outcomes. Although patients have the right to refuse medical and nursing care, be sure to document on the progress notes behavior that runs counter to medical instructions as well as the fact that you informed the patient of the possible consequences of his actions.

| 8/31/05 | 0800 | Pt. up and walking in hall without antiembolism stockings on. Reminded pt. that stockings need to be put on before getting out of bed, before edema develops, to be most effective. Pt. stated, "It's too early. I'll put them on after breakfast." Dr. Somers notified and told of situation. No orders given. Dr. Somers will talk with pt. this afternoon. ———————— Casey Adams, RN |

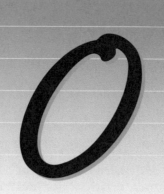

ORGAN DONATION

A federal requirement enacted in 1998 requires facilities to report deaths to the regional organ procurement organization (OPO). This regulation was enacted so that no potential donor would be missed. The regulation ensures that the family of every potential donor will understand the option to donate.

Collection of most organs, including the heart, liver, kidney, and pancreas, requires that the patient be pronounced brain dead and kept physically alive until the organs are harvested. Tissue, such as eyes, skin, bone, and heart valves, may be taken after death.

Follow your facility's policy for identifying and reporting a potential organ donor. Contact your local or regional OPO when a potential donor is identified. Typically, a specially trained person from your facility along with someone from your regional OPO will speak with the family about organ donation. The OPO coordinates the donation process after a family consents to donation.

ESSENTIAL DOCUMENTATION

Your documentation will vary depending on the stage of, and your role in, the organ donation process. You'll need to write a separate note for each stage. Make sure that you record the date and time of each note. Record the date and time that the patient is pronounced brain dead and the doctor's discussions with the family about the prognosis. (See "Brain death," page 48.) If the patient's driver's license or other documents indicate his wish to donate organs, place copies in the medical record and document that you have done so. The individual who contacts the regional OPO must document the conversation, including the date and time, the name of the person he spoke with, and instructions given. If you were part of the discussion about organ donation with the family, document who was present, what the family was told and by whom, and their response. Record your nursing care of the donor until the time he is taken to the operating room for organ procurement. Chart teaching, explanations, and emotional support given to the family.

11/12/05	0900	Dr. Silverstone explained at 0815 that pt. was brain dead
		and the prognosis. Mary Hubbard, wife, Ron Hubbard,
		son, Mary Rundell, daughter, and I were present.
		Family asked about organ donation. Wife stated, "My
		husband had spoken about donating his organs if this
		type of situation ever occurred. I believe his driver's
		license says he's an organ donor." Driver's license located
		with pt.'s belongings and removed from wallet by wife.
		License confirms pt.'s request for organ donation. Copy
		of license placed in medical record. Dr. Silverstone
		explained the criteria for organ donation and the
		process to the family. Mrs. Hubbard stated she would
		like more information from the regional OPO. OPO was
		contacted by this nurse at 0830. Intake information
		was taken by Rhonda Tierney. Appointment made for
		today at 1100 for OPO coordinator to meet with family
		in conference room on nursing unit. Family also re-
		quested to speak with a chaplain. Chaplain was paged,
		and Fr. Stone will be here at 0915 to meet with family.
		Family given use of private waiting room on the unit
		for privacy. Checking with family every hour to see if
		there is anything they need, to answer questions, and
		to provide support. —————— Patty Fisher, RN

OSTOMY CARE

An ostomy is a surgically created opening used to replace a normal physiologic function. Ostomies are used to facilitate the elimination of solid or liquid waste or to support respirations if placed in the trachea. The type and amount of care an ostomy requires depend on the output and location of the stoma. The nurse is responsible for providing ostomy care and assessing the condition of the stoma. The nurse may also need to help the patient adapt to the care and wearing of an appliance while helping him accept the body change.

ESSENTIAL DOCUMENTATION

Record the date and time of ostomy care. Describe the location of the ostomy and the condition of the stoma, including size, shape, and color. Chart the condition of the peristomal skin, noting any redness, irritation, breakdown, bleeding, or other unusual conditions. Note the character of drainage, including color, amount, type, and consistency. Record the type of appliance used, appliance size, and type of adhesive used. Document patient teaching, describing the teaching content. Record the patient's response to self-care, and evaluate his learning progress. Some facilities use a patient-teaching record to document patient teaching.

6/11/05	1000	Ostomy located in ⓛ upper abdomen. Appliance removed, minimal amount of dark brown fecal material in bag. Stoma 4 cm in diameter, round, beefy red in color; no drainage or bleeding. Skin surrounding stoma is pink and intact. Karaya ring applied to skin surrounding stoma after applying skin adhesive. New appliance snapped onto ring. Pt. helped measure stoma and applied skin adhesive. Pt. currently reading material on ostomy care. Discussed proper measurement of stoma and cutting hole in skin barrier to proper size. Pt. understands and agrees to cut skin barrier with next change. ————— Dawn March, RN

OVERDOSE, DRUG

Consumption of drugs in an amount that produces a life-threatening response is a drug overdose. The overdose can be intentional, such as a suicide gesture or attempt, or accidental such as overmedicating with pain medicine. Either situation requires your prompt and skilled actions. If you suspect that your patient has taken a drug overdose, immediately contact the doctor and take measures to ensure the patient's airway, breathing, and circulation. Other interventions focus on identifying, removing, neutralizing, and enhancing excretion of the drug.

ESSENTIAL DOCUMENTATION

Record the date and time of your entry. Chart a brief medical history, including allergies, current drugs, and history of substance abuse, if possible. Record the type and amount of drug taken, route of ingestion, and signs and symptoms exhibited. Document vital signs, noting the character of respirations and strength of pulses. Note the patient's mental status, including level of consciousness, orientation, and ability to follow commands. Document your neurologic assessment, including pupillary reaction, cranial nerve assessment, fine and gross motor activity, sensory functioning, and reflexes. Record the findings of your cardiopulmonary assessment.

Record interventions implemented before to arrival at your facility. Note the name of the doctor notified, time of notification, and orders given. Document your interventions, such as administering reversal agents (naloxone [Narcan] and flumazenil [Romazicon]) or GI decontaminants (activated charcoal, ipecac syrup, gastric lavage, cathartics, and whole-bowel irrigation) as well as supportive therapies. Include the patient's response to your interventions. If gastric emptying is performed, document the character and contents of the emesis. Use flow sheets to record your frequent assessments, vital signs, intake and output, I.V. therapy, and laboratory values. Record your patient teaching, including strategies to prevent future drug overdose.

9/17/05	0200	Pt. admitted to ED by ambulance with suspected opioid
		overdose. EMTs said friend of pt.'s at the scene said
		pt. may have taken "pain killers prescribed to treat his
		cancer pain." Lab called for stat toxicology screen, CBC
		BUN, creatinine, electrolytes, and ABGs. Pt. unresponsive
		to painful stimulation. HR 56, BP 100/50, tympanic
		T 96.8° F. Pupils pinpoint and nonreactive to light.
		Muscle tone in extremities flaccid, deep tendon reflexes
		absent. Pt. was intubated in the field and is receiving
		rescue breathing via AMBU with 100% FIO₂. Bilateral
		breath expansion present and breath sounds clear. Dr.
		Castro called at 0145 and orders given. I.V. access
		established in Ⓡ antecubital vein with 18G catheter on
		second attempt. 1000 ml NSS infusing at 100 ml/hr.
		Naloxone I.V. push administered. See MAR. Pt. immediately
		began moving extremities and coughing. He reached for
		the endotracheal tube and attempted to remove it. Pt.
		was calmed and instructed regarding treatment. He
		nodded his head yes to acknowledge understanding
		instructions. See flow sheets for frequent VS, I/O, I.V.
		therapy, and labs. ———————— Anthony Gasso, RN

OXYGEN ADMINISTRATION

A patient will need oxygen therapy when hypoxemia results from a respiratory or cardiac emergency or an increase in metabolic function. The adequacy of oxygen therapy is determined by arterial blood gas (ABG) analysis, oximetry monitoring, and clinical assessments. The patient's disease, physical condition, and age will help determine the most appropriate method of administration.

ESSENTIAL DOCUMENTATION

Record the date and time of oxygen administration. Document the oxygen delivery device used and oxygen flow rate. Record your assessment findings, including vital signs, skin color and temperature, respiratory effort, use of accessory muscles, breath sounds, and level of consciousness (LOC). Signs of hypoxia may include a decreased LOC, increased heart rate, arrhythmias, restlessness, dyspnea, use of accessory muscles, flared nostrils, cyanosis, and cool, clammy skin. Record ABG or oximetry values. If a doctor was notified, include the name of the doctor, time notified, orders given, and whether the doctor came to see the patient. Record the patient's response to oxygen therapy and include any patient and family teaching and emotional support given.

2/16/05	1152	When walking in room at 1130 to bring pt. his lunch tray,
		noted pt. sitting upright, pale, diaphoretic, taking deep
		labored respirations using accessory muscles with nasal
		flaring. O₂ currently at 2 L by nasal cannula. Pt. only able
		to speak 1-2 words at a time, stated his breathing has been
		"getting short" over the last hour. P 124 regular, BP 134/88,
		RR 32 and labored, tymp temp 97.2° F. Skin cool and pale,
		cyanosis noted around lips. Normal heart sounds, wheezes
		heard posteriorly on expiration. Pt. alert and oriented to
		time, place, and person, but appears anxious and restless.
		Pulse oximetry 87%. Dr. Desmond notified of findings at
		1140 and came to see pt. at 1145. Orders given. O₂ in-
		creased to 4 L by nasal cannula. Albuterol 2 puffs admin-
		istered by inhaler. 1145 pt. stated he's "breathing easier."
		P 92 and regular, BP 128/82, RR 24 and unlabored. Pulse
		oximetry 96%. No use of accessory muscles noted, skin
		warm and pink. Lungs clear. Pt. resting comfortably in bed.
		Explained to pt the importance of immediately reporting
		SOB to the nurse. Pt. verbalized understanding. Per orders,
		O₂ to be titrated to keep O₂ sat greater than 92%. 1150
		O₂ sat by pulse oximetry 96%, O₂ reduced back to 2 L. Will
		recheck O₂ sat in 10 min. ———— Mindy Pressler, RN

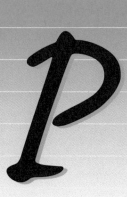

PACEMAKER, CARE OF PERMANENT

A pacemaker is implanted when the heart's natural pacemaker fails to work properly. It provides electrical impulses to the cardiac muscle as a means to stimulate contraction and support cardiac output.

Many types of pacemakers are available for use; the majority can be programmed to perform various functions. When caring for a patient with a pacemaker, it's important to know what type of pacemaker he has, what its rate is, and how it works. This information will help you ensure that the pacemaker is functioning properly and detect complications more quickly. The patient should have a manufacturer's card with pacemaker information; his medical records may also contain this information. You can obtain this information from the patient or his family.

ESSENTIAL DOCUMENTATION

Record the date and time of your entry. Chart the date of insertion, type of pacemaker (demand or fixed rate), rate of pacing, chambers paced, chambers sensed, how the pulse generator responds, and whether it's rate-responsive. If the patient knows the three or four-letter pacemaker code, record it. (See *Pacemaker codes,* page 276.) Document your patient's apical pulse rate, noting whether it's regular or irregular. If the patient is on a cardiac monitor, place a rhythm strip in the chart. Note the presence of pacemaker spikes, P waves, and QRS complexes and their relationship to each other. Ask the patient about and record symptoms of pacemaker malfunction, such as dizziness, fainting, weakness, fatigue, chest pain, and prolonged hiccups. Check the pacemaker insertion site and describe its

PACEMAKER CODES

A permanent pacemaker's three-letter (or sometimes five-letter) code refers to how it's programmed. The first letter represents the chamber that's paced; the second letter, the chamber that's sensed; and the third letter, how the pulse generator responds. The fourth and fifth letters describe special functions, as listed below.

First letter (chamber paced)
A = atrium
V = ventricle
D = dual (both chambers)
O = not applicable

Second letter (chamber sensed)
A = atrium
V = ventricle
D = dual (both chambers)
O = not applicable

Third letter (mode of response to sensing)
I = inhibited
T = triggered
D = dual (inhibited and triggered)
O = not applicable

Fourth letter (programmability)
R = rate responsiveness, or pacing rate that
varies in response to physiologic variables
such as skeletal muscle activity; an R is
added in the fourth position only if the
pacemaker is rate-responsive.
P = simple programmable
M = multiprogrammable
C = communicating
O = none

Fifth letter (antitachycardia and shock functions)
Letter codes in this position refer to functions
of implantable cardioverter-defibrillator
devices.

condition. Assess and document your patient's understanding of his pacemaker.

| 11/24/05 | 1500 | Pt. admitted to unit for treatment of exacerbation of ulcerative colitis. Pt. reports having a permanent DDD pacemaker with low rate set at 60, high rate set at 125, and AV interval of 200 msec. Pacemaker inserted 1998. AP 72 and regular, BP 132/84, RR 18, oral T 97.0° F. Pace-maker site in ® upper chest w/ healed incision. Pt. denies any dizziness, fainting spells, chest pain, or hiccups. Has been feeling weak and fatigued recently but states he feels this is due to a flare-up of his ulcerative colitis. Pt. able to explain pacemaker function, how to take his pulse, signs and symptoms to report, and need to avoid electromagnetic interference. ——————————————————— Thomas Harkin, RN |

PACEMAKER, CARE OF TRANSCUTANEOUS

Completely noninvasive and easily applied, a transcutaneous pacemaker proves especially useful in an emergency. Large skin electrodes are placed on the patient's anterior and posterior chest; then they're connected to a pulse generator to initiate pacing.

Nursing care of the patient receiving temporary transcutaneous pacing includes proper lead placement and attachment, application of conduction gel to the electrodes, cleaning the skin where the electrodes are applied, assessment of the patient's response, and monitoring for possible pacemaker malfunction. Because external pacing may be uncomfortable for the conscious patient, a sedative may be given.

ESSENTIAL DOCUMENTATION

Record the date and time. Chart the patient's heart rate and rhythm. Note the pacemaker rate and the output, in milliamperes (mA), at which capture occurs. Place a rhythm strip showing pacemaker function in the chart, if available. Describe the condition of the skin at the electrode sites and any skin care performed. Record your assessment of the patient, including skin color and temperature, mental status, and urine output. Document measures to reduce anxiety and provide comfort as well as the patient's response to these measures. Record patient teaching and emotional support given.

8/25/05	1800	Transcutaneous pacing continues with pacemaker set at
		rate of 68 and output 50 mA. BP 88/50, RR 16. Pt.
		fully paced and awaiting placement of transvenous
		pacemaker. Skin around electrodes slightly red and
		intact. Pt. c/o some burning at electrodes with each
		paced beat. Pt. given Valium 5 mg P.O. for anxiety and
		discomfort. Reassuring pt. that he's being monitored
		closely in CCU and that he'll be receiving transvenous
		pacemaker shortly. ——————— Karen Forbes, RN

PACEMAKER, CARE OF TRANSVENOUS

Transvenous pacing is accomplished by threading a pacing wire through a vein, such as the subclavian, antecubital, femoral, or jugular vein, to the right atrium (for atrial pacing), right ventricle (for ventricular pacing), or both (for dual chamber pacing). Some pulmonary artery catheters have a lumen for a transvenous pacing electrode. The pacing wire is then connected to a pulse generator outside the body.

If your patient has a transvenous pacemaker, you'll need to monitor him for complications, such as pneumothorax, hemothorax, cardiac perforation and tamponade, diaphragmatic stimulation, pulmonary embolism, thrombophlebitis, and infection. Also, if the doctor threads the electrode through the antecubital or femoral vein, venous spasm, thrombophlebitis, or lead displacement may occur. Nursing interventions also focus on protecting the patient from microshock, preventing and detecting pacemaker malfunction, and patient education.

ESSENTIAL DOCUMENTATION

Record the date and time of pacemaker care. Chart the pacemaker's settings. Document the patient's vital signs and include a rhythm strip in your note. Place a rhythm strip in the chart whenever pacemaker settings are changed or when the patient is treated for a complication caused by the pacemaker. Document interventions to prevent shock and pacemaker malfunction. Chart your assessment of the pacemaker insertion site, noting drainage, redness, and edema. Describe site care and document dressing changes. Include signs and symptoms of other complications, the name of the doctor notified, the time of notification, orders given, your interventions, and the patient's response. Record patient education and emotional support rendered.

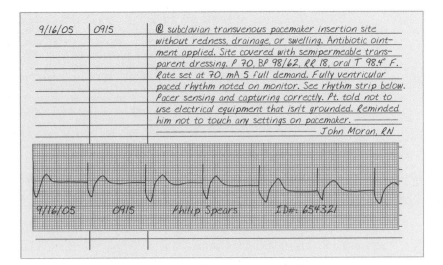

| 9/16/05 | 0915 | ® subclavian transvenous pacemaker insertion site without redness, drainage, or swelling. Antibiotic ointment applied. Site covered with semipermeable transparent dressing. P 70, BP 98/62, RR 18, oral T 98.4° F. Rate set at 70, mA 5 full demand. Fully ventricular paced rhythm noted on monitor. See rhythm strip below. Pacer sensing and capturing correctly. Pt. told not to use electrical equipment that isn't grounded. Reminded him not to touch any settings on pacemaker. ————————————————————— John Moran, RN |

9/16/05   0915   Philip Spears   ID#: 654321

PACEMAKER, INITIATION OF TRANSCUTANEOUS

A temporary pacemaker is usually inserted in an emergency. In a life-threatening situation, when time is critical, a transcutaneous pacemaker is the best choice. This device sends an electrical impulse from the pulse generator to the patient's heart by way of two electrodes, which are placed on the front and back of the patient's chest. Transcutaneous pacing is quick and effective, but it's used only until a doctor can establish transvenous pacing.

ESSENTIAL DOCUMENTATION

Chart the date and time of the procedure. Record the reason for transcutaneous pacing and the location of the electrodes. Chart the pacemaker settings. Note the patient's response to the procedure along with complications and interventions. If possible, obtain rhythm strips before, during, and after pacemaker use; whenever settings are changed; and when the patient is treated for a complication caused by the pacemaker. As you monitor the patient, record his response to temporary pacing and note changes in his condition. Record patient teaching, emotional support, and comfort measures provided.

2/15/05	1420	Pt. with AP 48, BP 84/50, RR 16, arousable with verbal
		and physical stimulation, speech incomprehensible. Skin
		pale and clammy, peripheral pulses weak. Monitor shows
		bradycardia. Transcutaneous pacing initiated until
		transvenous pacing can be initiated. Posterior pacing
		electrode placed on Ⓛ back, below scapula and to the Ⓛ
		of the spine. Anterior electrode placed on Ⓛ anterior
		chest over V₂ to V₅. Output set at 40 mA, rate at 60.
		AP 60, BP 94/60, RR 18. Pt. alert and oriented; no c/o
		chest pain, dyspnea, or dizziness. Peripheral pulses
		strong; skin warm and dry. Explained to pt. that he may
		feel a thumping or twitching sensation during pacing
		and to let nurse know if discomfort is intolerable so
		that meds can be given. Pt. states he can feel twitching
		and doesn't feel the need for meds at this time. ——
		———————————————— Sally Hanes, RN

PACEMAKER, INSERTION OF PERMANENT

A permanent pacemaker is a self-contained unit designed to operate for 3 to 20 years. In an operating room or cardiac catheterization laboratory, a surgeon implants the device in a pocket under the patient's skin.

A permanent pacemaker allows the patient's heart to beat on its own but prevents pacing from falling below a preset rate. Pacing electrodes can be placed in the atria, the ventricles, or both. Pacemakers may pace at a rate that varies in response to intrinsic conditions such as skeletal muscle activity, and may also have antitachycardia and shock functions.

Candidates for permanent pacemakers include patients with myocardial infarction and persistent bradyarrhythmia and patients with complete heart block or slow ventricular rates stemming from congenital or degenerative heart disease or cardiac surgery. Patients who suffer Stokes-Adams attacks and those with Wolff-Parkinson-White syndrome may also benefit from a permanent pacemaker.

ESSENTIAL DOCUMENTATION

Record the date and time of your entry. Record the time that your patient returned to the unit. Document the type of pacemaker used, pacing rate, and doctor's name. Verify that the chart contains information on the pacemaker's serial number and its manufacturer's name. Note whether the pacemaker reduces or eliminates the arrhythmia and include other pertinent observations such as the condition of the incision site. Chart the patient's vital signs and level of consciousness every 15 minutes for the first hour, every hour for the next 4 hours, every 4 hours for the next 48 hours, and then once every shift, or according to facility policy or doctor's order. You may record these frequent assessments on a critical care or frequent vital signs flow sheet. Assess for and record signs and symptoms of complications, such as infection, lead displacement, perforated ventricle, cardiac tamponade, or lead fracture and disconnection. Record the name of the doctor notified, the time of notification, interventions, and the patient's response. Document your patient teaching. This may be recorded on a patient-teaching flow sheet.

1/28/06	1445	Pt. returned from OR at 1430 following insertion of
		DDD pacemaker by Dr. Fleur. Upper rate limit of 125
		bpm and lower rate limit of 60 bpm. See attached
		rhythm strip. No arrhythmias noted on monitor. AP 71,
		BP 128/74, RR 18, oral T 97.4° F. Pt. alert and oriented
		to time, place, and person. Skin warm and dry, periph-
		eral pulses strong. Lungs clear, normal heart sounds.
		Dressing over ® subclavian insertion site dry and intact.
		No c/o discomfort. Saline lock in ® forearm. Told pt.
		to report any weakness, palpitations, chest pain, dyspnea,
		or prolonged hiccups. ————— Nancy Spencer, RN

1/28/06 1445
David Menda ID#: 987654

PACEMAKER, INSERTION OF TRANSVENOUS

A transvenous pacemaker is usually inserted in an emergency by thread-ing an electrode catheter through a vein, such as the brachial, femoral, subclavian, or jugular vein, into the patient's right atrium, right ventricle, or both. The electrodes are then attached to an external battery-powered pulse generator. Some pulmonary artery catheters have transvenous pac-ing electrodes.

ESSENTIAL DOCUMENTATION

Record the date and time that the pacemaker was inserted, the reason for pacing, and the location of the insertion site. Chart the pacemaker set-tings. Document the patient's level of consciousness and cardiopulmo-nary assessment, including vital signs. Note the patient's response to the procedure, complications, and interventions. Include a rhythm strip in your note. Document your assessment of the insertion site and your neu-rovascular assessment of the involved limb, if appropriate. Record your patient teaching and the support you gave.

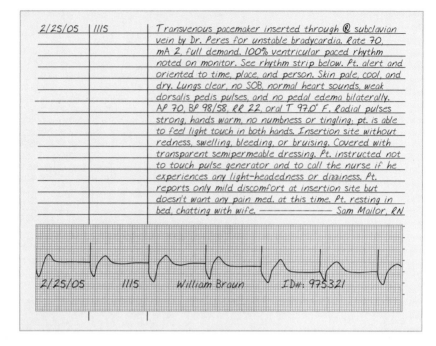

2/25/05	1115	*Transvenous pacemaker inserted through ® subclavian*
		vein by Dr. Peres for unstable bradycardia. Rate 70,
		mA 2, full demand. 100% ventricular paced rhythm
		noted on monitor. See rhythm strip below. Pt. alert and
		oriented to time, place, and person. Skin pale, cool, and
		dry. Lungs clear, no SOB, normal heart sounds, weak
		dorsalis pedis pulses, and no pedal edema bilaterally.
		AP 70, BP 98/58, RR 22, oral T 97.0° F. Radial pulses
		strong, hands warm, no numbness or tingling; pt. is able
		to feel light touch in both hands. Insertion site without
		redness, swelling, bleeding, or bruising. Covered with
		transparent semipermeable dressing. Pt. instructed not
		to touch pulse generator and to call the nurse if he
		experiences any light-headedness or dizziness. Pt.
		reports only mild discomfort at insertion site but
		doesn't want any pain med. at this time. Pt. resting in
		bed, chatting with wife. —————— Sam Mailor, RN

PACEMAKER MALFUNCTION

Occasionally, a pacemaker fails to function properly. To determine whether your patient's pacemaker is malfunctioning, you'll need to know its mode of function and its settings. If a malfunction occurs, you'll need to notify the doctor immediately, obtain a 12-lead ECG, call for a stat chest X-ray, begin continuous ECG monitoring, and prepare for temporary pacing.

ESSENTIAL DOCUMENTATION

Record the date and time of the malfunction. Record your patient's signs and symptoms, such as dizziness, syncope, irregular pulse, pale skin, dyspnea, chest pain, hypotension, heart rate below the pacemaker's set rate, palpitations, hiccups, and chest or abdominal muscle twitching. Place a cardiac rhythm strip in the chart, if possible. Note the name of the doctor notified, the time of notification, and the orders given, such as obtaining a stat ECG, placing a magnet over a permanent pacemaker, and preparing for temporary pacing. If a temporary pacemaker malfunctions, chart your troubleshooting actions, such as repositioning the patient and checking connections and battery settings; the results of these efforts; and the patient's response. Be sure to include patient education and emotional support provided.

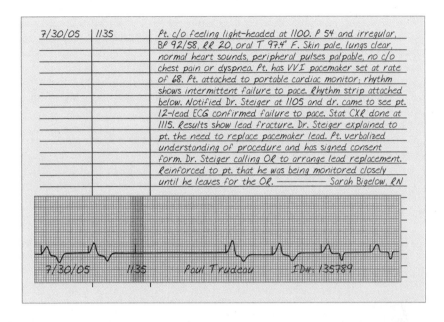

7/30/05	1135	Pt. c/o feeling light-headed at 1100. P 54 and irregular,
		BP 92/58, RR 20, oral T 97.4° F. Skin pale, lungs clear,
		normal heart sounds, peripheral pulses palpable, no c/o
		chest pain or dyspnea. Pt. has VVI pacemaker set at rate
		of 68. Pt. attached to portable cardiac monitor; rhythm
		shows intermittent failure to pace. Rhythm strip attached
		below. Notified Dr. Steiger at 1105 and dr. came to see pt.
		12-lead ECG confirmed failure to pace. Stat CXR done at
		1115. Results show lead fracture. Dr. Steiger explained to
		pt. the need to replace pacemaker lead. Pt. verbalized
		understanding of procedure and has signed consent
		form. Dr. Steiger calling OR to arrange lead replacement.
		Reinforced to pt. that he was being monitored closely
		until he leaves for the OR. ————— Sarah Bigelow, RN

7/30/05   1135   Paul Trudeau   ID#: 135789

PAIN MANAGEMENT

When a person feels severe pain, he typically seeks medical help not only because he wants relief, but also because he believes the pain signals a serious problem. This perception produces anxiety, which in turn increases the patient's pain. Your primary goal is to eliminate or minimize your patient's pain; however, determining its severity can be difficult because pain is subjective. You can use a number of tools to assess pain. Always document the results of your assessments. (See *Assessing and documenting pain,* page 284.)

Interventions to manage pain include administering analgesics, providing emotional support and comfort measures, and using cognitive techniques to distract the patient. Patients with severe pain usually require an opioid analgesic. Invasive measures, such as epidural or patient-controlled analgesia, may also be required.

AᴄᴄᴜCʜᴀʀᴛ

ASSESSING AND DOCUMENTING PAIN

Used appropriately, standard assessment tools, such as the McGill-Melzack Pain Questionnaire and the Initial Pain Assessment Tool (developed by McCaffery and Beebe), provide a solid foundation for your nursing diagnoses and care plans. If your health care facility doesn't use standardized pain questionnaires, you can devise other pain measurement tools, such as the pain flow sheet or the visual and graphic rating scales that appear below. Whichever pain assessment tool you choose, remember to document its use and include the graphic record in your patient's chart.

PAIN FLOW SHEET
Possibly the most convenient tool for pain assessment, a flow sheet provides a standard for reevaluating a patient's pain at regular intervals. It's also beneficial for patients and families, who may feel too overwhelmed by the pain experience to answer a long, detailed questionnaire.

   If possible, incorporate the pain assessment into the flow sheet you're already using. Generally, the easier the flow sheet is to use, the more likely you and your patient will be to use it.

PAIN FLOW SHEET					
Date and time	Pain rating (0 to 10)	Patient behaviors	Vital signs	Pain rating after intervention	Comments
1/16/06 0800	7	Wincing, holding head	186/88 98–22	5	Dilaudid 2 mg I.M. given
1/16/06 1200	3	Relaxing, reading	160/80 84–18	2	Tylox ÷ P.O. given

VISUAL ANALOG PAIN SCALE
In a visual analog pain scale, the patient marks a linear scale containing words or numbers that correspond to his perceived degree of pain. Draw a scale to represent a continuum of pain intensity. Verbal anchors describe the pain's intensity; for example, "no pain" begins the scale and "pain as bad as it could be" ends it. Ask the patient to mark the point on the continuum that best describes his pain.

VISUAL ANALOG SCALE

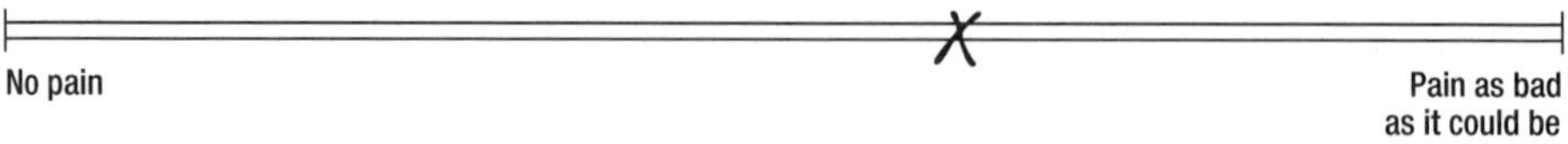

⊢————————————————————X————————————————————⊣

No pain   Pain as bad as it could be

GRAPHIC RATING SCALE
Other rating scales have words that represent pain intensity. Use one of these scales as you would the visual analog scale. Have the patient mark the spot on the continuum.

GRAPHIC RATING SCALE

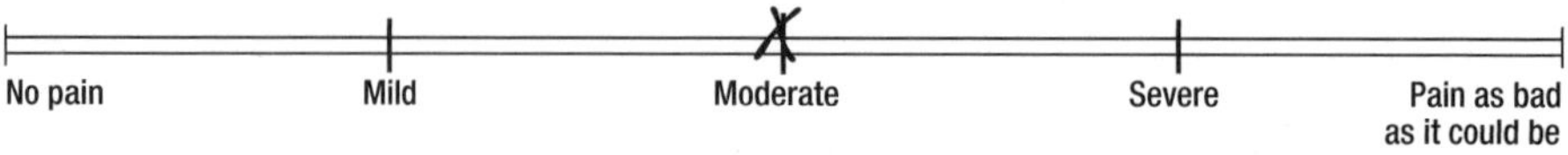

⊢————————|————————X————————|————————⊣

No pain   Mild   Moderate   Severe   Pain as bad as it could be

ESSENTIAL DOCUMENTATION

When charting pain levels and characteristics, describe the location of the pain and note if it's internal, external, localized, or diffuse. Record whether the pain interferes with the patient's sleep or activities of daily living. In the chart, describe what the pain feels like in the patient's own words. Chart the patient's description of how long the pain lasts and how often it occurs. Record the patient's ranking of his pain using a pain rating scale.

Describe the patient's body language and behaviors associated with pain, such as wincing, grimacing, or squirming in bed. Note sympathetic responses commonly associated with mild to moderate pain, such as pallor, elevated blood pressure, dilated pupils, skeletal muscle tension, dyspnea, tachycardia, and diaphoresis. Record parasympathetic responses commonly associated with severe, deep pain, including pallor, decreased blood pressure, bradycardia, nausea and vomiting, dizziness, and loss of consciousness.

Chart the positions that relieve or worsen the pain. Record measures that relieve or heighten the pain, including heat, cold, massage, or drugs.

Document interventions taken to alleviate your patient's pain and the patient's responses to these interventions. Also, note patient teaching and emotional support provided.

3/19/05	1600	Pt. admitted to room 304 at 1545 with diagnosis of pancreatic cancer and severe pain in LLQ. Pt. states, "It feels like my insides are on fire." Pt. rates pain as 6 on a scale of 0 to 10, w/ 10 being the worst pain imaginable. States pain keeps him from sleeping and eating. States he's been taking Percocet 2 tabs q4hr at home, but it's no longer providing relief. Pt. alert and oriented to time, place, and person. Curled in bed on ① side, with arms wrapped around abdomen and softly moaning. Skin pale and diaphoretic, pupils dilated. Dr. Martin notified at 1550. Dilaudid 2 mg ordered and given I.V. P 92, BP 110/64, RR 22, oral T 99.0° F. Pt. resting at present, no longer moaning or curled in a ball. Explained pain medication schedule to pt. and reassured him that staff will work with him to find medications and schedule that reduce his pain to a tolerable level. ———————————————————— Kaylee Compton, RN

PARACENTESIS

Paracentesis is a bedside procedure in which fluid from the peritoneal space is aspirated through a needle, trocar, or cannula inserted in the abdominal wall. Paracentesis is used to diagnose and treat massive ascites when other therapies have failed. Additionally, it's used as a prelude to other procedures, including radiography, peritoneal dialysis, and surgery. It's also used to detect intra-abdominal bleeding after traumatic injury and to obtain a peritoneal fluid specimen for laboratory analysis.

ESSENTIAL DOCUMENTATION

Document that the procedure and its risks have been explained to the patient and that a consent form has been signed. Chart what you taught the patient about the procedure. Your facility may require you to document patient education on a patient-teaching flow sheet. Record baseline vital signs, weight, and abdominal girth. Indicate that the abdominal area measured was marked with a felt-tipped marking pen.

Record the date and time of the procedure. Describe the puncture site and record the amount, color, viscosity, and odor of the aspirated fluid. Also, record the amount of fluid aspirated in the fluid intake and output record. Record the number of specimens sent to the laboratory. Note whether the wound was sutured and the type of dressing that was applied.

Record the patient's tolerance of the procedure, vital signs, and signs and symptoms of complications (such as shock and perforation of abdominal organs) that occur during the procedure. If peritoneal fluid leakage occurs, document that you notified the doctor, any orders given, your actions, and the patient's response.

Keep a running record of the patient's vital signs and nursing activities related to drainage and dressing changes. Document drainage checks and the patient's response to the procedure every 15 minutes for the first hour, every 30 minutes for the next 2 hours, every hour for the next 4 hours, and then every 4 hours for the next 24 hours (or according to your facility's policy). Continue to document drainage characteristics, including color, amount, odor, and viscosity. Document daily patient weight and abdominal girth measurements after the procedure.

2/12/05	0920	Procedure explained to pt. and consent obtained. Dr.
		Novello performed paracentesis in RLQ, as per protocol.
		1500 ml of cloudy pale-yellow fluid drained and sent to
		lab as ordered. Site sutured with one 3-0 silk suture.
		Sterile 4" X 4" gauze pad applied. No leakage noted at
		site. Abdomen marked at level of umbilicus with black
		felt-tipped pen for measurements. Abdominal girth 44"
		preprocedure and 42³/₄" postprocedure. VS and weight
		before and after procedure as per flow sheet. Before
		procedure pt. stated, "I am afraid of this procedure."
		Reinforced teaching related to the procedure and offered
		reassurances during the procedure. Pt. still anxious but
		resting comfortably in bed. ————— Carol Barsky, RN

PARENTERAL NUTRITION ADMINISTRATION, LIPIDS

Lipid emulsions are a source of calories and essential fatty acids. A deficiency in essential fatty acids can hinder wound healing, adversely affect the production of red blood cells, and impair prostaglandin synthesis. Typically given as separate solutions in conjunction with parenteral nutrition, lipid emulsions may also be given alone. They can be administered through a peripheral or central venous line.

ESSENTIAL DOCUMENTATION

Record the date and time of your entry. Note the type of lipid solution, its volume, and the infusion rate. Document whether the lipids are being given peripherally or centrally, and note the location of the line. Record vital signs before starting the infusion, at regular intervals during the infusion (according to your facility's policy), and following the infusion. In the intake and output record, chart the amount of lipids infused. Document site care and describe the condition of the insertion site, cleaning the site, and the type of dressing applied. Also, record tubing and lipid solution changes. Monitor the patient for adverse reactions, and document your observations, interventions, and the patient's response. Record what you teach the patient about lipids.

5/30/05	1200	*P 92, BP 118/70, RR 23, oral T 98.4° F. 500 ml of*
		10% lipids hung using new tubing c̄ a 1.2 micron in-
		line filter at a rate of 60 ml/hr via infusion pump.
		Infusing via Ⓡ subclavian CV line. See flow sheet
		for frequent VS assessments and I/O. Lips and nail
		beds pink, lungs clear. Transparent dressing intact,
		site without redness, drainage, swelling, or discom-
		fort. Instructed pt. to report any pain or discom-
		fort at insertion site. ————— David Felding, RN

PARENTERAL NUTRITION ADMINISTRATION, TOTAL

Total parenteral nutrition (TPN) is the administration of a solution of dextrose, proteins, electrolytes, vitamins, and trace elements in amounts that exceed the patient's energy expenditure, thereby achieving anabolism. Because this solution has about six times the solute concentration of blood, it requires dilution by delivery into a high-flow central vein to avoid injury to the peripheral vasculature. Typically, the solution is delivered to the superior vena cava through an indwelling subclavian vein catheter. Generally, TPN is prescribed for any patient who can't absorb nutrients through the GI tract for more than 10 days.

Because TPN solution supports bacterial growth and the central venous (CV) line gives systemic access, contamination and sepsis are always a risk. Strict surgical asepsis is required during solution, dressing, tubing, and filter changes. Site care and dressing changes should be performed according to your facility's policy, usually at least three times per week (once per week for transparent dressings) and whenever the dressing becomes wet, soiled, or nonocclusive. Tubing and filter changes should be performed every 24 to 48 hours, according to your facility's policy.

ESSENTIAL DOCUMENTATION

Record the date and time of your entry. Document the type and location of the CV line and the volume and rate of the solution infused. Record the amount of TPN infused on the intake and output record. Document site care, describing the condition of the insertion site, cleaning of the site, and the type of dressing applied. Many facilities document all this information on an I.V. flow sheet. (See *I.V. flow sheet,* page 244.) Monitor a patient receiving TPN for adverse reactions, such as air embolism, extravasation, phlebitis, pneumothorax, hydrothorax, septicemia, and thrombosis, and document your observations, interventions, and the patient's response to them. Record what you teach the patient about TPN.

When you discontinue a CV or peripheral I.V. line for TPN, record the date and time and the type of dressing applied. Also, describe the appearance of the infusion site.

8/31/05	2020	2-L bag of TPN hung at 2000. Infusing at 65 ml/hr
		via infusion pump through ® subclavian CV line. Trans-
		parent dressing intact, and site is without redness,
		drainage, swelling, or tenderness. See I/O flow sheet
		for intake and output. Told pt. to call nurse if dress-
		ing becomes loose or soiled, site becomes tender or
		painful, or tubing or catheter becomes dislodged. Re-
		viewed reasons for TPN and answered pt.'s questions
		about its purpose. ———————— Meg Callahan, RN

PATIENT-CONTROLLED ANALGESIA

Some patients receive opioids by way of a patient-controlled analgesia (PCA) infusion pump that allows patients to self-administer boluses of an opioid analgesic I.V., subcutaneously, or epidurally within limits prescribed by the doctor. To avoid overmedication, an adjustable lockout interval inhibits premature delivery of additional boluses. PCA increases the patient's sense of control, reduces anxiety, reduces drug use over the postoperative course, and gives enhanced pain control. Indicated for patients who need parenteral analgesia, PCA therapy is typically given to trauma patients postoperatively, terminal cancer patients, and others with chronic diseases.

ESSENTIAL DOCUMENTATION

Be sure to document the name of the opioid used, lockout interval, maintenance dose, amount the patient receives when he activates the device, and amount of opioid used during your shift. Record the patient's assessment of pain relief and patient teaching you perform. Document your patient's vital signs and level of consciousness according to your facility's policy. Record your observations of the insertion site. See *PCA flow sheet,* page 290, for an example of documentation.

PCA FLOW SHEET

The form shown below is used to document the use of patient-controlled analgesia (PCA). PCA allows the patient to self-administer an opioid analgesic as needed within limits prescribed by the doctor.

Patient name: _Martin Smith_ **Medical record #:** _1234567_ **Date:** _3/22/05_

Medication (Circle one) Meperidine 300 mg in 30 ml (10 mg/1 ml)
(Morphine 30 mg in 30 ml (1 mg/ml))

	7–3 Shift				3–11 Shift				11–7 Shift			
Time (enter in box)	1200	1400			1600							
New cartridge inserted	OR											
PCA settings Lockout interval 7 (minutes)		7			7							
Dose volume / (ml/dose)												
Four-hour limit 30												
Continuous settings / (mg/hr)												
Respiratory rate	18	20			20							
Blood pressure	150/70	130/62			128/10							
Sedation rating 1. Wide awake 2. Drowsy 3. Dozing, intermittent 4. Mostly sleeping 5. Only awakens when stimulated	1	2			3							
Analgesia rts (1–10) Minimal pain – 1 Maximum pain – 10	7	8			6							
Additional doses given (optional doses)	3ml/OR											
Total ml delivered (total from ampule)	3	6			15							
ml remaining	27	24			15							

RN SIGNATURE (7–3 SHIFT) _Janet Green, RN_ Date _3/22/05_

RN SIGNATURE (3–11 SHIFT) _Karen Singleton, RN_ Date _3/22/05_

RN SIGNATURE (11–7 SHIFT) _____ Date _____

PATIENT REQUESTING ACCESS TO MEDICAL RECORDS

According to the Health Insurance Portability and Accountability Act (HIPAA) of 1996, the patient has the right to view and obtain copies of his medical records. Many states have since enacted laws allowing patients access to such records, and health care providers are required to honor such requests. Psychologists, however, may deny a patient access to his psychotherapy records.

When a patient requests to see his medical record, assess why he wants to see it. He may simply be curious, or his request may reflect hidden fears about his treatment that you or another member of the health care team may be able to address. Be sure to follow facility policies for a patient viewing his own medical record. These policies may dictate that you notify your nursing supervisor or office manager of the request and that you notify the risk manager to alert administrative staff and legal counsel, if necessary.

Explain the procedure for accessing medical records, and provide the patient with the appropriate forms to use. Advise him when you expect the records to be available (typically, copies are available within 30 days of the request). Also, let him know whether the facility charges a fee for copying the records.

When the medical record is available, be sure to properly identify the patient and remain with him while he reads the record. Explain to the patient that he has the right to request that incorrect information be changed or that missing information be added. If the doctor or health care facility believes that the medical record is correct, the patient can note his disagreement in the medical record. Observe how the patient responds while he reads. Offer to answer any questions he may have; assure him that the doctor will also answer questions. While the patient reads, help him interpret the abbreviations and jargon used in medical charting.

ESSENTIAL DOCUMENTATION

If your patient asks to see his medical record, use your facility's form or have the patient draft a written request to see his medical record, according to your facility's policy. Chart the parts of the medical record that the patient requested and whether copies were given to the patient. Record the names of the nursing supervisor, risk manager, legal counsel, and doctor who were notified of the patient's request. Record the date and time that the patient reviewed his record and the name of the person who stayed with the patient while he read it. Document the patient's response to reading his record and whether he had questions or concerns.

6/3/05	1400	Pt. stated, "I want to look at my chart." Pt. informed that he needed to make request in writing. Appropriate forms given to pt. for requesting medical records. Pt. complied and request sent to medical records. When asked why he wanted to see his medical record, pt. stated, "I just want to be sure the doctors haven't been hiding anything from me." Notified Bruce Wallins, RN, nursing supervisor; Loretta Reilly, RN, risk manager; and Dr. Felbin of pt.'s request. Identity confirmed by checking ID band. Dr. Felbin and I were in attendance while pt. read record. Pt. asked questions regarding terms and abbreviations. Pt. appeared calm and relaxed after reading his medical record. ————— Monica Lutz, RN

PATIENT SEARCH, LEGALLY NECESSARY

The fourth amendment to the Constitution protects individuals from unreasonable searches of their person, house, office, or vehicle. A search is justified when there are reasonable grounds to believe that the search will produce evidence of a violation of the law or rules of the institution. It's generally accepted that the police may not enter a person's home without a search warrant. Typically, this applies to the patient's hospital room as well.

If a patient's belongings are to be searched by law enforcement authorities, immediately notify the nursing supervisor, facility administrator, and legal affairs department. No search or seizure should occur until it's ensured that the patient's legal rights are protected and a search warrant is presented by the law enforcement agency that would like to perform the search. The facility is required to cooperate with law enforcement agencies in the preservation or collection of evidence involving patients in accordance with appropriate medical ethics and legal statutes.

ESSENTIAL DOCUMENTATION

Record the date and time of your entry. Document the presentation of a search warrant by law enforcement agents. Chart the time of the presentation of a search warrant and the names of the nursing supervisor, hospital administrator, and doctor who witnessed the presentation. Record the rationale for searching the patient's belongings. Document compliance with your facility and local law enforcement policies and procedures before instituting the search. Record the time that the search occurred, the name of the person conducting the search, and the names of others present.

6/22/05	1700	Presented with search warrant by police officers
		M. Stark (badge #1234) and D. Witmer (badge #5678) at
		1630 to search patient's belongings for crime evidence.
		Notified Margo Kaufman, RN, nursing supervisor; Alan
		White, hospital administrator; and Dr. Chaddha of search
		warrant at 1635. Ms. Kaufman and Mr. White arrived
		on unit at 1640 to review search warrant. Search took
		place at 1645 by officers Stark and Witmer, with Ms.
		Kaufman, Mr. White, and I in attendance. Yellow watch,
		brown wallet, and yellow necklace with clear stone
		removed from pt.'s jacket. ———— Casey Logan, RN

PATIENT SELF-DOCUMENTATION OF CARE

Self-documentation can be effective for patients who must perform considerable self-care (those with diabetes, for example) or for those trying to discover what precipitates a problem such as chronic headaches.

By using self-documentation, a patient with diabetes may record information about his diet, insulin dose, self-tested blood glucose levels, and activity level. This information can help him avoid insulin reactions and delay, prevent, or even reverse complications of hyperglycemia or hypoglycemia. Self-documentation may provide valuable information for the doctor or nurse as well.

A patient with chronic headaches may be asked to chart, among other things, when a headache occurred, what warning signs he noticed, and

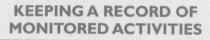

KEEPING A RECORD OF MONITORED ACTIVITIES

In many situations, your patient can provide information more accurately than a member of the health care team (case in point: a patient who wears a Holter monitor to evaluate the effect of medication on his heart and his daily activities).

Keeping this in mind, some health care facilities prepare patient instructional materials to be used in conjunction with a diary-like chart (such as the one below), which the patient refers to and completes for the medical record.

Date	Time	Activity	Feelings
1/15/06	10:30 a.m.	Rode home from hospital in cab	Legs tired, felt short of breath
	11:30 a.m.	Watched TV in living room	Comfortable
	12:15 p.m.	Ate lunch, took propranolol	Indigestion
	1:30 p.m.	Walked next door to see neighbor	Felt short of breath
	2:45 p.m.	Walked home	Very tired, legs hurt
	3:00 to 4:00 p.m.	Urinated, took nap	Comfortable
	5:30 p.m.	Ate dinner slowly	Comfortable
	7:20 p.m.	Had bowel movement	Felt short of breath
	9:00 p.m.	Watched TV, drank one beer	Heart beating fast for about 1 minute, no pain
	11:00 p.m.	Took propranolol, urinated, and went to bed	Tired
1/16/06	8:15 a.m.	Woke up, urinated, washed face and arms	Very tired, rapid heartbeat for about 30 seconds
	10:30 a.m.	Returned to hospital	Felt better

what pain-relief measures he tried. Analyzing this information may help ward off the headaches.

The patient can document entries on preprinted forms or in a journal. Such records can be used in both inpatient and outpatient care settings. Depending on your facility's policy, these entries may or may not become a permanent part of the medical record. (See *Keeping a record of monitored activities.*)

ESSENTIAL DOCUMENTATION

Record the date and time that you taught the patient about self-documentation. In your note, describe what you instructed the patient to measure or time or the symptoms to record and how frequently this should be done. Record that the patient knows how to chart his findings. Describe the type of record keeping he's using. Document that the patient is able to verbalize understanding or give a return demonstration. Include any written materials given to the patient. Record that the patient knows who to call with questions or for emergency services.

11/14/05	1030	Pt. being discharged tomorrow morning. Taught pt.
		how to record his antihypertensive meds and daily BP
		readings. Wife brought in pt.'s electronic BP equipment
		from home. Readings correlate well with cuff readings.
		Pt. demonstrated proper technique for taking BP. Pt.
		correctly recorded date, time, BP reading, his position
		(seated or standing), any associated symptoms, and times
		meds taken in a notebook. Explained that home health
		nurse will review his notebook at each home visit.
		Reminded him to bring his notebook to his doctor for
		follow-up visits. Pt. verbalized understanding of calling
		doctor for SBP greater than 180 and DBP greater than
		110 and to call EMS for s/s of stroke, such as difficulty
		speaking, numbness, difficulty moving, or weakness in
		arms or legs. —————————— Carolyn Buyers, RN

PATIENT SELF-GLUCOSE TESTING

A patient with an established diagnosis of diabetes may prefer to use his own glucose meter to test his daily glucose levels. Per policy, your facility will require a doctor's order stating that the patient may use his own glucose meter.

If your patient is permitted to use his own FDA approved glucose meter, you must verify his competency by having him demonstrate the procedure to ensure that he's performing it correctly and using the meter properly. Advise the patient to perform quality control testing on the meter each day. If the patient is using the meter for the first time during this

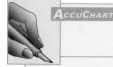

AccuChart

KEEPING A RECORD OF BLOOD GLUCOSE LEVELS

Recommendations for the best time of day to test your blood glucose level depend on your medicine, meal times, and glucose control. On the chart below, your doctor will check the times when you should test your glucose level. Your doctor may also suggest different goals, depending on your situation.

Name: *John Nichols*

Time to test:	Fasting, before breakfast	1 to 2 hours after breakfast	Before lunch	1 to 2 hours after lunch	Before dinner	1 to 2 hours after dinner	Bedtime	3 a.m.
Target goal ranges:*	90-130 mg/dl	<180 mg/dl	90-130 mg/dl	<180 mg/dl	90-130 mg/dl	<180 mg/dl		
Doctor's recommendation	90-110 mg/dl	160 mg/dl	90-110 mg/dl	160 mg/dl	90-110 mg/dl	160 mg/dl	100-130 mg/dl	70-100 mg/dl
Monday	93	159	95	147	97	158	118	84
Tuesday	88	158	98	143	101	161	112	81
Wednesday	89	161	103	156				
Thursday								
Friday								
Saturday								
Sunday								

*The target goals are based on recommendations from the American Diabetes Association. Talk with your doctor about what changes to make if your blood glucose levels are not within this range.

admission, correlate the first glucose result from his meter with a fasting blood glucose level drawn by your facility's laboratory.

Confirm with the patient how to record his blood glucose levels, and stress the importance of bringing results to all follow-up appointments. (See *Keeping a record of blood glucose levels*.) Review blood glucose levels that should be reported immediately. Frequency of testing is determined by whether the patient has type 1 or type 2 diabetes as well as his individual goals.

ESSENTIAL DOCUMENTATION

Verify the doctor's order allowing the patient to use his glucose meter as well as the patient's ability to use his meter by demonstration. Compare the patient's first glucose meter reading with the fasting blood glucose level drawn by your facility's laboratory to correlate the patient's glucose meter accuracy. Then, record the date and time that the patient performs self-glucose monitoring. Be sure to document how often the patient tests the quality control of his meter. Also, document the results of the patient's glucose testing as ordered or per your facility's policy.

2/15/05	1000	Pt. uses his own glucose meter to monitor glucose levels per order by Dr. James Wells using an Optium glucose meter. Pt. demonstrated his ability to properly use his meter. 0800 fasting blood glucose drawn by lab confirmed with pt.'s glucose meter results. Laboratory 0800 fasting blood glucose level was 93 mg/dl. Pt.'s glucose meter reading was 90 mg/dl. Pt. states he checks the quality of the meter every day in the morning and checks his blood glucose every day before meals, 2 hours after meals, and at bedtime and 0300 per dr.'s orders. Pt. verbalized how to record glucose levels and when to call the dr. or emergency services. ———————————— Nancy Cooper, RN

PATIENT TEACHING

Patient and caregiver teaching is essential for maintaining the patient's health, preventing or detecting early signs of complications, and promoting self-care and independence. Patient teaching is every patient's right in any setting. Teaching is most effective when it's specific to the patient's and family's physical, financial, emotional, intellectual, cultural, and social circumstances and when the patient and family are ready to learn, mentally alert, and free from discomfort and distraction.

Keep teaching sessions short, and reinforce all instructions using verbal explanations, demonstrations, videos, and written materials. Evaluate the patient's understanding by asking him to restate material, answer your questions, or give a return demonstration.

Documentation of your teaching is important and lets other health care team members know what the patient has been taught and what materials need to be reinforced. It also serves as a record to back you up if

DOCUMENTING WHAT YOU TEACH

Always document what you teach the patient and his family and their understanding of what you taught. The court in *Kyslinger v. United States (1975)* addressed the nurse's liability for patient teaching. In this case, a veterans administration (VA) hospital sent a hemodialysis patient home with an artificial kidney. He eventually died (apparently while on the hemodialysis machine) and his wife sued, alleging that the hospital and its staff failed to teach either her or her late husband how to properly use and maintain a home hemodialysis unit.

After examining the evidence, the court ruled against the patient's wife, as follows: "During those 10 months that plaintiff's decedent underwent biweekly hemodialysis treatment on the unit (at the VA hospital), both plaintiff and decedent were instructed as to the operation, maintenance, and supervision of said treatment. The Court can find no basis to conclude that the plaintiff or plaintiff's decedent were not properly informed on the use of the hemodialysis unit."

the patient files a lawsuit claiming he was injured because he didn't receive instruction. (See *Documenting what you teach*.)

ESSENTIAL DOCUMENTATION

Check your facility's policies and procedures regarding when, where, and how to document your teaching. Despite their similar content, patient-teaching forms vary according to the health care facility. The forms may ask you to document information by filling in blanks, checking boxes, or writing brief narrative notes. Typically, you'll need to document information about the patient's learning abilities, barriers to learning, goals to be met, equipment or supplies used, specific content taught, response to teaching, and skills to be acquired by the time of discharge. You'll also need to chart how you evaluated the patient's learning, such as by return demonstration or verbalization of understanding. Before discharge, document the patient's remaining learning needs, and note whether you provided him with printed material or other patient-teaching aids.

See *Patient-teaching record* for an example of how to document patient education.

(Text continues on page 302.)

AccuChart

PATIENT-TEACHING RECORD

Use the model patient-teaching form below— for a patient with diabetes mellitus— as a guideline for documenting your teaching sessions clearly and completely.

PATIENT TEACHING
Instructions for Patients with Diabetes

County Hospital, Waltham, MA

Bernard Miller
7 Main St.
Waltham, MA 04872

Admission date: *1/3/06*   **Anticipated discharge:** *1/8/06*   **Diagnosis:** *TIA, type 2 DM*

Educational assessment
Comprehension level
Ability to grasp concepts
☑ High
☐ Average
☐ Needs improvement
Comments: _____

Motivational level
☑ Asks questions
☐ Eager to learn
☐ Anxious
☐ Uncooperative
☐ Disinterested
☐ Denies need to learn
Comments: _____

Knowledge and skill levels
Understanding of health condition
and how to manage it
☐ High (> 75% working knowl-
edge)
☐ Adequate (50% to 75% work-
ing knowledge)
☑ Needs improvement (25% to
50% working knowledge)
☐ Low (< 25% working knowl-
edge)
Comments: _____
_____
_____

Learning barriers
☐ Language (specify: foreign, im-
pairment, laryngectomy, other):
_____
☐ Vision (specify: blind, legally
blind, other): _____
☐ Hearing (impaired,) deaf) _____
  Need to speak loudly
☐ Memory
  ☐ Change in long-term
  memory (specify): _____
  _____
  ☐ Change in short-term
  memory (specify): _____
  _____
☐ Other (specify): _____
  _____
☐ No learning barriers noted
Instructor's initials: *CW*

Anticipated outcomes
Patient will be prepared to perform self-care at the following level:
  ☑ High (total self-care)   ☐ Moderate (self-care with minor   ☐ Minimal (self-care with more
                                    assistance)   than 50% assistance)

(continued)

PATIENT-TEACHING RECORD *(continued)*

Key

P	=	Patient taught	N/A	=	Not applicable	C	=	Expressed denial, resistance
F	=	Caregiver or family taught	A	=	Asked questions	D	=	Verbalized recall
R	=	Reinforced	B	=	Nonattentive, poor concentration	E	=	Demonstrated ability

Date	1/4/06	1/5/06	1/5/06	1/5/06	1/6/06	1/7/06	1/7/06	1/8/06	
Time	1900	0800	1330	1830	1000	0800	1830	0800	
Assessed educational needs									
Assessment of patient's (or caregiver's) current knowledge of disease (include medical, family, and social histories)	A/CW								
Assessment of learner's reaction to diagnosis (verbal and nonverbal responses)	A/CW								
General diabetic education goals The patient (or caregiver) will:									
▪ define diabetes mellitus.	P/A/CW	R/EG	D/ME					D/EG	
▪ state hormone produced in the pancreas.	P/A/CW	R/EG	D/ME					D/EG	
▪ identify three signs and symptoms of diabetes.	P/CW	R/EG	D/ME					D/EG	
▪ discuss risk factors associated with diabetes.	P/CW	R/EG	D/ME					D/EG	
▪ differentiate between type 1 and type 2 diabetes.	P/A/CW	R/EG	D/ME					D/EG	
Survival skill goals The patient (or caregiver) will:									
▪ identify the name, purpose, dose, and time of administration of medication ordered.		P/EG	R/ME	D/LT				D/EG	
▪ properly administer insulin.	N/A								
– draw up insulin properly.	N/A								
– discuss and demonstrate site selection and rotation.	N/A								
– demonstrate proper injection technique with needle angled appropriately.	N/A								
– explain correct way to store insulin.	N/A								
– demonstrate correct disposal of syringes.	N/A								
▪ distinguish among types of insulin.	N/A								
– species (pork or recombinant DNA)	N/A								
– regular	N/A								
– NPH/Ultralente (longer acting)	N/A								

PATIENT-TEACHING RECORD *(continued)*

Key

P	=	Patient taught	N/A	=	Not applicable	C	=	Expressed denial, resistance
F	=	Caregiver or family taught	A	=	Asked questions	D	=	Verbalized recall
R	=	Reinforced	B	=	Nonattentive, poor concentration	E	=	Demonstrated ability

Date	1/4/06	1/5/06	1/5/06	1/5/06	1/6/06	1/7/06	1/7/06	1/8/06	
Time	1900	0800	1330	1830	1000	0800	1830	0800	
▪ properly administer mixed insulins.	N/A								
— demonstrate injecting air into vials.	N/A								
— draw up mixed insulin properly (regular before NPH).	N/A								
▪ demonstrate knowledge of oral antidiabetic agents.									
— identify name of medication, dose, and time of administration.		P/EG	A/ME		D/EG	F/EG	R/LT	D/EG	
— identify purpose of medication.		P/EG	A/ME		D/EG	F/EG	R/LT	D/EG	
— state possible adverse effects.		P/EG	A/ME		D/EG	F/EG	R/LT	D/EG	
▪ list signs and symptoms, causes, implications, and treatments of hyperglycemia and hypoglycemia.		P/EG	A/ME			F/EG		D/EG	
▪ monitor blood glucose levels satisfactorily.									
— demonstrate proper use of blood glucose monitoring device.				P/LT	E/EG	E/EG	R/LT	E/EG	
— perform fingerstick.				P/LT	E/EG	E/EG	R/LT	E/EG	
— obtain accurate blood glucose reading.				P/LT	E/EG	E/EG	R/LT	E/EG	
Healthful living goals The patient (or caregiver) will:									
▪ consult with the nutritionist about meal planning.			P/ME	R/LT	A/EG			D/EG	
▪ follow the diet recommended by the American Diabetes Association.			P/ME	R/LT	A/EG			D/EG	
▪ state importance of adhering to diet.			P/ME	R/LT	A/EG			D/EG	
▪ give verbal feedback on 1-day meal plan.			P/ME	D/LT	A/EG			D/EG	
▪ state the effects of stress, illness, and exercise on blood glucose levels.			P/ME	D/LT	A/EG			D/EG	
▪ state when to test urine for ketones and how to address results.			P/ME	D/LT	A/EG			D/EG	
▪ identify self-care measures for periods when illness occurs.			P/ME	D/LT	A/EG			D/EG	
▪ list precautions to take while exercising.			P/ME	D/LT	A/EG			D/EG	
▪ explain what steps to take when patient doesn't want to eat or drink on proper schedule.			P/ME	D/LT	A/EG			D/EG	
▪ agree to wear medical identification (for example, a Medic Alert bracelet).			P/ME	A/LT				D/EG	

(continued)

PATIENT-TEACHING RECORD *(continued)*

Key

P	=	Patient taught	N/A	=	Not applicable	C	=	Expressed denial, resistance
F	=	Caregiver or family taught	A	=	Asked questions	D	=	Verbalized recall
R	=	Reinforced	B	=	Nonattentive, poor concentration	E	=	Demonstrated ability

	1/4/06	1/5/06	1/5/06	1/5/06	1/6/06	1/7/06	1/7/06	1/8/06	
Date	1/4/06	1/5/06	1/5/06	1/5/06	1/6/06	1/7/06	1/7/06	1/8/06	
Time	1900	0800	1330	1830	1000	0800	1830	0800	
Safety goals The patient (or caregiver) will:									
▪ state the possible complications of diabetes.	P/CW	R/EG		D/LT		F/EG		D/EG	
▪ explain the importance of careful, regular skin care.	P/CW	R/EG		D/LT		F/EG		D/EG	
▪ demonstrate healthful foot care.	P/CW	R/EG		D/LT		F/EG		D/EG	
▪ discuss the importance of regular eye care and examinations.	P/CW	R/EG		D/LT					
▪ state the importance of oral hygiene	P/CW	R/EG		D/LT					
Individual goals									

Initial	Signature								
CW	Carol Witt, RN, BSN								
EG	Ellie Grimes, RN, MSN								
ME	Marianne Evans, RN								
LT	Lynn Tata, RN, BSN								

PATIENT TEACHING, PATIENT'S REFUSAL OF

Although the Patient's Bill of Rights clearly outlines a patient's right to receive information about his condition and treatment, and the Joint Commission on Accreditation of Healthcare Organizations (JCAHO) requires that the patient and his family be provided with education, occasionally you'll come across a patient who doesn't want to be taught. If possible, try to determine the reason for your patient's refusal. You may be able to help the patient overcome some of his barriers to learning or provide instruction to other members of his family.

ESSENTIAL DOCUMENTATION

If a patient doesn't want to be taught, be sure to document the incident. Include the patient's exact words in quotes. If the patient gives you a reason for not wanting to be taught, include that information as well. Note whether you were able to teach another family member or caregiver. Describe specifically what you taught, how you taught it, and the person's response to your teaching. Record the name of the doctor you notified of the patient's refusal to be taught.

7/22/05	1320	When giving pt. his meds at 1230, attempted to tell him
		what each one was for. Pt. waved me away with his hands
		stating, "Tell my wife when she comes in. That's her
		department." Wife came in to visit at 1300 and was
		willing to learn about pt.'s meds. Gave her written
		information for each drug the pt. is taking. Reviewed
		indications for each drug, the dose, frequency, and
		adverse effects. Wife verbalized understanding of each
		med. and made out an appropriate schedule for giving
		her husband his meds at home. Notified Dr. Smith of
		pt.'s unwillingness to be taught. ——— Thomas Daily, RN

PATIENT THREAT OF SELF-HARM

A threat of self-harm may come as a refusal of care, a threat to injure oneself, or a threat to commit suicide. The best way to prevent self-harm is early recognition and treatment of depression and other mental illnesses, including substance abuse. (See "Suicidal intent," page 397, for specific clues to watch for in a hospitalized patient who is at risk for self-harm or suicide.)

When a patient threatens or tries to harm himself, you have a duty to protect him from harm. Use your communication skills to try to calm the patient. Keep talking with him, and ask him to tell you what's bothering him. Let him know you care about him. If possible, remove potentially harmful objects from the immediate area. If the patient is holding a dangerous object and is threatening to harm himself, send a coworker to call security, the nursing supervisor, and the patient's doctor. Don't turn your back on the patient, and stay with him until assistance arrives. If constant observation is ordered, someone must stay with the patient at all times. Administer medications, as ordered. Restraints should be used as a last resort, according to your facility's policy.

ESSENTIAL DOCUMENTATION

Record the date and time of your entry. Record, in the patient's own words, his threat to harm himself. Objectively describe any behaviors that indicate a desire for self-harm. Note all steps taken immediately to protect the patient from harm, such as one-to-one observation and removal of any potential weapons from the immediate environment. Chart the names of the doctor, nursing supervisor, security officer, and risk manager notified and the time of notification. Document their responses, your interventions, and the patient's response. Record any explanations given to the patient and efforts to reduce anxiety.

1/1/06	1655	*Heard thumping noise in room at 1625 and found pt.*
		beating his fist against wall. Asked pt. to stop beating Ⓡ
		fist and tell nurse what was bothering him. Pt. replied,
		"I'm better, and my wife doesn't visit. If I was hurt,
		maybe she would visit." Asked pt. to sit on his bed and
		he complied. Sat on chair across from pt. and listened
		as he spoke of family problems. Pt. agreed to talk with
		social worker. Pt. able to move fingers of Ⓡ hand, no
		bruising noted, no c/o pain. Called Meg Watkins, CNA, to
		sit with pt. and talk to him while doctor was called.
		Spoke with Dr. Sterling at 1635 who agreed to referral
		to social worker. Dr. Sterling will be by to see pt. at
		1700. Andrew O'Toole, social worker, called at 1640
		and will be by immediately to see pt. Will have CNA stay
		with pt. until social worker and doctor arrive. CNA
		instructed to speak calmly with pt. and to call nurse
		immediately if pt. resumes harmful behaviors. ———
		——————————————————— *Maria Perez, RN*

PATIENT THREAT TO HARM ANOTHER

When a patient threatens to harm someone else — whether verbally or by making threatening gestures — quick action is needed because a threat can turn to violence. Follow your facility's policy for dealing with a patient who threatens to harm someone else. Remove the person being threatened from the immediate area. Use your communication skills to calm the patient and reduce agitation. Call the doctor, nursing supervisor, security, and risk manager to inform them of the patient's threats. Stay with the patient. If your own safety is threatened, have another coworker stay with you if necessary. Assess your patient for physical and psychosocial triggers to violence. Share your findings with the doctor and nursing supervisor.

ESSENTIAL DOCUMENTATION

Record the date and time in your nurse's note. Chart the location of the incident. Describe the threat, quote exactly what the patient said, and record threatening behaviors or gestures. Record your immediate interventions and the patient's response. Chart the names of the people you notified, such as the doctor, nursing supervisor, security, and risk manager; the time of notification; and their responses. Include your assessment results and the people with whom you shared the results. Record any changes in the care plan. Don't name another patient in your patient's chart; this violates confidentiality. Use the word "roommate" or "visitor," or give a room and bed number to describe the person threatened.

Complete an incident report, repeating the exact information that is in your nurse's note. Include names, addresses, and telephone numbers of witnesses. This is the place to document the name of the threatened person.

5/29/05	0315	Pt. pacing back and forth in room at 0300, muttering
		phrases such as "I'll take care of it my way. I'll take care
		of him real good," while punching one hand into the other.
		Pt.'s roommate awoke and moved to another room. At 0310
		Dr. Chi, nursing supervisor Ron Hardy, RN, and security
		officer Tom Gulden were notified of pt.'s threats toward
		his roommate. Message left on voice mail of risk manage-
		ment dept. Pt. alert, not oriented to time and date, states
		when asked his name, "I'm going to get him." c/o "bad smell
		in here." No foul odor noted. Face red, diaphoretic, draws
		away from touch. Trying to open sealed window to "let the
		bad smell out." Breathing easily, skin color other than face
		is pink. Extremities moving well. Chart shows meds taken as
		prescribed, pt. admitted to r/o seizure disorder. ————
		—————————————— Carla Aiken, RN
	0345	Dr. Chi, Mr. Hardy, and Mr. Gulden arrived on unit at
		0320. Assessment findings shared with them. Pt. less
		agitated. No longer punching his palm. Assisted back to bed.
		P 88 and regular, BP 136/94, RR 32. I.V. line started in Ⓡ
		forearm with #20 angiocath on first attempt. 1000 ml
		NSS running at 30 ml/hr. Dilantin 100 mg given as slow
		I.V. bolus by Dr. Chi. Lab called to draw Dilantin level in a.m.
		Order for Dilantin 100 mg P.O. t.i.d. transcribed to MAR.
		Pt. now sleeping. Will check pt. q15min. —— Carla Aiken, RN

PATIENT THREAT OF LAWSUIT

A patient who threatens to sue a facility or health care provider usually perceives a potential or actual threat to his health, rights, or safety. All implied threats of a lawsuit should be taken seriously and should be reported to your nursing supervisor or your employer's legal department or attorney. (See *Reducing the risk of a lawsuit,* page 306.) Without admitting wrong-doing, talk to your patient about his concerns. Use therapeutic communication skills and, if appropriate, provide teaching or other interventions as necessary. Assess his physical and emotional status.

REDUCING THE RISK OF A LAWSUIT

Patients who are more likely to file lawsuits against nurses share certain personality traits and behaviors. Additionally, nurses who are more likely to be named as defendants also have certain characteristics in common.

BEWARE OF THESE PATIENTS

Although not all persons displaying the behaviors listed below will file a lawsuit, a little extra caution in your dealings with them won't hurt. Providing professional and competent care to such patients will lessen their tendency to sue.

A patient who is likely to file a lawsuit may:

- persistently criticize all aspects of the nursing care provided
- purposefully not follow the care plan
- overreact to any perceived slight or negative comment, real or imagined
- unjustifiably depend on nurses for all aspects of care and refuse to accept any responsibility for his own care
- openly express hostility to nurses and other health care personnel
- project his anxiety or anger onto the nursing staff, attributing blame for all negative events to health care providers
- have previously filed lawsuits.

NURSES AT RISK

Nurses who are most likely to be named as defendants in a lawsuit display certain characteristic behaviors. If you recognize any of these attributes within yourself, changing your behavior will reduce your risk of liability.

A nurse who is likely to be a defendant in a lawsuit may:

- be insensitive to the patient's complaints or fail to take them seriously
- fail to identify and meet the patient's emotional and physical needs
- refuse to recognize the limits of her nursing skills and personal competency
- lack sufficient education for the tasks and responsibilities associated with a specific practice setting
- display an authoritarian and inflexible attitude when providing care
- inappropriately delegate responsibilities to subordinates.

ESSENTIAL DOCUMENTATION

Follow your facility's policy, and document the following information in your nurse's note or on another appropriate form such as an incident report:

- date and time that the patient made the threat of a lawsuit; record the patient's threat using his own words in quotes
- patient's mental and physical condition before, during, and after he threatened to sue
- your actions in response to the threat and your assessment

- names of witnesses (including family members, visitors, and other staff members) who overheard the discussion
- names of people that you notified of the patient's threat to sue and the date and time of notification
- any actions that may have contributed to the incident.

1/26/06	1000	Pt. states, "I plan to file a lawsuit against this facility for causing my bed sores." Pt. very agitated and refusing to discuss issue any further. Dr. Collins and risk manager Judy Robbins, RN, notified. ———— Carol Moore, RN

PATIENT TRANSFER TO ASSISTED LIVING FACILITY

Many care and service options are available to elderly people to help them function at their highest level of independence. Assisted living provides the elderly person with meals, assistance with activities of daily living (ADLs), health care, 24-hour supervision, and other supportive systems.

Transfer to an assisted living facility requires preparation and careful documentation. Preparation includes explaining the transfer to the patient and his family, discussing the patient's condition and care plan with the assisted living staff, and arranging for transportation, if necessary. Documentation of the patient's condition before transfer and adequate communication between nursing staffs ensure continuity of nursing care and provide legal protection for the transferring facility and its staff.

ESSENTIAL DOCUMENTATION

Record the date and time of the transfer in your nurse's note. Include the doctor's name, and indicate that transfer orders have been written. Record the name of the assisted living facility to which the patient will be discharged and the name of the nurse who received your verbal report. Indicate that discharge instructions were written and that a copy was given to and discussed with the patient. Have the patient sign a personal belongings form acknowledging that he has all his belongings. In your note, record that the form was completed and placed in the medical record. Describe the condition of your patient at discharge. Be sure to include vital signs and descriptions of wounds as well as tubes and other equipment still in place. Chart the time of discharge, who accompanied the patient, the mode of transportation, and the name of the person at the assisted living facility who will be receiving the patient. Indicate that the medical record was copied and sent with the patient.

Document that transfer forms have been completed and one copy is being sent to the receiving facility. (See *Referral form.*) Although details may vary, the transfer form may contain the following information:

- demographic patient information
- financial information
- receiving facility information
- medical information, including diagnoses, surgeries, allergies, laboratory test values, and advance directives
- family contacts
- services needed, such as physical, occupational, or speech therapy; dialysis; or wound management
- doctor's information and orders
- medication information, including last dose given
- assessment of body systems
- ability to perform ADLs.

3/4/05	1100	Pt. transferred to The Oaks Assisted Living Facility at
		1030. Pt. transported to front door in wheelchair,
		accompanied by pt.'s daughter, Evelyn Tomin, and me.
		Pt. assisted into car and transported by her daughter.
		Personal belongings sheet completed and signed by pt.
		Personal belongings packed by daughter and placed in
		suitcase to be transported with pt. Transfer orders
		written by Dr. Chang. Verbal report given to Cathy
		O'Rourke, RN, who will be receiving pt. Transfer forms
		completed by health care team members, copy sent with
		pt. to The Oaks. Copy of medical record also sent with
		pt. Discharge instruction sheet completed and reviewed
		with daughter and pt. Copy given to pt. Pt. and daughter
		verbalized understanding of med schedule, times, doses,
		and adverse effects to report to Dr. Chang. On dis-
		charge, pt. is alert and oriented to time, place, and
		person. P 88, BP 148/84, RR 22, oral T 97.0° F. Lungs
		clear, normal heart sounds, positive bowel sounds in all 4
		quadrants, urinating without problems, skin warm, dry,
		and intact. On no-added-salt diet, ambulating on own
		with walker. Wears glasses and bilateral hearing aids.
		———————— Thomas Corrigan, RN

(Text continues on page 312.)

AccuChart

REFERRAL FORM

Documentation of the patient's condition before transfer and adequate communication between nursing staffs ensure continuity of nursing care and provide legal protection for the transferring facility and its staff. Referral forms such as the one below contain basic information about the patient and his care.

REFERRAL FORM

PATIENT INFORMATION

Last Name: *Tomlin*   MR#: *1234*

First Name: *Vera*   MR#:

Address: *123 Main St.*

City: *Newtown*   State: *VA* Zip: *22222*

County: Marital Status: *W*

Telephone: *(123) 456-7890* S.S. #: *111-22-3333*

Age: *90* Sex: *F* Height: *5'3"* Weight: *126#* DOB: *2/8/16*

Adm. date: *2/26/05*   Discharge date: *3/4/05*

FINANCIAL INFORMATION

Primary: Medicare #:

Medicaid: County:

Policy #:   Group #:

Secondary:

Precert #:

Level of Care: ☐ CORF   ☐ ICF   ☐ SNF   ☐ Rehab Hospital
              ☑ Assisted ☐ Home Health   ☐ ICF-MR

MEDICAL INFORMATION

Primary Dx: (date) *Fx @ arm*   *2/26/05*

Secondary Dx: *Type 2 DM*

Surgery: (date) *2/27/05 open reduction*

Allergies: *none*

Prior functional status: *independent*

Advance Directives: ☑ Living Will   ☑ Power of Attorney
                       ☑ DNR   ☐ Legal Guardian
                       ☐ PASSAR   ☐ Level of Care

FAMILY or GUARDIAN

Last Name: *Tomlin*

First Name: *Evelyn*

Relationship: *daughter*

(H)#: *(123) 456-7890*   (W)#:

SERVICES REQUIRED

☑ PT   ☐ OT   ☐ ST   ☐ I.V. Therapy ☐ Hook Up

☐ Skilled Nursing ☐ Social Services ☐ Pain Management

☐ Home Health Aid ☐ RT   ☐ Wound Management

☐ Enteral Fdgs. ☐ TPN ☐ Nut. Tx.   ☐ Palliative Care ☐ Hospice

☐ Dialysis: ☐ Peritoneal ☐ Hemo   ☐ Ventilator Weaning/
                                      Maintenance
Day/week:

Location:

Established Post Hospital LOS: ☐ Other
☑ < 30 days   ☐ > 30 days

AGENCY ACCEPTING REFERRAL

Name: *The Oaks Assisted Living Facility*

Contact: *Cathy O'Rourke, RN*

Phone: *(123) 987-6543*   FAX:

Name:

Contact:

Phone: FAX:

PHYSICIAN

MD ordering: *Dr. Chang*   Phone:

MD to follow: *Dr. Meadows*   Phone:

Other   Phone:

Prognosis *good*

To the best of my knowledge, all information provided about the individual is a true and accurate reflection of the patient's needs. I certify that inpatient care is required at: Level: ☐ Skilled ☑ Intermediate

Physician Signature: *Dr. Chang*

Date signed: *3/5/05*

(continued)

REFERRAL FORM *(continued)*

Patient Name: *Vera Tomlin*

LAB ORDERS

Labs: _____   Labs: _____

_____   _____

Call or FAX results to: _____   Call or Fax results to: _____

Phone: _____ FAX: _____   Phone: _____ FAX: _____

GENERAL PHYSICIAN ORDERS

PT to Ⓛ arm

1800-cal ADA diet

DNR

Home Medications	Last Dose Given	Dosage	Route	Frequency	Dosing Times	Start Date	End Date
Glucotrol	*0730*	*5 mg*	*PO*	*daily*	*0730*		
Lasix	*0730*	*10 mg*	*PO*	*daily*	*0730*		

☐ HIVAT (see Final HIVAT Script)

Comments/Delivery: _____

PHYSICAL THERAPY NOTES/PLAN

Assist for transfers supine to sit: ☐ Max ☐ Mod ☐ Min ☐ Contact Guard ☐ Superv ☐ Verbal Cue ☐ Tactile Cue ☑ Independ

Assist for transfers sit to stand: ☐ Max ☐ Mod ☐ Min ☐ Contact Guard ☐ Superv ☐ Verbal Cue ☐ Tactile Cue ☑ Independ

Ambulated _____ feet with: ☐ Walker ☐ Crutches ☐ Quad cane ☐ Straight cane ☐ W/o device ☐ Nonambulatory
☐ W/wheels ☐ W/platform attachments

With assistance needed: ☐ Max ☐ Mod ☐ Min ☐ Contact Guard ☐ Superv ☐ Verbal Cue ☐ Tactile Cue ☑ Independ

Weight Bearing Status: ☐ NWB ☐ TDNWB ☐ TDWB ☐ PWB ☐ WBAT ☐ FWB ☐ On which leg: ☐ Right ☐ Left ☐ Both

Plan: *strengthen Ⓛ arm* ☐ Therapy EX ☐ Bed Mobility Plan ☐ Transfer Training ☐ Gait Training

Goal: *regain function Ⓛ arm* Demonstrates understanding of home safety precautions ☑ Yes ☐ No

PT Additional Comments: _____

Signature: *Mary Jones*   Title: *PT*   Phone: *(123) 234-8290*   Date: *3/4/05*

REFERRAL FORM *(continued)*

Patient Name: _Vera Tomlin_

ASSESSMENT

Cardio-pulmonary				
BP _148/84_	☐ Oxygen		☐ Chest Tube(s)	☐ CXR (date):
Pulse _88_	Rate _____ Method _____		☐ Vent Settings	☐ TB (date):
Temp _97.0° F_	☐ Secretions (describe):			
Resp _22_	☐ Tracheostomy Size: _____ Type: _____			

Nutrition and Hydration

Diet _1800 cal ADA_ ☑ Feeds self   ☐ Dehydration   Access device: _____
Consistency _regular_   ☐ Assist feed ☐ Total feed   ☐ Edema
☐ Teeth ☐ No teeth   ☐ Hyperalimentation   ☐ Nausea   Insertion date: _____
☑ Dentures type _____   ☐ Feeding tube type _____ ☐ Vomiting   Last flushed: _____
   upper/lower   ☐ Dysphagia
☐ Dentures with patient   Date inserted _____   ☐ Poor appetite

Sensory-Comfort

	VISION	HEARING	SPEECH	COMFORT	COMMENTS
	☑ Adequate	☑ Adequate	☑ Good	Pain? ☐ Yes ☑ No	
	☐ Poor	☐ Poor	☐ Difficult	Where? When?	
	☐ Blind	☐ Deaf	☐ Unable		
	☑ Glasses	☐ Aid in _____ ear	Language: _____		
	☐ Contacts				

Pyschosocial

	MENTAL STATUS	BEHAVIOR	SUPPORTS
	☑ Alert	☐ Wanders	Supports:
	☐ Lethargic	☑ Cooperative	
	☐ Comatose	☐ Combative	_daughter – Evelyn Tomlin_
	☐ Oriented	☐ Forgetful	
	☐ Disoriented	☐ Sleep Problems	Safety:
	☐ Confused	☐ Other (specify)	
	☐ Anxious		

Elimination

	BLADDER	BOWEL	TOILETING	
	☑ Continent	☑ Continent	☑ Independent	☐ Bedpan
	☐ Incontinent	☐ Incontinent	☐ Dependent	☐ Catheter
	☐ Retention	☐ Constipation	☐ Toilet	Type _____
	☐ Frequency	☐ Diarrhea	☐ Ostomy	Size _____
	☐ Dribbling	☐ Last BM: _3/4/05_	Type _____	Date inserted: _____
			Appliance _____	

Skin

Skin intact? ☑ Yes ☐ No
Describe any impairments: _Incision ⓛ upper arm intact, healing well_

	INDEPENDENT	ASSIST	TOTAL DEPENDENT	EQUIPMENT/# PERSONS USED
Hygiene Oral Care	✓			
Bathing		✓		_needs help of 1 until arm heals_
Dressing		✓		
Wheelchair				
Mobility Transfer	✓			
Ambulation	✓			
	☐ Amputation ☐ Contractures ☐ Paralysis ☐ Paresis ☐ Other			

Labs

Test	Date	Result	Test	Date	Result	Test	Date	Result	Isolation Precautions?
									Last culture date:
									Results:

PATIENT TRANSFER TO LONG-TERM CARE FACILITY

Most older adults are cared for at home, either by themselves or by their families. However, as many as 25% will need long-term care (LTC) assistance in their later years.

Several types of LTC facilities are available. An assisted living facility provides meals, sheltered living, and some medical monitoring. This type of facility is appropriate for someone who doesn't need continuous medical attention.

An intermediate care facility provides custodial care for individuals unable to care for themselves due to mental or physical infirmities. Intermediate care facilities provide room, board, and regular nursing care. Physical, social, and recreational activities are provided, and some facilities have rehabilitation programs.

A skilled nursing facility provides medical supervision, rehabilitation services, and 24-hour nursing care by registered nurses, licensed practical nurses, and nurses' aides for patients who have the potential to regain function.

ESSENTIAL DOCUMENTATION

In your note, record the date and time of the transfer, the doctor's name, and that transfer orders were written. Note the long-term care facility's name and the name of the nurse who received your verbal report. Note that discharge instructions were written and that a copy was discussed with the patient and given to him. You'll need to have the patient sign a personal belongings form acknowledging that he has all his belongings. Remember to record that the form was completed and placed in the medical record. In your note, describe the condition of your patient at discharge, including vital signs, descriptions of wounds, and tubes or other equipment that's still in place. Record the time of discharge, who accompanied the patient, the mode of transportation, and the name of the person at the long-term care facility who will be receiving him. Indicate that the medical record was copied and sent with the patient.

Document that transfer forms have been completed. Also, indicate that one copy is being sent to the receiving facility.

The transfer form may contain the following information:

- demographic patient information
- financial information
- receiving facility information
- medical information, including diagnoses, surgeries, allergies, laboratory test values, and advance directives
- family contacts
- services needed, such as physical, occupational, or speech therapy; dialysis; or wound management
- doctor's information and orders
- medication information, including last dose given
- assessment of body systems
- ability to perform activities of daily living.

5/11/05	1300	Pt. transferred to Aristocrat Skilled Nursing Facility at
		1230. Pt. transported by stretcher via Metro ambulance.
		Personal belongings list completed and placed in chart.
		Copy placed with belongings sent with pt. Transfer
		orders written by Dr. Desai. Verbal report given to
		Rachel Peters, RN, who will be receiving pt. Transfer
		forms completed, copy sent with pt. Copy of medical
		records also sent with pt. At the time of discharge, pt.
		alert and oriented to person but not to place, date, and
		time. P 72, BP 128/70, RR 18, oral T 98.2° F. Lungs clear
		with diminished breath sounds at bases, normal heart
		sounds, positive bowel sounds in all 4 quadrants, incontinent
		of bladder and bowels. Skin warm, dry, pedal pulses
		palpable, no edema. Has stage 2 ulcer on coccyx, 2 cm X
		2 cm and approximately 2 mm deep, red granulation
		tissue at base, transparent dressing covering wound. See
		referral form for treatments. ——— Kristen Rice, RN

PATIENT TRANSFER TO SPECIALTY UNIT

Specialty units provide continuous and intensive monitoring of patients and constant and spontaneous care to persons who have limited tolerance for delay. Specialty units include perioperative units, labor and delivery units, burn units, and the many types of intensive care units.

Specialty units rely on close and continuous assessment by registered nurses as well as multiple uses of technological monitoring. Medication administration is complex and frequent; measurements are performed hourly or more frequently.

ESSENTIAL DOCUMENTATION

Record the date and time of the transfer and the name of the unit receiving the patient. Document that you received transfer orders. Describe the patient's condition at the time of transfer, including vital signs, descriptions of incisions and wounds, and locations of tubes or medical devices still in place. Report significant events that occurred during the hospital stay. Be sure to note whether the patient has advance directives and include special factors, such as allergies, special diet, sensory deficits, and language or cultural issues. List medications, treatments, and teaching needs. Note which goals were and weren't met. Chart that you gave a report to the receiving unit, and include the name of the nurse who received the report. Note how the patient was transported to the specialty unit and who accompanied him. Include patient teaching given that related to the transfer such as explaining to the patient why he's being transferred. Some facilities may use a transfer form to record this information.

5/24/05	1430	Pt. is 63 y.o. white English-speaking female, with early
		Alzheimer's disease, being transferred from medical unit
		to MICU by stretcher accompanied by her daughter and
		medical resident. Report given to Sue Riff, RN. Advance
		directives in chart. Pt. unresponsive to verbal stimuli,
		opens eyes to painful stimuli. Prior to this episode,
		daughter reports pt. was alert and oriented to person but
		not always to place and time. Daughter states that pt.'s
		forgetfulness and confusion have recently gotten worse.
		Found alone in her apartment 2 days ago, unresponsive,
		no food eaten or dishes used since last groceries
		purchased for pt. 5 days ago. Pt. is severely dehydrated
		despite 2000 ml over last 24 hr. Currently NPO. I.V.
		infusion with 18G catheter in Ⓡ antecubital vein with 0.45%
		NSS at 75 ml/hr. AP 124 irregular, BP 84/palp, RR 28,
		rectal T 100.0° F, weight 78 lb, height 64". Allergies to
		molds, pollen, and mildew. Lungs clear, normal heart
		sounds. Skin intact, pale, cool, poor skin turgor. Radial
		pulses weak, pedal pulses not palpable. Foley catheter in
		place draining approx. 30 ml/hr. Dr.'s orders written.
		Medical record, MAR, and nursing Kardex transferred
		with pt. ———————————————— Diana Starr, RN

PATIENT'S BELONGINGS, AT ADMISSION

Encourage patients to send home their money, jewelry, and other valuable belongings. If a patient refuses to do so, make a list of his possessions and store them according to your facility's policy.

Place valuable items in an envelope and other personal belongings in approved containers; then label them with the patient's identification number. Never use garbage containers, laundry bags, or other unauthorized receptacles for valuables because they could be discarded accidentally.

ESSENTIAL DOCUMENTATION

Make a list of the patient's valuables and include a description of each one. Most facilities provide an area on the nursing admission form to list the belongings. To protect yourself and your employer, ask the patient (or a responsible family member) to sign or witness the list that you compile so that you both understand the items for which you're responsible.

Use objective language to describe each item, noting its color, approximate size, style, type, and serial number or other distinguishing features. Don't assess the item's value or authenticity. For example, you might describe a diamond ring as a "clear, round stone set in a yellow metal band."

Besides jewelry and money, include dentures, eyeglasses or contact lenses, hearing aids, prostheses, and clothing on the list.

3/9/05	1500	*Pt. admitted to room 318 with one pair of brown glasses, upper and lower dentures, a yellow metal ring with a red stone on 4th ⓛ finger, a pink bathrobe, and a black radio. —————————— Paul Cullen, RN*

PATIENT'S BELONGINGS, MISSING

Patients admitted into health care facilities will undoubtedly bring personal items, ranging from clothing to eyeglasses, hearing aids, and electronic devices. Because of the number of health care employees providing care to a patient, coupled with the lack of locks on patient rooms and furniture, personal items can be misplaced or lost. When items are lost, patients may hold the facility responsible.

Upon admission, encourage patients to send belongings home with a family member or to lock valuables in the facility's safe, and document that you told them to do so. That way, if items are missing later, you'll have documentation to support your facility's case.

Some facilities no longer use checklists and now instruct the patient to send personal belongings home with family members. The patient is then expected to assume responsibility for his own personal items left behind at the hospital.

When a patient believes an item is missing, check the list of his belongings and ask family members if they took the item home. Help the patient search his room. If the item can't be found, notify security and the nursing supervisor.

ESSENTIAL DOCUMENTATION

Depending on your facility's policy, you may have a special form on which to document missing items or you may have to complete an incident report. Chart the date and time you learned about the missing item, and objectively describe it. Record whether the item was on the list of belongings made upon admission. Note that you asked family members if they took the item home. Include the last time and place the item was seen. Describe how you helped the patient search for the item. Document the names of the people that you notified, such as security and the nursing supervisor, the time of notification, and their actions.

7/15/05	0900	At 0815 pt. reported his electric razor missing. Item
		was on belongings list made at admission. Pt. called wife
		at home who said she didn't take it home. Pt. last
		remembers using razor prior to surgery. Pre-op unit
		called. Razor found in bathroom of pt.'s previous room.
		Volunteer will bring pt. his razor. ——— Sandy Kelly, RN

PATIENT'S CONDITION, CHANGE IN

One of your major responsibilities is to document any change in a patient's condition. You'll also need to record the name of the doctor you notified and his response. Unless you properly document your conversation, the doctor could claim he wasn't notified should a patient's care subsequently come into question.

Nurses often write "Notified doctor of patient's condition." This statement is too vague. In the event of a malpractice suit, it allows the plain-

COMMUNICATING A CHANGE IN THE PATIENT'S CONDITION

To ensure clear communication when discussing a patient's care with a doctor on the phone, remember to keep the following points in mind:

■ If you don't know the doctor, ask him to state and spell his full name.

■ Include the exact time you contacted the doctor. To establish proof, you could have another nurse listen in and then cosign the time of notification. If you don't note the time you called, allegations may be made later that you failed to obtain timely medical treatment for the patient.

■ Always note in the chart the specific change, problem, or result you reported to the doctor, along with the doctor's orders or response. Use his own words, if possible.

■ If you're reporting a critical laboratory test result (for example, a serum potassium level of 3.2 mEq/L but don't receive an order for intervention (such as potassium replacement therapy), be sure to verify with the doctor that he doesn't want to give an order. Then document this fact in the progress notes. For example, you'd write: "Dr. Jones informed of potassium level of 3.2 mEq/L. No orders received."

■ If you think a doctor's failure to order an intervention puts your patient's health at risk, follow the chain of command and notify your supervisor. Then be sure to document your action.

tiff's lawyer (and the doctor) to imply that you didn't communicate the essential data. The chart should include exactly what you told the doctor. (See *Communicating a change in the patient's condition*.)

ESSENTIAL DOCUMENTATION

Your note should include the date and time that you notified the doctor, the doctor's name, and what you reported. Record the doctor's response and orders given. If no orders are given, document that also.

| 3/29/05 | 0900 | Pt. had moderate-sized, soft, dark brown stools positive for blood by quaiac test. Abdomen soft, nontender, positive bowel sounds heard in all 4 quadrants. Skin warm, pink, capillary refill less than 3 sec. P 92, BP 128/68, RR 28, oral T 97.2° F. Dr. Rodriguez notified at 0915. Added hemoglobin and hematocrit to morning blood work. Doctor in to discuss with pt. the need for colonoscopy. Pt. agreed to procedure, which is scheduled for 0800 on 3/30/05. Explained bowel prep procedure to pt. —————————— Jackie Paterno, RN |

PERIPHERAL PULSE, ABSENT

If not quickly resolved, loss of a peripheral pulse compromises blood flow to the limb, leading to ischemia and infarction. The most common cause of acute loss of a peripheral pulse is embolization of thrombi from the heart and from atherosclerotic plaque. Other diseases and conditions that may lead to loss of peripheral pulse include diabetes mellitus with peripheral vascular disease, aortic aneurysm, peripheral artery trauma, certain drugs, infection, invasive procedures, and devices, such as casts, splints, or braces.

Your assessments and prompt interventions can save your patient's limb, and even his life, when arterial pulses are absent. Notify the doctor immediately, and anticipate administering such drugs as vasodilators, anticoagulants, and thrombolytic therapy.

ESSENTIAL DOCUMENTATION

Record the date and time of your entry. Document your assessment findings of the affected and unaffected limbs, such as pain, absent pulses, numbness, tingling, weakness or paralysis, slow capillary refill, and pale, cool skin. Describe any lesions on the affected limb. Note whether a pulse can be heard by Doppler. Record the name of the doctor notified, the time of notification, and orders given, such as administering a vasodilator, an anticoagulant, or thrombolytic drugs or preparing the patient for embolectomy or thrombectomy. Record your interventions, such as administering drugs, providing for comfort, proper positioning, relieving pressure, and protecting the affected limb. Chart your patient's response to these interventions. Flow sheets may be used to document frequent assessments, vital signs, intake and output, I.V. therapy, and laboratory test values, such as partial thromboplastin time (PTT), prothrombin time, and International Normalized Ratio. Document patient teaching and emotional support rendered.

11/30/05	1115	Called to pt.'s room at 1040 by pt. who reported
		sudden onset of pain in Ⓛ calf and numbness of Ⓛ
		foot. Ⓛ foot and calf cool to touch and pale; upper
		leg warm and pink. Ⓛ femoral pulse palpable; unable
		to palpate popliteal and dorsalis pedis pulses. Faint
		popliteal pulse heard by Doppler. Ⓛ leg movement weak.
		Ⓡ leg warm and pink over entire length, capillary refill
		less than 3 sec., strong femoral, popliteal, and dorsalis
		pedis pulses. No c/o pain or numbness in Ⓡ leg and
		foot. Able to move Ⓡ leg and foot, good strength. Skin
		intact both legs. P 98, BP 140/84, RR 28, oral T 98.2° F.
		Dr. Hensley called at 1050 and notified of assessment
		findings. Doctor came to see pt. at 1100. Heparin
		5000-unit bolus given I.V. in Ⓡ forearm, followed
		by 1000-unit/hr infusion. PTT to be drawn at 1700.
		Positioned pt. with Ⓛ leg flat in bed, footboard in place.
		See flow sheets for documentation of frequent VS,
		I/O, and PTT. Explained reason for heparin to pt., who
		verbalized understanding. Reviewed s/s to report
		immediately, such as increased pain, numbness, or
		tingling. ————————————Steve Bates, RN

PERIPHERALLY INSERTED CENTRAL CATHETER, INSERTION OF

For a patient who needs central venous (CV) therapy for 1 to 6 months or requires repeated venous access, a peripherally inserted central catheter (PICC) may be the best option. Made of silicone or polyurethane, a PICC is soft and flexible with increased biocompatibilty and is available in single and double lumens. The doctor may order a PICC if the patient has suffered trauma or burns resulting in chest injury or if he has respiratory compromise due to chronic obstructive pulmonary disease, a mediastinal mass, cystic fibrosis, or pneumothorax. With any of these conditions, a PICC helps avoid complications that may occur with a CV line.

PICCs are being used increasingly for patients receiving home care. The device is easier to insert than other CV devices and provides safe, reliable access for drug administration and blood sampling.

Infusions commonly given by PICC include total parenteral nutrition, chemotherapy, antibiotics, opioids, and analgesics.

Some state nurse practice acts permit nurses to insert PICC lines; those that do require that nurses receive certification after mandatory course work and successful supervised practice. Nurses may also need to demonstrate their skills in PICC line insertion and care on a yearly basis to remain certified.

ESSENTIAL DOCUMENTATION

Record the date and time of insertion, and note that the procedure has been explained to the patient and all questions have been answered. Document the entire procedure, including problems with catheter placement. Also, chart the size, length, and type of catheter as well as the insertion site. Record flush solutions. Describe the dressing applied. Document that a chest X-ray verified tip placement before initial use. Record the patient's tolerance of the procedure.

6/30/05	1200	PICC insertion procedure explained to pt. and husband.
		After asking many questions about PICC care, pt. and
		husband verbalized understanding of the procedure.
		Antecubital–shoulder–sternal notch measurement 20¼".
		Using sterile technique, PICC cut to 23¼". Extension
		tubing and catheter flushed w/NSS. Ⓛ basilic vein site
		prepared with povidone-iodine. With pt. in supine
		position and Ⓛ arm at 90-degree angle, catheter
		introducer inserted into vein at 10-degree angle; blood
		return noted. Catheter introduced and advanced to
		shoulder. Instructed pt. to turn head Ⓛ and place chin
		on chest. Catheter then advanced until only 4" remained.
		Introducer sheath removed, and catheter advanced
		until completely inserted. Catheter flushed with NSS
		followed by heparin. See MAR. 2" X 2" gauze pad placed
		over site, covered by sterile transparent semipermeable
		dressing. CXR done at 1150 to check tip placement;
		results pending. Following procedure, pt. sitting up
		in bed talking with husband. No c/o pain, except for
		"minor" discomfort at insertion site. — Anita Cain, RN

PERIPHERALLY INSERTED CENTRAL CATHETER SITE CARE

Proper site care and dressing changes are vital to preventing infection. Follow your facility's policy for the procedure and frequency of site care. Keep in mind, though, that a dressing should be changed any time it becomes wet or soiled or it loses integrity.

After the initial insertion, apply a new sterile, transparent, semipermeable dressing without using gauze because gauze may hold moisture, be a haven for bacteria, and promote skin maceration. Thereafter, change the dressing every 3 to 7 days, according to your facility's policy, or as needed.

Assess the catheter insertion site through the transparent semipermeable dressing every 24 hours, or per your facility's policy. Look at the catheter and cannula pathway, and check for bleeding, redness, drainage, and swelling. Question the patient about pain at the site.

ESSENTIAL DOCUMENTATION

Record the date and time of site care. Note that you have explained the procedure to the patient and answered his questions. Describe the condition of the site, noting any bleeding, redness, drainage, and swelling. Document pain or discomfort reported by the patient. Note the name of the doctor notified of complications, the time of notification, orders given, your interventions, and the patient's response. Record how the site was cleaned and the type of dressing applied. Chart the patient's tolerance of the procedure and any patient teaching you provide.

10/31/05	1100	Explained dressing change and site care for PICC to
		pt. Pt. verbalized understanding. Placed pt. in seated
		position with ℚ arm at 45-degree angle from body. Old
		dressing removed, no redness, bleeding, drainage, or
		swelling. No c/o pain at site. Using sterile technique,
		site cleaned with alcohol, followed by povidone-iodine.
		Sterile, transparent, semipermeable dressing applied
		and tubing secured to edge of dressing with tape. Pt.
		reports no pain or tenderness following the dressing
		change. Reminded pt. to report pain or discomfort at
		insertion site or in ℚ arm to nurse. — Lillian Mott, RN

PERITONEAL DIALYSIS

Peritoneal dialysis is indicated for patients with chronic renal failure who have cardiovascular instability, vascular access problems that prevent hemodialysis, fluid overload, or electrolyte imbalances. In this procedure, dialysate – the solution instilled into the peritoneal cavity by a catheter – draws waste products, excess fluid, and electrolytes from the blood across the semipermeable peritoneal membrane. After a prescribed period, the dialysate is drained from the peritoneal cavity, removing impurities with it. The dialysis procedure is then repeated, using a new dialysate each time until waste removal is complete and fluid, electrolyte, and acid-base balances have been restored. Peritoneal dialysis may be performed manually or by using an automatic or semiautomatic cycle machine.

ESSENTIAL DOCUMENTATION

Record the date and time of dialysis. During and after dialysis, monitor and document the patient's response to treatment. Record his vital signs every 10 to 15 minutes for the first 1 to 2 hours of exchanges and then every 2 to 4 hours or as often as necessary. If you detect any abrupt changes in the patient's condition, document them, notify the doctor, and document your notification.

Record the amount of dialysate infused and drained and medications added. Be sure to complete a peritoneal dialysis flow chart every 24 hours. Keep a record of the effluent's characteristics and the assessed negative or positive fluid balance at the end of each infusion-dwell-drain cycle. Also, record each time you notify the doctor of an abnormality.

Chart the patient's weight (immediately after the drain phase) and abdominal girth daily. Note the time of day and variations in the weighing-measuring technique. In addition, document physical assessment findings and fluid status daily.

Keep a record of equipment problems, such as kinked tubing or mechanical malfunction, and your interventions. Also, note the condition of the patient's skin at the dialysis catheter site, the patient's reports of unusual discomfort or pain, and your interventions.

1/15/06	0700	Pt. receiving exchanges q2hr of 1500 ml 4.25 dialysate with
		500 units heparin and 2 mEq KCL. Dialysate infused over
		15 min. Dwell time 75 min. Drain time 30 min. Drainage
		clear, pale-yellow fluid. Weight 135 lb, abdominal girth 40"
		after drain phase. Lungs clear, normal heart sounds, mucous
		membranes moist, no skin tenting when pinched. VSS (See
		flow sheets for fluid balance and frequent VS assessments.)
		No c/o cramping or discomfort. Skin warm, dry at RLQ
		catheter site, no redness or drainage. Dry split 4" X 4"
		dressing applied after site cleaned per protocol. —————
		————————————————————— Liz Schaeffer, RN

PERITONEAL DIALYSIS, CONTINUOUS AMBULATORY

Continuous ambulatory peritoneal dialysis (CAPD) requires the insertion of a permanent peritoneal catheter to continuously circulate dialysate in the peritoneal cavity. Inserted when the patient is under local anesthetic, the catheter is sutured in place and its distal portion tunneled subcutaneously to the skin surface. There it serves as a port for the dialysate, which flows in and out of the peritoneal cavity by gravity. The bag of dialysate is attached to the tube entering the patient's abdominal area. The fluid flows into the peritoneal cavity over a period of 5 to 10 minutes. The dialysate remains in the peritoneal cavity, usually 4 to 6 hours. The patient can roll up the bag and place it under his shirt. After the prescribed dwell time is completed, the bag is unrolled and suspended below the pelvis, which allows the dialysate to drain from the peritoneal cavity back into the bag by gravity.

CAPD is used most commonly for patients with end-stage renal disease. It provides more patient independence, reduces travel for treatment, and helps stabilize fluid and electrolyte levels. Patients and family members can usually learn to perform CAPD after only 2 weeks of training.

ESSENTIAL DOCUMENTATION

Record the type and amount of fluid instilled and returned for each exchange, the time and duration of the exchange, and drugs added to the dialysate. Be sure to complete a peritoneal dialysis flow chart every 24 hours. Note the color and clarity of the returned exchange fluid, and check it for mucus, pus, and blood. Also, note discrepancies in the balance of fluid intake and output as well as signs or symptoms of fluid imbalance, such as weight changes, decreased breath sounds, peripheral edema, ascites, and changes in skin turgor. Record the patient's weight, blood pressure, and pulse rate after his last fluid exchange of the day.

12/2/05	2200	2-L dialysate bag connected to peritoneal catheter for
		CAPD at 2145 using sterile technique, infused over 10
		min., dwell time 6 hr. Empty dialysate bag rolled up and
		placed under pt.'s shirt. Drain clamp closed. Reinforced
		need to report fever, abdominal pain, and tenderness.
		———————————— Louise Falconi, RN
12/3/05	0400	Drain clamp opened, bag unfolded. 2300 ml of clear
		peritoneal fluid returned to the dialysate bag. Fluid is
		clear and free of mucus, pus, or blood. Weight 135.2 lb,
		wt. unchanged. Clear breath sounds, no edema, no skin
		tenting when pinched. No c/o abdominal pain. P 80, BP
		130/74, RR 22, oral T 98.6° F. — Louise Falconi, RN

PERITONEAL LAVAGE

Used as a diagnostic procedure in a patient with blunt abdominal trauma, peritoneal lavage helps detect bleeding in the peritoneal cavity. The test may proceed through several steps. Initially, the doctor inserts a catheter through the abdominal wall into the peritoneal cavity and aspirates the peritoneal fluid with a syringe. If he can't see blood in the aspirated fluid, he then infuses a balanced saline solution and siphons the fluid from the cavity. He inspects the siphoned fluid for blood and also sends fluid samples to the laboratory for microscopic examination.

ESSENTIAL DOCUMENTATION

Record the date and time of the procedure. Chart teaching done to prepare the patient for the procedure. Frequently monitor and document the patient's vital signs and signs and symptoms of shock (for example, tachycardia, hypotension, diaphoresis, or dyspnea).

Note whether an indwelling urinary catheter or nasogastric (NG) tube were inserted prior to the procedure. Record the size and type of urinary catheter or NG tube, and describe the amount, color, and other characteristics of the urine or NG drainage.

Keep a record of the incision site's condition, and document the type and size of peritoneal dialysis catheter used, the type and amount of solution instilled and withdrawn from the peritoneal cavity, and the amount and color of fluid returned. Note whether the fluid flowed freely into and out of the abdomen. Record which specimens were obtained and sent to the laboratory. Note the patient's tolerance of the procedure. Also, note complications that occurred and the nursing actions you took to manage them.

| 1/2/06 | 1500 | NG tube inserted at 1445 via ℗ nostril and connected to low continuous suction, draining small amount of greenish colored fluid; hematest negative. #16 Fr. Foley catheter inserted to straight drainage. Drained 200 ml clear amber urine, negative for blood. Dr. Fisher inserted #15 peritoneal dialysis catheter below umbilicus via trocar. Clear fluid withdrawn. 700 ml warm NSS instilled as ordered and clamped. Pt. turned from side to side. NSS dwell time of 10 min. NSS drained freely from abdomen. Fluid samples sent to lab, as ordered. Peritoneal catheter removed and incision closed by Dr. Fisher. 4" X 4" gauze pad with povidone-iodine ointment applied to site. Pt. resting comfortably in semi-Fowler's position. No c/o pain or cramping. Breathing comfortably. Preprocedure P 92, BP 110/64, RR 24. Postprocedure P 88, BP 116/66, RR 18. ———————————— Angela Novack, RN |

PERITONITIS

Peritonitis develops from a local or general inflammatory process in the peritoneal cavity caused by chemical irritation or infection. It may be an acute or chronic condition. Although the peritoneum is sterile, in peritonitis, bacteria and chemicals may enter the peritoneum as a result of such conditions as appendicitis, diverticulitis, peptic ulcer, ulcerative colitis, volvulus, strangulated obstruction, abdominal neoplasm, penetrating wound, peritoneal dialysis, rupture of the fallopian tube or the bladder, or released pancreatic enzyme. Untreated, peritonitis can lead to complications, such as septicemia, septic shock, abscess formation, and total body organ failure. Mortality is 10%, with death usually resulting from bowel obstruction.

If you suspect that your patient has peritonitis, immediately contact the doctor and anticipate administering I.V. fluids and antibiotics, assisting with the insertion of a nasogastric (NG) tube, and preparing the patient for surgery to repair organ perforation.

ESSENTIAL DOCUMENTATION

Record the date and time of your entry. Document your assessment findings, such as sudden and severe abdominal pain, rebound tenderness, abdominal rigidity and spasm, abdominal distention, nausea or vomiting, fever, tachycardia, tachypnea, hypotension, pallor, cold skin, diaphoresis, decreased bowel sounds, and signs of dehydration. Note the name of the doctor notified, the time of notification, and orders given, such as to obtain abdominal X-rays and blood work, insert an NG tube, and administer I.V. fluids, electrolytes, and antibiotics. Record your interventions, such as administering drugs and I.V. fluids, positioning for comfort and improved ventilation, providing analgesics and other comfort measures, keeping the patient from eating or drinking anything, preparing the patient for surgery, monitoring gastric decompression, and inserting a urinary catheter. Chart your patient's responses to these interventions. Use flow sheets to record your frequent assessments, vital signs, intake and output, I.V. therapy, and laboratory test values. Document patient teaching and emotional support rendered.

11/1/05	1000	Postop day #3 status post exploration and repair
		following gunshot wound to Ⓛ lower abdomen. Pt. c/o
		severe pain in Ⓛ lower abdomen at 0930, rated as 6 on
		scale of 0 to 10, w/10 being the worst pain imaginable.
		Noticed pt. guarding abdomen with arms and moaning.
		Pt. placed on Ⓛ side with legs flexed. No c/o nausea.
		Abdomen is rigid and distended, bowel sounds hypo-
		active. No rebound tenderness noted. Skin cool, diapho-
		retic, and pale. Skin tents when pinched. Abdominal
		incision has purulent drainage, skin around wound red.
		P 118, BP 92/68, RR 24 and shallow, oral T 101.5° F. Dr.
		Fromm notified at 0940 and came to see pt.; orders
		given. Pt. made NPO, radiology called for stat abdominal
		X-ray, lab called for stat CBC w/diff, electrolytes, BUN,
		creatinine. Culture of wound drainage sent to lab. I.V.
		line started in Ⓡ antecubital space with 20G catheter on
		first attempt. 1000 ml D₅W at 150 ml/hr infusing via
		infusion pump. Gentamicin 80 mg I.V. q8hr ordered,
		with first dose given at 0953. Receiving O₂ at 2 L by
		NC, with O₂ sat. by pulse oximetry 96%. NG tube inserted
		by Dr. Fromm and attached to low intermittent suction.
		Drained 100 ml dark green fluid, negative for blood.
		Morphine sulfate 2 mg given I.V. at 0955. See flow
		sheets for documentation of frequent vital signs, I/O,
		I.V., and lab values. Explaining all procedures to pt.
		Helping him to take slow deep breaths. Diane Smith, RN

PHOTOGRAPHING OR VIDEOTAPING PATIENT

Each patient is entitled to privacy and may not be photographed or videotaped without his informed consent. Using a photograph or videotape of a patient without his written consent violates his right to privacy and may lead to legal action against the health care facility. Before you let anyone photograph or videotape your patient, make sure the person has your facility's authorization. Follow your facility's policy for photographing or videotaping a patient. If your facility doesn't have a policy or if you have questions, contact your nursing supervisor. Commonly, the public affairs office handles consent for photographing or videotaping a patient.

Photographs and videotapes are frequently used in publications and for the purpose of educating health care workers. Before signing the consent form, the patient must be fully informed as to why the photograph or videotape is being taken as well as how, when, and where the photograph or videotaped will be used. Patients should be advised against signing consents that speak to disguising their identity because there's always the possibility that recognition may occur.

Accu**C**hart

CONSENT TO PHOTOGRAPH
OR VIDEOTAPE

A form such as the sample below can be used to obtain consent to videotape or photograph a patient.

CONSENT TO PHOTOGRAPH OR VIDEOTAPE

I, _____ *Barry Arnold* _____ , consent to have my surgical procedure
                (patient's name)
_____ *coronary artery bypass* _____ videotaped and photographed by _____
      (name of the procedure)   (Person/facility requesting permission)
for the purpose of educating nursing or medical students. I understand that the photographs or videotape
will be used in nursing and medical publications.

Barry Arnold _____   *4/21/05*
Patient signature   Patient address   Patient phone number   Date

Angela Steiner _____   *4/21/05*
Witness signature   Date

ESSENTIAL DOCUMENTATION

Most health care facilities use a consent form that includes the patient's name, address, telephone number; the name of the person requesting permission for the photographs or videotapes; and the manner in which the photographs or videotapes will be used. The person signing must be of legal age, competent, and not taking any mind-altering drugs. One copy of the signed consent form should be given to the patient, and a second copy should be placed in the patient's medical record. The person requesting permission to photograph or videotape should also receive a copy of the consent.

A notation should be made in the patient's record regarding the date and time that the request was signed, the person's name who made the request, and the patient's response.

See *Consent to photograph or videotape* for documenting a request to photograph or videotape your patient.

PNEUMONIA

An acute infection of the lung parenchyma, pneumonia often impairs gas exchange. The prognosis is generally good for people who have normal lungs and adequate host defenses before the onset of pneumonia; however, pneumonia is the sixth leading cause of death in the United States.

If your patient has pneumonia, administer antibiotics, as ordered, and provide for good respiratory hygiene.

ESSENTIAL DOCUMENTATION

Record the date and time of your entry. Document your assessment findings, such as coughing, sputum production, pleuritic chest pain, shaking, chills, fever, malaise, anorexia, weakness, tachypnea, tachycardia, dyspnea, use of accessory muscles, abnormal breath sounds, pleural friction rub, dullness to percussion over consolidated areas, and tactile fremitus. Note the name of the doctor notified, time of notification, and orders given, such as to obtain a chest X-ray and blood and sputum cultures, administer antibiotics, administer humidified oxygen therapy, and provide mechanical ventilation, if necessary.

Record your interventions, such as administering antibiotics and oxygen therapy, providing a high-calorie diet, promoting rest, and providing comfort measures and analgesics. Chart your patient's responses to these interventions. Use flow sheets to record your frequent assessments, vital signs, intake and output, I.V. therapy, and laboratory test values. Record what you teach the patient, including coughing and deep-breathing exercises, controlling the spread of infection, taking antibiotics properly, and encouraging vaccinations for influenza and pneumonia.

12/24/05	0900	Pt. has cough productive for large amount of thick
		yellow sputum. Breath sounds diminished to base of ℚ
		lower lung, crackles throughout all lung fields bilaterally.
		Dullness to percussion and tactile fremitus heard over
		base of ℚ lung. Pt. is SOB, using accessory breathing
		muscles. P 112, BP 152/88, RR 32 and shallow, rectal T
		102.4° F. Pulse oximetry 91%. Pt. is shaking and c/o of
		chills, weakness, and malaise. Normal heart sounds. Skin
		hot, dry, peripheral pulses palpable, no edema. Pt. alert
		and oriented to time, place, and person. Notified Dr.
		Landers at 0845 of assessment findings. Per dr.'s
		orders, chest X-ray and blood cultures ordered. Sputum
		sent for culture and sensitivity. Placed pt. on 2 L
		humidified O₂ by NC. Pulse oximetry 96%. Explained all
		procedures to pt. Showed pt. how to perform cough and
		deep-breathing exercises and encouraged him to
		perform them q2hr. Pt. able to give proper return
		demo. ————————————— Henry Porter, RN

PNEUMOTHORAX

Pneumothorax is an accumulation of air in the pleural space, which leads to partial or complete lung collapse. Pneumothorax may be closed or open. A closed pneumothorax has no associated external wound. It's commonly caused by the rupture of small blebs in the lung's visceral pleural space. An open pneumothorax develops when air enters the pleural space through an opening in the external chest wall; it's commonly associated with a stab or gunshot wound. With a tension pneumothorax, the intrathoracic pressure increases, causing the lung to collapse and the mediastinum to shift toward the side opposite the pneumothorax. These anatomic changes result in decreased venous return and compression of the great vessels, which decreases cardiac output. The respiratory and cardiovascular systems are affected, thus creating an emergency situation.

If you suspect your patient has a pneumothorax, contact the doctor immediately and anticipate insertion of a chest tube.

ESSENTIAL DOCUMENTATION

Record the date and time of your entry. Document your assessment findings of pneumothorax, such as asymmetrical chest wall movement, shortness of breath, cyanosis, and sudden, sharp pleuritic pain exacerbated by movement. If the pneumothorax is moderate to severe, you may assess and record such findings as profound respiratory distress, weak and rapid pulse, pallor, neck vein distention, shifting of the trachea and point of maximal impulse to the unaffected side, and anxiety. Note the name of the doctor notified, time of notification, and orders given. Record your interventions, such as assisting with insertion of a chest tube or large-bore needle, managing the chest tube, close monitoring of vital signs and cardiopulmonary assessments, administering oxygen, and encouraging coughing and deep-breathing exercises. Chart your patient's responses to these interventions. Use flow sheets to record your frequent assessments, vital signs, intake and output, I.V. therapy, and laboratory values. Include patient teaching and emotional care given.

7/12/05	0200	Pt. entered ED at 0130 with c/o difficulty breathing and
		Ⓛ-sided chest pain that worsened with movement; has
		history of COPD. Breath sounds absent on Ⓛ side, clear
		breath sounds on Ⓡ. Skin pale, cool. Normal heart sounds;
		however, PMI is shifted to Ⓡ of midclavicular line. P 128
		and weak, BP 112/62, RR 32, axillary T 99.0° F. Pulse
		oximetry 84% on room air. Dr. Hall in to see pt. at 0140
		and orders given. Portable CXR done and reveals Ⓛ pneu-
		mothorax. O₂ applied at 30% via facemask. Chest tube
		inserted by Dr. Hall and placed to water seal drainage
		with 20 cm water suction with Pleurevac. Chest tube
		sutured to chest wall. Airtight dressing applied. I.V.
		line inserted in Ⓡ forearm on first attempt using 18G
		catheter. 500 ml NSS infusing at 30 ml/hr. Pt. states
		he's breathing easier, appears more comfortable P 110
		and strong, BP 118/60, RR 24. See flow sheets for docu-
		mentation of frequent VS, I/O, I.V. therapy, and lab
		values. ————————————— Sue Jones RN

POISONING

Poisoning occurs after accidental or intentional contact with a harmful substance. Approximately 1 million poisonings occur in the United States every year. In children, accidental poisoning usually involves ingestion of salicylates, acetaminophen, cleaning agents, insecticides, paints, or cosmetics. In adults, common workplace poisonings take place in companies that use chlorine, carbon dioxide, hydrogen sulfide, nitrogen dioxide, and ammonia and in companies that ignore safety standards. Other causes of poisoning in adults involve improper cooking, canning, and storage of food; ingestion of or skin contamination by plants; and drug overdose.

If you suspect that your patient has been exposed to a poison, immediately notify the doctor and provide emergency resuscitation and support, prevention of further poison absorption, continuing supportive or symptomatic care and, when possible, administration of a special antidote. Specific interventions are based on the type of poison and the route of contact or ingestion, so every effort should be made to identify the poison involved. Consultation with a poison control center will clarify the specific interventions.

ESSENTIAL DOCUMENTATION

Record the date and time of your entry. Record the type and amount of poison, route of poisoning, signs and symptoms exhibited, and interventions implemented before the patient's arrival at your facility. Chart a brief medical history, including allergies and current drugs. Document continued assessments of the patient, administration of an antidote or GI decontaminant (such as activated charcoal, ipecac syrup, gastric lavage, cathartics, and whole-bowel irrigation), and supportive therapies. Include the patient's response to your interventions. Use flow sheets to record your frequent assessments, vital signs, intake and output, I.V. therapy, and laboratory test values. Record your patient teaching, including strategies to prevent future poison exposure.

7/14/05	1700	3 y.o. girl admitted to pediatric ED at 1645 accompanied by
		her grandparents, Robert and Linda Fowler, who report
		that they discovered the child playing on the floor with a
		Tylenol bottle. Stated that they didn't know how many
		tablets the child may have consumed but did see a white
		powder around her mouth. Grandmother recalls that
		bottle was approximately ½ full, as she had taken 2
		Tylenol for a headache earlier in the afternoon. The
		bottle contained 33 tablets remaining from a 60 total
		count bottle. Grandparents report that the incident
		occurred approximately 30 minutes ago. "Jessica walked
		to the kitchen to get a glass of water. She loves to drink
		the water from our new refrigerator. I never should
		have left the bottle on the table after taking the Tylenol
		for my headache." Child is sleepy but responsive to ques-
		tions. Child states that "They tasted bad. I only tasted
		them." P 100, BP 90/60, RR 24, tympanic T 98.4° F. Wt.
		30 lb. Grandparents report no previous medical hx for
		child, no known allergies, and taking no drugs. Dr. Greene
		examined pt. at 1650 and ordered acetylcysteine 1904 mg
		P.O. now, followed by 952 mg P.O. q4hr X 17 doses. Blood
		for LFTs and drug tox. drawn by lab. See flow sheets
		for documentation of frequent VS, I/O, and lab values.
		Explained all procedures to grandparents and child. Re-
		inforced the need to keep all drugs out of reach of
		children and to use child-resistant bottles. Grandparents
		verbalized understanding. ————— Joyce Tomlin, RN

POLICE CUSTODY OF PATIENT

A patient in police custody may be admitted voluntarily for medical or surgical treatment or involuntarily for psychiatric assessment and care. Follow your facility's policy for caring for a patient in police custody. Safety considerations include removal of objects that the patient could use to harm himself or others.

The accompanying police officer isn't permitted to make decisions regarding the patient's medical care and treatment. The patient is afforded the rights of confidentiality, informed consent, refusal of treatment, and review of documents that describe his condition and care. All care must be delivered without discrimination against the patient. The nurse serves as the patient's advocate, protecting his rights to health care as she would the rights of any other patient. As the patient advocate, the nurse must protect him from physical, spiritual, or mental harm. The patient in police custody, if determined competent, also has the right to make his treatment decisions and such decisions must be respected. (See *When a prisoner refuses treatment*.)

If blood, urine, or other samples are collected, make sure they aren't left unattended. Follow your facility's guidelines for using a chain of custody form. The form should serve as an uninterrupted log of the whereabouts of the evidence.

LEGAL CASEBOOK

WHEN A PRISONER REFUSES TREATMENT

Several courts have stated that individuals have a constitutional right to privacy based on a high regard for human dignity and self-determination. That means any competent adult may refuse medical care, even lifesaving treatments. A suspected criminal may refuse unwarranted bodily invasions. However, an arrested suspect or convicted criminal doesn't have the same right to refuse lifesaving measures. In *Commissioner of Correction v. Myers* (1979), a prisoner with renal failure refused hemodialysis unless he was moved to a minimum-security prison. The court disagreed, saying that although the defendant's imprisonment didn't divest him of his right to privacy or his interest in maintaining his bodily integrity, it did impose limitations on those constitutional rights.

As a practical matter, any time a patient refuses lifesaving treatments, inform your facility's administration. In the case of a suspect or prisoner, notify law enforcement authorities as well.

ESSENTIAL DOCUMENTATION

Documentation of care should be equivalent to that provided for any patient. Special attention is required for documentation related to the presence of the police officer and visitors. Record the name and badge number of the officer guarding your patient.

Be especially careful and precise in documenting medical and nursing procedures when you care for a suspected criminal. Document that the patient's rights were protected. Note blood work done, and list all treatments and the patient's responses to them.

If you turn anything over to the police or administration, record what it is and the name of the person receiving it. Record a suspect's statements that are directly related to his care. If a suspect says, "I shot a cop in the arm tonight," that isn't related to his care. However, if he says, "I think I was shot in the leg by a cop," it relates directly to his care.

When the patient is discharged, document all specific instructions given for follow-up home care. Such documentation may be critical, especially if the patient claims he was mistreated. Give a copy of the discharge instructions to the patient and the police officer.

8/2/05	0800	Pt. admitted to ED at 0730 with head laceration from
		MVA accompanied by San Antonio police officer B. Starr,
		badge #4532. Pt. placed in private exam room for
		privacy and safety. Officer in attendance at all times.
		Pt. alert, oriented to time, place, and person. Speech
		clear and coherent. PERRLA. Lungs clear, normal heart
		sounds, all peripheral pulses palpable. P 82, BP 138/74,
		RR 18 and unlabored, oral T 97.7° F. Moves all extremities
		on own, no deformities noted. No c/o nausea, vomiting,
		dizziness, diplopia, pain, except for sore forehead. Dr.
		Lawson in to see pt at 0740. Cleaned head wound
		and applied sterile 4" X 4" dressing to 2-cm cut on
		® side of forehead. Orders written for pt. discharge.
		Explained wound care to pt. and police officer, s/s to
		report to doctor. Written instructions for wound care
		and head injury given to pt. and police officer. Both
		pt. and police officer verbalized understanding of
		instructions.——————————— Joshua Jones, RN

POSTOPERATIVE CARE

When your patient recovers sufficiently from the effects of anesthesia, he can be transferred from the postanesthesia care unit (PACU) to his assigned unit for ongoing recovery and care. Your documentation should reflect your frequent assessments and interventions.

ESSENTIAL DOCUMENTATION

Record the date and time of each entry. Avoid block charting. The frequency of your assessments depends on your facility's policy, doctor's orders, and your patient's condition. Compare your assessments to preoperative and PACU assessments. Your documentation should include the following information:

- time the patient returned to your nursing unit
- assessment of airway and breathing, including breath sounds, positioning to maintain a patent airway, use of oxygen, and respiratory rate, rhythm, and depth
- vital signs
- neurologic assessment, including level of consciousness
- wound assessment, including the appearance of dressing, drainage, bleeding, and skin around site (Note the presence of drainage tubes and amount, type, color, and consistency of drainage; chart the type and amount of suction, if applicable.)
- cardiovascular assessment, including heart rate and rhythm, peripheral pulses, skin color and temperature, and Homans' sign
- renal assessment, including urine output, patency of catheter, and bladder distention
- GI assessment, including bowel sounds, abdominal distention, and nausea or vomiting
- pain assessment, including the use of 0 to 10 rating scale, need for analgesics and patient's response, and use of other comfort measures
- safety measures, such as call bell within reach, bed in low position, proper positioning, and use of side rails
- fluid management, including intake and output, type and size of I.V. catheter, location of I.V. line, I.V. solution, flow rate, and condition of I.V. site

- use of antiembolism stockings, sequential compression device, early ambulation, and prophylactic anticoagulants
- patient education, such as turning and positioning, coughing and deep breathing, splinting the incision, pain control, and the importance of early ambulation, as well as emotional support given.

Document drugs given; the dosage, frequency, and route; and the patient's response. Record the name of the doctor whom you notified of changes in the patient's condition, the time of notification, orders given, your actions, and the patient's responses. Use flow sheets to record your frequent assessments, vital signs, intake and output, I.V. therapy, and laboratory values.

| 12/8/05 | 1100 | Pt. returned from PACU at 1030 S/P laparoscopic laser cholecystectomy. P 88 and regular, BP 112/82, RR 18 deep, regular, tympanic T 98.2° F. Pt. breathing comfortably, breath sounds clear on room air, skin pink and warm, capillary refill less than 3 sec. Sleeping but easily arousable and oriented to time, place, and person. Speech clear and coherent. PERRLA. Normal heart sounds, strong radial and dorsalis pedis pulses bilaterally. Bladder nondistended, no indwelling urinary catheter, doesn't feel urge to void, positive bowel sounds in all 4 quadrants. Abdomen slightly distended, no c/o nausea. Has 4 abdominal puncture wounds covered with 4" X 4" gauze. Dressings without blood or drainage. Pt. c/o of abdominal discomfort rated as 3 on a scale of 0 to 10, w/10 being the worst pain imaginable, refusing analgesics at this time. Pt. placed in semi-Fowler's position, bed in low position, call bell within reach and pt. verbalized understanding of its use. I.V. of 1000 ml D₅/0.45 NS infusing at 75 ml/hr in Ⓡ forearm via infusion pump. See flow sheets for documentation of frequent VS, I.V. therapy, and I/O. Explained coughing and deep-breathing exercises to pt. and showed how to splint abdomen with pillow when coughing. Pt. able to give return demo. Told her to call if she feels she needs pain medication. ——————————— Christina Gault, RN |

PREOPERATIVE CARE

Effective nursing documentation during the preoperative period focuses on two primary elements – the baseline preoperative assessment and patient teaching. Documenting these elements encourages accurate communication among caregivers. Most facilities use a preoperative checklist to verify that the required data have been collected, preoperative teaching has occurred, and prescribed procedures and safety precautions have been executed.

ESSENTIAL DOCUMENTATION

To use the preoperative checklist, place a check mark in the appropriate column to indicate that a procedure has been performed (for example, checking that the patient is wearing an identification band or that the informed consent form has been signed). If an item doesn't apply to your patient, write "N/A," indicating that the item isn't applicable (such as the use of antiembolism stockings in a patient undergoing a minor surgical procedure). Place your initials in the appropriate column to indicate that an item has been completed. Make sure your full name, credentials, and initials appear on the form. Chart the patient's baseline vital signs on the form. Before the patient leaves for surgery, check the appropriate boxes to indicate that the patient has been properly and positively identified. (See "Surgical site identification," page 404.)

Be sure to document the name of the person you notified of abnormalities that could affect the patient's response to the surgical procedure or deviations from facility standards.

See *Preoperative checklist and surgical identification form* for an example of preoperative documentation.

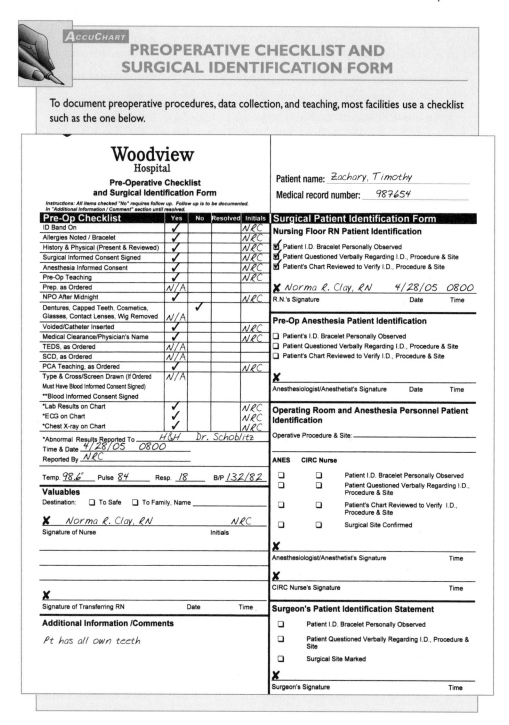

AccuChart

PREOPERATIVE CHECKLIST AND SURGICAL IDENTIFICATION FORM

To document preoperative procedures, data collection, and teaching, most facilities use a checklist such as the one below.

Woodview
Hospital

**Pre-Operative Checklist
and Surgical Identification Form**

Instructions: All items checked "No" requires follow up. Follow up is to be documented. In "Additional Information / Comment" section until resolved.

Patient name: Zachary, Timothy

Medical record number: 987654

Pre-Op Checklist	Yes	No	Resolved	Initials
ID Band On	✓			NRC
Allergies Noted / Bracelet	✓			NRC
History & Physical (Present & Reviewed)	✓			NRC
Surgical Informed Consent Signed	✓			NRC
Anesthesia Informed Consent	✓			NRC
Pre-Op Teaching	✓			NRC
Prep. as Ordered	N/A			
NPO After Midnight	✓			NRC
Dentures, Capped Teeth, Cosmetics, Glasses, Contact Lenses, Wig Removed	N/A	✓		
Voided/Catheter Inserted	✓			NRC
Medical Clearance/Physician's Name	✓			NRC
TEDS, as Ordered	N/A			
SCD, as Ordered	N/A			
PCA Teaching, as Ordered				NRC
Type & Cross/Screen Drawn (If Ordered Must Have Blood Informed Consent Signed)	N/A			
**Blood Informed Consent Signed				
*Lab Results on Chart	✓			NRC
*ECG on Chart	✓			NRC
*Chest X-ray on Chart	✓			NRC

*Abnormal Results Reported To __H&H___ Dr. Schoblitz__
Time & Date _4/28/05___ 0800_____
Reported By _NRC___

Temp. _98.6°_ Pulse _84_____ Resp. _18___ B/P _132/82_

Valuables

Destination: ☐ To Safe ☐ To Family, Name _____

X __Norma R. Clay, RN_____ NRC
Signature of Nurse   Initials

_____

_____

X _____
Signature of Transferring RN   Date   Time

Additional Information /Comments

Pt has all own teeth

Surgical Patient Identification Form

Nursing Floor RN Patient Identification

☑ Patient I.D. Bracelet Personally Observed
☑ Patient Questioned Verbally Regarding I.D., Procedure & Site
☑ Patient's Chart Reviewed to Verify I.D., Procedure & Site

X _Norma R. Clay, RN_____ 4/28/05___ 0800_
R.N.'s Signature   Date   Time

Pre-Op Anesthesia Patient Identification

☐ Patient's I.D. Bracelet Personally Observed
☐ Patient Questioned Verbally Regarding I.D., Procedure & Site
☐ Patient's Chart Reviewed to Verify I.D., Procedure & Site

X _____
Anesthesiologist/Anesthetist's Signature Date Time

Operating Room and Anesthesia Personnel Patient Identification

Operative Procedure & Site: _____

ANES	CIRC Nurse	
☐	☐	Patient I.D. Bracelet Personally Observed
☐	☐	Patient Questioned Verbally Regarding I.D., Procedure & Site
☐	☐	Patient's Chart Reviewed to Verify I.D., Procedure & Site
☐	☐	Surgical Site Confirmed

X _____
Anesthesiologist/Anesthetist's Signature   Time

X _____
CIRC Nurse's Signature   Time

Surgeon's Patient Identification Statement

☐ Patient I.D. Bracelet Personally Observed
☐ Patient Questioned Verbally Regarding I.D., Procedure & Site
☐ Surgical Site Marked

X _____
Surgeon's Signature   Time

PRESSURE ULCER ASSESSMENT

Pressure ulcers develop when pressure impairs circulation, depriving tissues of oxygen and life-sustaining nutrients. This process damages skin and underlying structures. The pressure may be of short duration with great force, or it may have been present for a longer period of time with lesser force.

Most pressure ulcers develop over bony prominences, where friction and shearing force combine with pressure to break down skin and underlying tissue. Common sites include the sacrum, coccyx, ischial tuberosities, and greater trochanters. In bedridden and relatively immobile patients, pressure ulcers develop over the vertebrae, scapulae, elbows, knees, and heels. Untreated pressure ulcers may lead to serious systemic infection.

To select the most effective treatment plan for pressure ulcers, the nurse first assesses the pressure ulcer and stages it based on the National Pressure Ulcer Advisory Panel and the Agency for Healthcare Research and Quality. (See *Stages of pressure ulcers.*)

In addition to assessing the pressure ulcer, perform an assessment to determine the patient's risk of developing pressure ulcers. The Braden scale is one of the most reliable instruments. The Braden scale assesses sensory perception, moisture, activity, mobility, nutrition, and friction and shear. The lower the score, the greater the risk. (See *Braden scale: Predicting pressure ulcer risk,* pages 340 and 341.)

Documentation of pressure ulcer assessments assists the nurse in detecting changes in a patient's skin condition, determining the response to treatment, identifying at-risk patients, and reducing the incidence of pressure ulcers through early independent interventions and treatment.

ESSENTIAL DOCUMENTATION

Documentation of your pressure ulcer assessment should include the patient's history and risk factors leading to the formation of a pressure ulcer, using a tool such as the Braden scale. In your note, describe the pressure ulcer, including its location, size and depth (in centimeters), stage, color, and appearance; presence of necrotic or granulation tissue, drainage, and

(Text continues on page 342.)

STAGES OF PRESSURE ULCERS

To select the most effective treatment for a pressure ulcer, you first need to assess the ulcer's characteristics. The pressure ulcer stages described below, used by the National Pressure Ulcer Advisory Panel and the Agency for Healthcare Research and Quality, reflect the anatomic depth of exposed tissue. Keep in mind that if the wound contains necrotic tissue, you won't be able to determine the stage until you can see the wound base.

STAGE 1
The heralding lesion of a pressure ulcer is persistent redness in lightly pigmented skin and persistent red, blue, or purple hues on darker skin. Other indicators include changes in temperature, consistency, or sensation.

STAGE 2
A stage 2 ulcer is marked by partial-thickness skin loss involving the epidermis, the dermis, or both. The ulcer is superficial and appears as an abrasion, a blister, or a shallow crater.

STAGE 3
A stage 3 ulcer constitutes a full-thickness wound penetrating the subcutaneous tissue, which may extend to—but not through—underlying fasciae. The ulcer resembles a deep crater and may undermine adjacent tissue.

STAGE 4
A stage 4 ulcer extends through the skin, accompanied by extensive destruction, tissue necrosis, or damage to muscle, bone, or supporting structures, such as tendons and joint capsules.

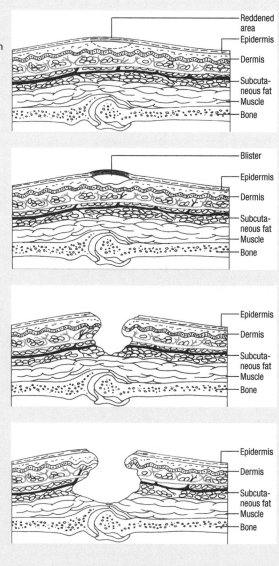

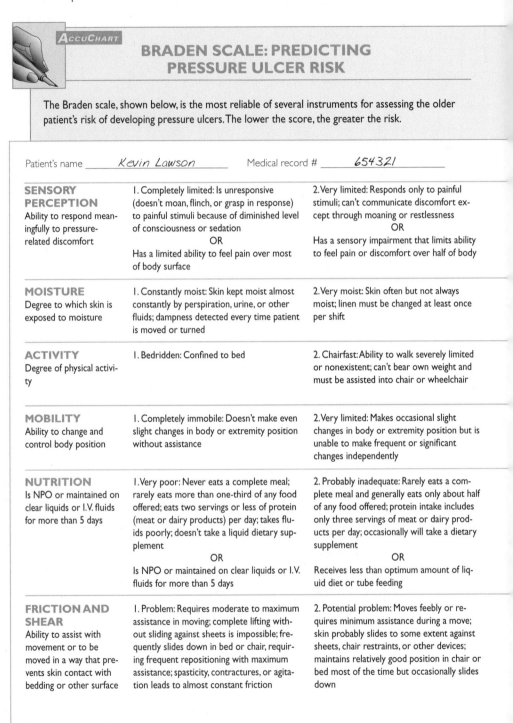

AccuChart

BRADEN SCALE: PREDICTING PRESSURE ULCER RISK

The Braden scale, shown below, is the most reliable of several instruments for assessing the older patient's risk of developing pressure ulcers. The lower the score, the greater the risk.

Patient's name ___Kevin Lawson___   Medical record # ___654321___

SENSORY PERCEPTION Ability to respond meaningfully to pressure-related discomfort	1. Completely limited: Is unresponsive (doesn't moan, flinch, or grasp in response) to painful stimuli because of diminished level of consciousness or sedation OR Has a limited ability to feel pain over most of body surface	2. Very limited: Responds only to painful stimuli; can't communicate discomfort except through moaning or restlessness OR Has a sensory impairment that limits ability to feel pain or discomfort over half of body
MOISTURE Degree to which skin is exposed to moisture	1. Constantly moist: Skin kept moist almost constantly by perspiration, urine, or other fluids; dampness detected every time patient is moved or turned	2. Very moist: Skin often but not always moist; linen must be changed at least once per shift
ACTIVITY Degree of physical activity	1. Bedridden: Confined to bed	2. Chairfast: Ability to walk severely limited or nonexistent; can't bear own weight and must be assisted into chair or wheelchair
MOBILITY Ability to change and control body position	1. Completely immobile: Doesn't make even slight changes in body or extremity position without assistance	2. Very limited: Makes occasional slight changes in body or extremity position but is unable to make frequent or significant changes independently
NUTRITION Is NPO or maintained on clear liquids or I.V. fluids for more than 5 days	1. Very poor: Never eats a complete meal; rarely eats more than one-third of any food offered; eats two servings or less of protein (meat or dairy products) per day; takes fluids poorly; doesn't take a liquid dietary supplement OR Is NPO or maintained on clear liquids or I.V. fluids for more than 5 days	2. Probably inadequate: Rarely eats a complete meal and generally eats only about half of any food offered; protein intake includes only three servings of meat or dairy products per day; occasionally will take a dietary supplement OR Receives less than optimum amount of liquid diet or tube feeding
FRICTION AND SHEAR Ability to assist with movement or to be moved in a way that prevents skin contact with bedding or other surface	1. Problem: Requires moderate to maximum assistance in moving; complete lifting without sliding against sheets is impossible; frequently slides down in bed or chair, requiring frequent repositioning with maximum assistance; spasticity, contractures, or agitation leads to almost constant friction	2. Potential problem: Moves feebly or requires minimum assistance during a move; skin probably slides to some extent against sheets, chair restraints, or other devices; maintains relatively good position in chair or bed most of the time but occasionally slides down

		DATE OF ASSESSMENT	3/21/05			

Evaluator's name ___*Joan Norris, RN*___

		3/21/05			
3. Slightly limited: Responds to verbal commands but can't always communicate discomfort or need to be turned	4. No impairment: Responds to verbal commands; has no sensory deficit that would limit ability to feel or voice pain or discomfort	3			
3. Occasionally moist: Skin occasionally moist, requiring an extra linen change approximately once per day	4. Rarely moist: Skin usually dry; linen only requires changing at routine intervals	3			
3. Walks occasionally: Walks occasionally during day, but for very short distances, with or without assistance; spends majority of each shift in bed or chair	4. Walks frequently: Walks outside room at least twice per day and inside room at least once every 2 hours during waking hours	2			
3. Slightly limited: Makes frequent though slight changes in body or extremity position independently	4. No limitations: Makes major and frequent changes in body or extremity position without assistance	2			
3. Adequate: Eats more than half of most meals; eats four servings of protein (meat and dairy products) per day; occasionally refuses a meal but will usually take a supplement if offered OR Is on a tube feeding or total parenteral nutrition regimen that probably meets most nutritional needs	4. Excellent: Eats most of every meal and never refuses a meal; usually eats four or more servings of meat and dairy products per day; occasionally eats between meals; doesn't require supplementation	2			
3. No apparent problem: Moves in bed and in chair independently and has sufficient muscle strength to lift up completely during move; maintains good position in bed or chair at all times		2			
	Total	14			

odor; length of any undermining; and condition of the surrounding tissue. A sketch of the wound may also be included. Assess the pressure ulcer with each dressing change or at least weekly for the patient at home.

| 1/18/06 | 1100 | Pt. admitted to 6 South from Green Brier Nursing Home. Pt. has stage 2 pressure ulcer on coccyx, approx. 2 cm X 1 cm X 0.5 cm. No drainage noted. Base has deep pink granulation tissue. Skin surrounding ulcer pink, intact, well-defined edges. Irrigated ulcer with NSS. Skin around ulcer dried and ulcer covered with transparent dressing. Pt. has h/o CVA with ①-sided weakness and dysphagia. Braden score 14 (see Braden Pressure Ulcer Risk Assessment Scale). ———————— Joan Norris, RN |
| | | |

PRESSURE ULCER CARE

Successful pressure ulcer treatment involves relieving pressure, restoring circulation and, if possible, resolving or managing related disorders. Typically, the effectiveness and duration of treatment depend on the pressure ulcer's characteristics.

Ideally, prevention is the key to avoiding extensive therapy. Preventive measures include ensuring adequate nourishment and mobility to relieve pressure and promote circulation.

When a pressure ulcer develops despite preventive efforts, treatment includes methods to decrease pressure, such as frequent repositioning to shorten pressure duration and the use of special equipment to reduce pressure intensity. Treatment may also involve special pressure-reducing devices, such as beds, mattresses, mattress overlays, and chair cushions. Other therapeutic measures include risk-factor reduction and the use of topical treatments, wound cleansing, debridement, and dressings to support moist wound healing.

Nurses usually perform or coordinate treatments according to facility policy. Always follow the standard precautions guidelines of the Centers for Disease Control and Prevention.

ESSENTIAL DOCUMENTATION

Record the date and time of initial and subsequent dressing changes and treatments. Note the specific treatment and the patient's response. Detail preventive strategies performed. Document the pressure ulcer's location and size (length, width, and depth in centimeters); color and appearance of the wound bed; amount, color, odor, and consistency of drainage; and condition of surrounding skin. Reassess ulcers with each dressing change and at least weekly.

Update the care plan as required. Note changes in the condition or size of the pressure ulcer and elevation of skin temperature on the clinical record. Document when the doctor was notified of pertinent changes. Record the patient's temperature daily on the graphic sheet to allow easy assessment of body temperature patterns. Chart patient education, such as your explanation of treatments, the need for turning and positioning every 2 hours, and proper nutrition.

4/20/05	1230	Pt. has stage 2 pressure ulcer on Ⓛ heel. Approx. 2 cm
		X 5 cm X 1 cm. Base of ulcer has necrotic tissue, no
		drainage. Skin around ulcer intact. P 82, BP 134/78, RR
		18, oral T 98.6° F. Wet-to-dry dressing removed and
		ulcer irrigated with NSS. Gauze moistened with NSS,
		placed in wound bed, and covered with dry sterile
		4" X 4" gauze. Pt. turned and repositioned. Heels
		elevated off bed with pillow placed lengthwise under
		legs. Dietitian in to see pt. High-protein, high-calorie
		shakes being encouraged with each meal. Explained
		importance of proper nutrition for wound healing.
		———— Harrriet Newman, RN

PSYCHOSIS, ACUTE

Acute psychosis is a psychiatric disorder characterized by an inability to recognize reality. The person suffering from acute psychosis experiences hallucinations (such as auditory, visual, tactile, and olfactory) and delusions. He may also show paranoia, disordered thinking, and catatonia.

Acute psychosis may result from a psychiatric disorder, such as schizophrenia, schizoaffective disorder, bipolar disorder, and personality disorders. Other conditions that can lead to acute psychosis include drug intoxication, drug withdrawal, and a host of endocrine, metabolic, and neurologic abnormalities.

If your patient exhibits manifestations of acute psychosis, notify the doctor immediately. Reassure the patient that he's in a safe and secure place. Ask him to describe his hallucinations. Acknowledge that you believe the patient is experiencing what he tells you he's experiencing. Administer antipsychotic drugs as ordered.

ESSENTIAL DOCUMENTATION

Record the date and time of your entry. Objectively document the patient's behavior. Describe what the patient tells you he's hearing or seeing (if auditory or visual hallucinations are present) and what the patient is being told to do if he's hearing voices. Record any delusions that the patient relates. Describe inappropriate behaviors or statements. Describe threats or thoughts of suicide or violence, your interventions, and the patient's response. Record a general assessment, vital signs, and history as best as you can obtain. Record the name of the doctor that you notified, the time of notification, orders given, your actions, and the patient's response to drugs administered, the environment, and caregivers.

9/3/05	1500	23 y.o. male brought to ED by police at 1430. Officers
		state that pt. was found walking in the middle of
		Route 1 waving his arms and conversing with himself.
		Pt. states, "An angry voice told me to stop all traffic.
		I'm getting very upset about all this, and I've been
		very upset all week." Pt. states he has been hearing
		voices the last several days. Pt. interrupts conversation
		frequently, turns his head and cups his hand to his
		ear. When asked what he's hearing, he shakes his head
		and only says, "Terrible, terrible." Told pt. that he was
		in the hospital and that he was safe. Dr. Clark in to see
		pt. at 1445 and orders written. Given oral liquid halo-
		peridol and lorazepam. See MAR. Pt. accepted meds. Pt.
		and belongings searched as per hospital policy and no
		weapons or sharp objects found. Pt. not allowing any-
		one to touch him to perform physical exam; will try
		again after meds begin to work. —— Marion Tuttle, RN

PULMONARY EDEMA

Pulmonary edema is a diffuse extravascular accumulation of fluid in the tissues and airspaces of the lungs due to increased pressure in the pulmonary capillaries. Normally, fluid that crosses the capillary membrane and enters the lung is removed by the pulmonary lymphatic system. If the left ventricle fails, blood backs up into the pulmonary vasculature, and capillary pressure increases. Fluid crosses the membrane in amounts greater than the lymphatics can drain. Fluid builds up in the interstitial tissues, then in the alveoli. Pulmonary edema can occur as a chronic condition, or it can develop quickly and rapidly become fatal.

Most cases of pulmonary edema are cardiogenic, and the causes include acute myocardial infarction, acute volume overload of the left ventricle, and mitral stenosis. Noncardiogenic pulmonary edema can also occur and is caused by increased capillary permeability, which also permits fluid leakage into the alveoli. Causes of noncardiogenic pulmonary edema include acute respiratory distress syndrome, increased intracranial pressure, shock, and disseminated intravascular coagulation.

If your patient shows signs of pulmonary edema, notify the doctor immediately. Administer oxygen by nasal cannula or facemask or, if respiratory distress develops, prepare for intubation and mechanical ventilation. Administer drugs as ordered, such as diuretics, nitrates, morphine, inotropics, vasodilators, and angiotensin-converting enzyme inhibitors. Anticipate assisting with the insertion of hemodynamic monitoring lines. Reassure the patient and family, and explain what's being done and the rationale.

ESSENTIAL DOCUMENTATION

Record the date and time of your entry. Document your assessment findings of pulmonary edema, such as dyspnea, orthopnea, use of accessory muscles, pink frothy sputum, diaphoresis, cyanosis, tachypnea, tachycardia, adventitious breath sounds (such as crackles, wheezing, or rhonchi), pleural rub, neck vein distention, and increased intensity of the pulmonic component of S_2 and S_3 heart sounds. Note the name of the doctor notified, time of notification, and orders given, such as oxygen and drug administration. Record your interventions, such as positioning the patient with legs dangling, inserting I.V. lines, administering oxygen and drugs, assisting with the insertion of hemodynamic monitoring lines, and suctioning. Chart your patient's responses to these interventions. Use flow sheets to record your frequent assessments, vital signs, hemodynamic measurements, intake and output, I.V. therapy, and laboratory test and arterial blood gas values. Include patient teaching and emotional care given.

9/17/05	0300	Pt. discovered lying flat in bed at 0230 trying to sit
		up and stating, "I can't breathe." Pt. coughing and
		bringing up small amount of pink frothy sputum. Skin
		pale, lips cyanotic, sluggish capillary refill, +1 ankle
		edema bilaterally. Lungs with crackles ½ way up
		bilaterally, S_3 heard on auscultation of heart. P 120 and
		irregular, BP 140/90, RR 30 and shallow, tympanic T
		98.8° F. Pt. restless, alert, and oriented to time, place,
		and person. Dr. Green notified of assessment findings
		at 0235 and came to see pt. at 0245. Pt. placed in
		sitting position with legs dangling. O_2 via NC at 2
		L/min changed to nonrebreather mask at 12 L/min.
		Explained to pt. that mask would give her more O_2 and
		help her breathing. O_2 sat. by pulse oximetry 81%. Stat
		portable CXR done. 12-lead ECG shows sinus tachycardia
		with occasional PVCs. CBC and electrolytes drawn and
		sent to lab stat. Morphine, furosemide, and digoxin I.V.
		ordered and given through intermittent infusion device
		in ® forearm. See MAR. Indwelling urinary catheter
		inserted to straight drainage, drained 100 ml on
		insertion. Pt. encouraged to cough and deep-breathe.
		Explained all procedures and drugs to pt. See flow
		sheets for documentation of frequent VS, I/O, and lab
		values. —————————————— Rachel Moreau, RN

PULMONARY EMBOLISM

The most common pulmonary complication in hospitalized patients, pulmonary embolism is an obstruction of the pulmonary arterial bed by a dislodged thrombus or foreign substance. It strikes an estimated 6 million adults each year in the United States, resulting in 100,000 deaths. Massive pulmonary embolism obstructing more than 50% of the pulmonary arterial circulation can be rapidly fatal. In fact, approximately 10% of patients die within the first hour.

Pulmonary embolism generally results from dislodged thrombi originating in the leg veins. More than half of such thrombi arise in the deep veins of the legs and are usually multiple. Other less common sources of thrombi are the pelvic veins, renal veins, hepatic vein, right side of the heart, and upper extremities. Such thrombus formation results directly from vascular wall damage, venostasis, or hypercoagulability of the blood.

Predisposing risk factors to pulmonary embolism include immobility, chronic pulmonary disease, heart failure, atrial fibrillation, thrombophlebitis, polycythemia vera, thrombocytosis, autoimmune hemolytic anemia, sickle cell disease, varicose veins, vascular injury, surgery, advanced age, pregnancy, lower extremity fractures or surgery, burns, obesity, malignancy, and use of hormonal contraceptives.

If you suspect that your patient has a pulmonary embolism, notify the doctor immediately. Prepare your patient for pulmonary angiography and a lung scan. Administer oxygen, and anticipate I.V. administration of heparin. With massive pulmonary embolism, anticipate fibrinolytic therapy.

ESSENTIAL DOCUMENTATION

Record the date and time of your entry. Document your assessment findings of pulmonary embolism, such as dyspnea, tachypnea, tachycardia, crackles on lung auscultation, chest pain, productive cough, mild fever, change in mental status, and feelings of apprehension and impending doom. Note the name of the doctor notified, the time of notification, and orders given, such as diagnostic testing, oxygen administration, and heparin and thrombolytic therapy. Record your interventions, such as positioning, inserting I.V. lines, giving drugs, administering oxygen, watching for bleeding, and monitoring coagulation studies. Chart your patient's responses to these interventions. Use flow sheets to record your frequent assessments, vital signs, intake and output, I.V. fluid therapy, and laboratory test and arterial blood gas (ABG) values. Include patient teaching and emotional care given.

4/19/05	0745	Answered call light at 0720 and found pt. SOB, pale,
		restless, and c/o chest pain described as "crushing." P 104,
		BP 150/90, RR 30 and shallow, oral T 99.9° F. Crackles
		heard in lower lobes bilaterally. Occasional productive
		cough with pink-tinged sputum. Alert and oriented but
		very anxious, stating "Help me, I'm going to die." Dr.
		Hope stat paged and came to see pt. immediately at
		0725. O₂ started via nonrebreather mask at 12 L/min.
		I.V. line started in ® forearm with 18G angiocath on
		first attempt. 500 ml NSS infusing at 30 ml/hr. Stat
		portable CXR done at 0735. ABGs, CBC, coagulation
		studies, and cardiac enzymes drawn and sent to lab stat.
		12-lead ECG shows ® axis deviation and tall peaked P
		waves. V/Q scan ordered stat. Heparin 5000 units given
		I.V. bolus, followed by 1000 units/hr continuous infusion.
		PTT due in 6 hours. See flow sheets for documentation
		of frequent VS, assessments, I/O, I.V. therapy, and lab
		values. Explaining all procedures to pt. as well as the
		need for lung scan. ——————— George Stein, RN

PULSE OXIMETRY

Pulse oximetry is a noninvasive procedure used to monitor a patient's arterial blood oxygen saturation (SpO_2) to detect hypoxemia. Lack of adequate oxygenation can cause permanent cellular damage and death.

A sensor containing two light-emitting diodes (LEDs) – one red and one infrared – and a photodetector placed opposite these LEDs across a vascular bed are attached to the skin with adhesive or clips. The sensor is placed across a pulsating arteriolar bed, such as a finger, toe, nose, or earlobe. Selected wavelengths of light are absorbed by hemoglobin and transmitted through tissue to the photodetector. The pulse oximeter computes SpO_2 based on the relative amounts of light that reach the photodetector. The normal value is between 95% and 100%. Pulse oximetry may be performed intermittently or continuously.

ESSENTIAL DOCUMENTATION

Record the date and time of each pulse oximetry reading. Frequent SpO_2 readings may be documented on a flow sheet. Document the reason for use of pulse oximetry and whether readings are continuous or intermittent. If SpO_2 readings are continuous, record the alarm settings. Chart whether the reading is obtained while the patient is breathing room air or receiving supplemental oxygen. If the patient is receiving oxygen, record the concentration and mode of delivery. Describe events precipitating acute oxygen desaturation, your actions, and the patient's response. Record activities or interventions affecting SpO_2 values. Document patient teaching related to pulse oximetry.

3/13/05	1100	At 1040 pt. gasping and SOB. P 128, BP 140/96, RR 34, tympanic T 97.3° F. Lips and nail beds cyanotic. Able to speak only 2 or 3 words between breaths due to dyspnea. O₂ NC resting on bedside table. Wife states, "He took it off because it hurts his ears." Pulse oximetry 86%. NC reapplied at 6 L/min. Pt. less dyspneic, able to speak in sentences. P 100, BP 136/90, RR 26. Pulse oximetry 93%. Pt. and wife instructed to leave NC in place in nostrils. Tubing padded around earpieces for comfort. Pt. instructed to call the nurse if tubing becomes uncomfortable rather than removing it. Pt. and wife verbalized understanding of the need for the oximetry monitoring. ——— Terry Delmonico, RN

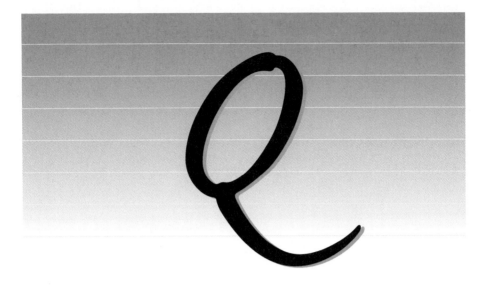

QUALITY OF CARE, FAMILY QUESTIONS ABOUT

At times, the family of a patient may have questions about the quality of care that a family member is receiving. These concerns should be taken seriously – ignoring them increases the risk of a lawsuit. Moreover, don't argue with the family, and avoid defending yourself, a coworker, the doctor, or the facility.

When family members question the quality of care, show that you're concerned and ask them to clarify what they believe to be the problem. Provide education about nursing routines, policies, procedures and, within the limits of confidentiality, the patient's care plan. If the concern isn't a nursing issue, help the family find the answers to their questions. Also, ask the doctor, nursing supervisor, or another appropriate person to speak with the family. Report all unresolved concerns about the quality of care to your nursing supervisor or risk manager.

ESSENTIAL DOCUMENTATION

Record the date and time of your initial conversation. Include the names of the family members present. Document the concerns using their own words, in quotes, if possible. Describe your answers and the family members' responses. Record the names of the people you notified of the family's concerns, including the doctor, nursing supervisor, and risk manager, and the time of notification. Document your conversation and their responses, in quotes.

6/22/05	1600	Pt.'s daughter, Emily Jones, verbalized concerns
		regarding mother's hygiene. She stated, "I don't think
		my mother is receiving her showers. Her hair and
		fingernails are dirty." After reviewing the shower
		schedule, explained to Mrs. Jones that her mother has
		been refusing 1 of her 2 scheduled showers each week
		since admission 2 weeks ago and has been receiving
		sponge baths instead. Nurses' notes indicate that
		resident stated, "I've never taken more than 1 shower
		per week in my entire life and I don't intend to
		start now." Records also show that for the last 2 days
		resident has been participating in planting flower boxes
		around the facility. Mrs. Jones spoke with her mother
		and reported that her mother will continue to shower
		once per week, sponge bathe on a daily basis, and have
		an appointment at the facility beauty salon once per
		week. Care plan amended to reflect this. ————
		———————————— Liz Mazerka, RN

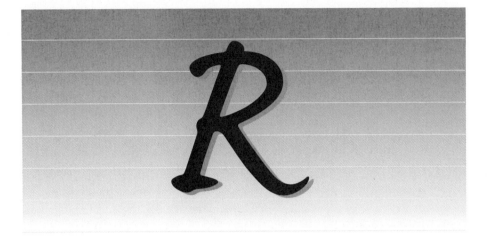

RAPE-TRAUMA SYNDROME

The term "rape" refers to nonconsensual sexual intercourse. Rape inflicts varying degrees of physical and psychological trauma. Rape-trauma syndrome typically occurs during the period following the rape or attempted rape. It refers to the victim's short- and long-term reactions and to the methods she uses to cope with the trauma. In most cases, the rapist is a man and the victim is a woman. However, rape does occur between persons of the same sex, especially in prisons, schools, hospitals, and other institutions. Children are also often victims of rape; most of the time these cases involve manual, oral, or genital contact with the child's genitalia. Usually, the rapist is a member of the child's family. In rare instances, a man or child is sexually abused by a woman.

The prognosis is promising if the rape victim receives physical and emotional support and counseling to help her deal with her feelings. The patient who articulates her feelings can cope with fears, interact with others, and return to normal routines faster than the patient who doesn't.

Be objective and precise when documenting care for a patient who was raped. Your notes may be used as evidence if the rapist is tried.

ESSENTIAL DOCUMENTATION

Record the date and time of each entry. Record the patient's statements, using her own words, in quotes. Also, document objective information provided by others. Include the time that the patient arrived at the facility, date and time of the alleged rape, and time that she was examined.

Ask the patient about allergies to penicillin and other drugs, recent illnesses (especially venereal disease), the possibility of pregnancy before the attack, the date of her last menstrual period, and details of her obstetric and gynecologic history. Describe the patient's emotional state and behaviors.

Make sure the doctor has obtained the patient's informed consent for treatment. Note whether she douched, bathed, or washed before coming to the facility. If the case comes to trial, specimens will be used for evidence, so accuracy is essential. Most emergency departments have special kits for rape victims, with containers for specimens. During the examination, make sure all specimens collected (including fingernail scrapings, pubic hair combings, semen, and gonorrhea culture) are labeled carefully with the patient's name, doctor's name, and location from which the specimen was obtained. Place all the patient's clothing in paper, not plastic, bags. If placed in plastic bags, secretions and seminal stains will become moldy, destroying valuable evidence. Label each bag and its contents. List all specimens in your note, and record to whom these specimens were given. Document whether photographs were taken and, if so, by whom.

This examination is typically very distressing for the rape victim. Reassure her and allow her as much control as possible. If the patient wishes, ask a counselor to stay with her throughout the examination, and remember to document the name of the individual. Counseling helps the patient identify new coping mechanisms. She may relate more easily to a counselor of the same sex. Before the patient's pelvic area is examined, take her vital signs and document them. If the patient is wearing a tampon, remove it, wrap it, and label it as evidence.

On the medication administration record, list all medications administered, such as antibiotics and birth control prophylaxis (for example, morning-after pills). Explain possible adverse effects, what to expect of the medication, and signs and symptoms to report. Document all teaching administered, and provide the patient with written instructions before discharge. Record care given to such injuries as lacerations, cuts, or areas of swelling. Document whether the patient was offered and received testing for human immunodeficiency virus (HIV) or hepatitides B and C. Include whether prophylaxis for hepatitis was given. Chart that you told the patient the importance of follow-up testing in 5 to 6 days for gonorrhea and syphilis. Record the names and telephone numbers of contact persons for local resources, including rape crisis centers, victims' rights advocates, and local law enforcement. Chart any other education and support that you give to the patient.

8/10/05	2250	Pt. admitted to ED accompanied by police officers John Hanson (badge #1234) and Teresa Collins (badge #5678). Pt. states, "I was attacked in the supermarket parking lot. I think it was about 9 p.m. He pulled me into the bushes and raped me. When he ran away, I called 911 from my cell phone." Pt. trembling and crying but able to walk into ED on her own. Placed in private room. Police officers waited in waiting room. Pt. denies being pregnant, drug allergies, and recent illnesses including venereal disease. LMP 7/28/05. States she didn't wash or douche before coming to the hospital. Chain of evidence maintained for all specimens collected (see flow sheet). After obtaining written consent and explaining procedure, Dr. Smith examined pt. Pt. has reddened areas on face and anterior neck and blood on lips. Bruising noted on inner aspects of both thighs; some vaginal bleeding noted. See dr.'s note for details of pelvic exam. Specimens for venereal disease, blood, and vaginal smears collected and labeled. Evidence from fingernail scraping and pubic hair combing collected and labeled. Photographs of injuries taken. Stayed with pt. throughout exam, holding her hand and offering reassurance and comfort. Pt. cooperated with exam but was often teary. After explaining the need for prophylactic antibiotics to pt., she consented and ceftriaxone 250 mg I.M. was administered in Ⓛ dorsogluteal muscle. Pt. declined morning-after pill. Pt. consented to blood screening for HIV and hepatitis. Blood samples drawn, labeled, and sent to lab. Pt. understands need for f/u tests for HIV, hepatitis, and venereal disease. States she will f/u with family dr. ———————— Susan Rose, RN
	2330	June Jones, MSW, spoke with pt. at length. Gave pt. information on rape crisis center and victims' rights advocate. Pt. states, "I'll call them. Ms. Jones told me they can help me deal with this." Pt. phoned brother and sister-in-law who will come to hospital and take pt. to their home for the night. Police officers interviewed pt. with her permission regarding the details of the event. At pt.'s request, Ms. Jones and myself remained with pt. ———————— Susan Rose, RN
	2350	Pt.'s brother, John Muncy, and his wife, Carol Muncy, arrived to take pt. to their house. Pt. will make appt. tomorrow to f/u with own dr. next week or sooner, if needed. Pt. has names and phone numbers for rape crisis counselor, victims' rights advocate, Ms. Jones, ED, and police dept. ———————— Susan Rose, RN

REFUSAL OF TREATMENT

Any mentally competent adult can refuse treatment. In most cases, the health care personnel responsible for the patient's care can remain free

RESPECTING A PATIENT'S RIGHT TO REFUSE CARE

Never ignore a patient's request to refuse treatment. A patient can sue you for battery — intentionally touching another person without authorization—for simply following a doctor's orders. To overrule the patient's decision, the doctor or your facility must obtain a court order. Only then are you legally authorized to administer the treatment.

from legal jeopardy as long as they fully inform the patient about his medical condition and the likely consequences of refusing treatment. The courts recognize a competent adult's right to refuse medical treatment, even when that refusal will clearly lead to his death. (See *Respecting a patient's right to refuse care.*)

When your patient refuses treatment, inform him of the risks involved in making such a decision. If possible, inform him in writing. If he continues to refuse treatment, notify the doctor, who will choose the most appropriate plan of action.

ESSENTIAL DOCUMENTATION

Record the date and time of the patient's refusal of treatment. Be sure to document the patient's exact words in the chart. To protect yourself legally, document that you didn't provide the prescribed treatment because the patient refused it. Then ask the patient to sign a refusal-of-treatment release form.

If the patient refuses to sign the release form, document this refusal in your progress note. For additional protection, your facility's policy may require you to ask the patient's spouse or closest relative to sign another refusal-of-treatment release form. Document which relative signs the form.

| 9/8/05 | 2000 | Pt. refusing to have I.V. line inserted, stating that he's "sick and tired of being stuck." Explained to pt. the need for I.V. fluids and antibiotics and the likely result of refusing treatment. Dr. Eisenberg notified at 1930 and came to see pt. Dr. Eisenberg spent 20 minutes with pt. explaining rationales for therapies and potential risks of refusing therapy. Pt. still refusing I.V. line. Pt. has agreed to drink at least 4 oz of fluid every hour and take oral antibiotics. Pt. verbalized understanding that oral antibiotics aren't as effective in treating his condition. Orders written for 4 oz of fluids P.O. q1hr; amoxicillin 250 mg P.O. q8hr. Repeat electrolytes in a.m. ————————————— Jack Bard, RN |

REFUSAL TO LEAVE, VISITOR'S

Visitors can be an important source of support for patients and may help the patient with his needs. On occasion, visitors may be unable to give support and may, in fact, be detrimental to the patient. This may be seen through objective measurement, or may even be verbalized by the patient to you privately, when the visitor isn't present. At times, visitors may interfere with patient care. At the time of admission, explain visiting policies to the family and ensure that they understand why it's necessary, referring to the needs of the patient (to conserve energy, to rest, or to reduce pain). Provide a telephone number for the family spokesperson to call at predetermined times to get updates and ask questions, within the limits of patient confidentiality.

There may be situations in which visitors may refuse to leave. This is commonly related to anxiety and concern about the patient. Ask the visitors to tell you what their concerns are, and show them that you care. Remember that family members react differently to stress and need to be encouraged to take care of themselves as well. Educate them about nursing routines and visiting policies, reiterating, as necessary, the reasons for limiting visitation.

In special circumstances, such as when a patient is critically ill, visitors may be permitted to stay or visit at times other than the scheduled visiting hours if the nurse caring for the patient or the nursing supervisor feels it's in the patient's or family's best interest.

If family members continue to refuse to leave despite all interventions, call the nursing supervisor and security. By all means, don't place yourself in a dangerous situation, such as arguing with the visitor or making physical contact.

ESSENTIAL DOCUMENTATION

On admission, document that visiting policies were explained to the patient and his family. Note whether written visiting policies were given to them.

When visitors refuse to leave, document what they tell you, using their own words. Note which family members are present. Also, record what you tell the family and their responses, objectively describing their behaviors. Chart the names of the nursing supervisor and security personnel notified, the time of notification, and any instructions given. If a supervisor or security comes to see the family, describe what was said to the visitors and their responses.

7/5/05	1945	Pt.'s roommate put on call light at 1915 and said that he was bothered by pt.'s 4 sons and their families all in the room visiting, totaling 14 visitors. Visiting guidelines reviewed with pt. and family. Reinforced that only 2 people may visit at a time and that visiting hours are from 1000 to 2000. Written guidelines also given to family members. Suggested that 2 family members stay with the pt. while others wait in the waiting room and that family members take turns in the pt.'s room. Also reminded them that visiting hours were over at 2000. Eldest son, Joshua said, "My father just had surgery. In our country, it's important for the family to take care of and respect their father. We have to be with him all the time." Explained to family that a nurse was responsible 24 hours per day for the care of their father. With pt.'s permission, reviewed 24-hour care plan with family. Son said he understood the care being given but still felt the family should stay. Nursing supervisor, Alicia Stevens, RN, called at 1930 and came to floor. Mrs. Stevens discussed the situation with the family. The family, Mrs. Stevens, and myself agreed that the son could stay all night with his father and the rest of the family would go home. The son would act as family spokesperson and would call them at bedtime and on awakening in the morning to give a progress report. The family would continue to come to the hospital but would wait in the waiting room and take turns visiting, 2 at a time. A cot was obtained for son. Curtain pulled around pt.'s bed for privacy. Care plan amended to reflect these changes. Security notified of the change in visiting procedures for this family. — Penny Woods, RN

REMOVAL OF MEDICAL RECORD BY DOCTOR REQUEST

The medical record is the property of the facility and may not be removed or copied without consent of the facility and the patient. The medical record must stay with the patient and may not be moved from the nursing unit by any member of the health care team unless the patient is moved as well. The medical record must accompany the patient to other departments in the facility (such as dialysis, radiology, and the operating room) and be returned with the patient when he returns to the nursing unit.

If a doctor attempts to remove a medical record from the nursing unit, remind him that the record may not be removed. If the doctor insists, notify the nursing supervisor immediately. Any attempt to remove a medical record from the nursing unit requires immediate follow-up to protect the patient and the facility.

If a medical record is removed and lost, serious legal consequences can occur. If a lost chart isn't found, the risk management team and legal affairs will spearhead efforts to create a secondary document that will reflect the care given to the patient. The secondary document will reflect that the original chart was lost and that documentation was done as a late entry substitution for the original lost document. Because laws and regulations may differ by state, follow legal and facility policies in amending a medical record. Make sure that the date reflects the actual date a retrospective note is written and the reason for the amended chart. Don't backdate a record under any circumstances.

Essential documentation

Record the date and time of your entry. Document the name of the doctor who attempted to remove the chart from the nursing unit, the location, and any comments made by the doctor. Record your insistence that the chart not be removed and the doctor's response. Write down the name of the nursing supervisor and risk manager that you notified and the time notification occurred. Record their instructions and your actions. If the nursing supervisor or risk manager came to the nursing unit to discuss the situation, record the discussion that ensued, and document the doctor's response. If the doctor left the unit with the record, chart the time that the record was taken and returned. Complete an incident report, according to your facility's policy.

| 11/26/05 | 1530 | Dr. Smith in to see pt. at 1430. At 1440, he picked up the chart and began to walk off the unit. This nurse followed him to the exit and reminded him that the chart couldn't leave the unit and must stay with the pt. at all times. He stated he needed to review it in his office and would return it shortly. I asked him to review it on the unit and when he refused, I asked him to discuss it with the nursing supervisor. He stated he didn't have time to wait and left the unit at 1445. Nursing supervisor, Tonya Haas, RN, notified of occurrence at 1447 and stated that she would contact the doctor. Medical record returned to the nursing unit at 1530 by Tonya Haas and Larry Brown, hospital administrator. —————— Brenda Murphy, RN |

RENAL FAILURE, ACUTE

Acute renal failure (ARF) is a clinical syndrome characterized by a rapid decline in renal function with progressive azotemia and increasing levels of serum creatinine in the blood. Obstruction, reduced circulation, and renal parenchymal disease can all cause the sudden interruption of renal function. Most commonly, ARF follows ischemic changes to renal cells due to severe, prolonged hypotension or hypovolemia, or renal cell changes due to contact with nephrotoxic agents. ARF is usually reversible with medical treatment; however, it may progress to end-stage renal disease, uremic syndrome, and death.

If you suspect your patient has ARF, contact the doctor immediately. Anticipate diuretic therapy, fluid restrictions, electrolyte monitoring, treatment of hyperkalemia, and a diet low in protein, sodium, and potassium.

ESSENTIAL DOCUMENTATION

Record the date and time of your entry. Document your assessment findings of ARF, such as oliguria, azotemia, anorexia, nausea, vomiting, bleeding, drowsiness, irritability, confusion, dry skin and mucous membranes, pruritus, Kussmaul's respirations, pulmonary edema, and hypotension early in ARF. Later in the disease, document such assessment findings as hypertension, arrhythmias, fluid overload, heart failure, systemic edema, anemia, and altered clotting. Note the name of the doctor notified, the time of notification, and orders given, such as diagnostic testing; diet high in calories and low in protein, sodium, and potassium; fluid restrictions; and treatment of hyperkalemia with such therapies as dialysis, hypertonic glucose and insulin infusions, or sodium polystyrene sulfonate. Record your interventions, such as cardiac monitoring, initiating an I.V. line, inserting an indwelling urinary catheter, monitoring daily weights, assessing for pericarditis, monitoring electrolytes and fluid balance, maintaining proper nutrition, reporting abnormal laboratory test values to the doctor, and monitoring for bleeding. Chart your patient's responses to these interventions. Use flow sheets to record your frequent assessments, vital signs, hourly intake and output, daily weight measurements, I.V. fluid therapy, drug administration, and laboratory test values. Chart all patient teaching and emotional care provided. Depending on your facility's policy, education may be recorded on a patient-teaching flow sheet.

12/18/05	1300	Answered call light at 1230 and found pt. SOB. Crackles
		and wheezes heard bilaterally, S₃ heart sound present,
		but no murmurs. Peripheral pulses palpable, skin warm
		and dry. Restless, moving about in bed. Drowsy, but alert
		and oriented to time, place, and person. No c/o nausea,
		vomiting, numbness, or tingling. P 118 and regular, BP
		92/58, RR 22 and deep, tympanic T 99.0° F, weight 187
		lb, up 3 lb since last weight on 12/17/05. Dr. Kirsch
		notified of assessment findings at 1240 and came to
		see pt. Orders given. Lab called to draw stat CBC w/diff.,
		BUN, creatinine, electrolytes, and coagulation studies.
		Urine sample sent to lab for UA. #18 French Foley
		catheter inserted w/o difficulty to gravity drainage,
		initially drained 40 ml straw-colored urine. Renal
		ultrasound scheduled for 1500. 1500 ml fluid
		restriction started. Dietary called and notified of fluid
		restriction and change to high-calorie, low-protein, Na,
		and K diet. Pharmacy also notified of fluid restriction
		and dietary change. See flow sheets for documentation
		of frequent VS, assessments, I/O, I.V. therapy, weights,
		and lab values. Furosemide 40 mg P.O. daily ordered
		and given at 1250. Explained fluid restriction, dietary
		change, and indications and action of furosemide to pt.
		and wife. ————————————— Bob Harkin, RN

REPORTS TO DOCTOR

Reports you need to communicate to the doctor include changes in the patient's condition, laboratory and other test results, and patient concerns. If this patient's care comes into question, the doctor could claim that he wasn't notified; that's why proper documentation of your conversation is essential.

Nurses often write, "Notified doctor of lab results." This statement is too vague. In the event of a malpractice suit, it allows the plaintiff's lawyer (and the doctor) to imply that you didn't communicate reports to the doctor. (See "Critical test values, reporting," page 84.)

ESSENTIAL DOCUMENTATION

Your note should include the date and time you notified the doctor, the means you used to communicate (such as telephone or fax), the doctor's name, and what you reported. If you left a message for the doctor or gave a result to someone else such as a receptionist, record that person's name as well. Record the doctor's response and any orders given. If no orders are given, document that as well.

9/13/05	2215	Called Dr. Spencer at 2200 to report increased serous
		drainage from pt.'s Ⓛ chest tube. Dr. Spencer's order
		was to observe the drainage for 1 more hr and then
		call him back. ———————— Danielle Bergeron, RN

REQUEST FOR PATIENT INFORMATION FROM MEDIA

You have a professional and ethical responsibility to protect your patient's privacy. The American Nurses Association's Code for Nurses states that you must safeguard the patient's right to privacy "by judiciously protecting information of a confidential nature." Moreover, the American Hospital Association's Patient's Bill of Rights upholds a patient's right to privacy. This means that you may not disclose any medical or personal information about the patient to the media, even the fact that the patient has been admitted to your facility. (See *The public's right to know.*)

Follow your facility's policy on handling requests from the media. Don't give out any information; instead, refer the media to the public affairs office. Contact your nursing supervisor to advise her of the event, and call security, if necessary, to escort the media from the unit.

ESSENTIAL DOCUMENTATION

If the media arrive on your unit requesting information on a patient, record the date and time, the name of the individuals, their organizations, and the information requested. Document what you told the media and

LEGAL CASEBOOK

THE PUBLIC'S RIGHT TO KNOW

The newsworthiness of an event or person can make disclosure acceptable. In such circumstances, the public's need for information may outweigh a person's right to keep his medical condition private. For example, newspapers routinely publish the findings of the president's annual physical examination in response to the public's demand for information.

Other events for which the public's right to know may outweigh the patient's right to privacy include breakthroughs in medical technology (the first successful hand transplant) and product tampering cases, for example. In 1999, the national media gave wide exposure to an incident in New York state in which nine people died from St. Louis encephalitis transmiited by mosquito bites.

their responses. Record the time security was notified, time security arrived on the unit, names of the security officers, and time security escorted the media from the unit. Chart the name of the nursing supervisor you notified of the event, the time of notification, and her response.

If the media call your unit requesting information about a patient, document the date and time of the call, the name of the individuals, their organizations, the information requested, and your response. Chart the name of the nursing supervisor that you notified of the telephone calls and the time of notification.

12/13/05	1745	Post Tribune reporter James Smith, appeared at the
		nurse's station at 1730 requesting information about pt.
		Agnes Jones. See attached business card. Told Mr. Smith
		that no information could be given out about any pt.,
		to contact the hospital's public affairs office in the
		morning, and to please leave the hospital immediately.
		Mr. Smith refused to leave. Security called at 1735.
		Security officer, Steven Tully, arrived on unit at 1737
		and escorted Mr. Smith off the unit. Nursing super-
		visor, Betty Blakemore, RN, notified of incident at 1740.
		Message also left on answering machine of public affairs
		office. ———————————————— Catherine Watts, RN

RESPIRATORY ARREST

Respiratory arrest is defined as the absence of respirations. If a patient is found without respirations, rapid intervention is critical because brain death occurs within 4 minutes after respirations cease. Immediately call for help and send a coworker to call the code team and the doctor. After assessing the patient's airway and breathing, check for a pulse. If you detect a pulse, begin rescue breathing (using a pocket facemask) and continue until respirations return spontaneously or ventilatory support via endotracheal intubation and mechanical ventilation can be instituted.

ESSENTIAL DOCUMENTATION

Most facilities use a code sheet to facilitate documentation. (For more on code sheets, see "Cardiopulmonary arrest and resuscitation," page 53.) Your charting should include the date and time that the patient was found unresponsive and without respirations and the name of the person who found the patient. Include whether the event was witnessed. Record the name of the person who initiated cardiopulmonary resuscitation (CPR) and the time CPR was initiated as well as the names of the other members of the code team. All members of the team should sign the flow sheet. Document all interventions (such as drugs administered, cardiac monitoring, endotracheal intubation, and arterial blood gas analysis), the time they occurred, and the patient's response. Describe the outcome of the code. For example, did the patient resume spontaneous respirations, is he receiving mechanical ventilation, or did he expire? Note whether the family was present or the time that the family was notified of the event.

In your note, record the events leading to the respiratory arrest, the assessment findings prompting you to call a code, and any other interventions performed before the code team arrived (such as the time that CPR was initiated). Include the patient's response to the interventions. Indicate in your note that a code sheet was used to document the events of the code.

10/3/05	1440	Found pt. unresponsive on floor next to his bed at
		1428. Airway opened using head-tilt, chin-lift maneuver;
		no respirations noted. Called for help. Carol Ross, RN,
		arrived and was sent to call code team at 1431. Venti-
		lation attempt via pocket facemask unsuccessful. Head
		repositioned but still unable to deliver breath. No
		foreign bodies noted in mouth. After delivery of 3rd
		abdominal thrust, piece of meat was expelled. Pt. still
		without respirations; carotid pulse palpable. Rescue
		breathing initiated via facemask. Code team arrived at
		1433 and continued resuscitative efforts. See code
		record. —————————————————— Fran Vitello, RN
	1450	Pt. resumed respirations and opened eyes. P 68,
		BP 102/52, RR 32 unlabored and deep. Placed on O_2
		2 L/min via NC. Pt. being transferred to ICU for
		observation. Report called to Peggy Wallace, RN, at 1445.
		Family notified of pt.'s condition and transfer to ICU.
		Family will call ICU in 1 hour to check on pt.'s condition.
		——————————————————— Fran Vitello, RN

RESPIRATORY DISTRESS

Respiratory distress occurs when abnormalities of oxygenation or carbon dioxide are severe enough to endanger the function of vital organs. Causes of respiratory distress may be pulmonary or nonpulmonary in origin and may be a failure of oxygenation, ventilation, or both. Common causes of respiratory distress include acute respiratory distress syndrome, pneumonia, cardiogenic pulmonary edema, pulmonary embolism, asthma, chronic obstructive pulmonary disease, sedative and opioid overdose, hypersensitivity pneumonitis, head injury, chest trauma, massive obesity, amyotrophic lateral sclerosis, phrenic nerve or cervical cord injury, Guillain-Barré syndrome, and multiple sclerosis.

Respiratory distress can develop suddenly or gradually and can quickly become a life-threatening emergency. If your patient develops respiratory distress, notify the doctor immediately. Anticipate interventions to treat the underlying condition and improve oxygenation, such as administering oxygen, mobilizing secretions, initiating endotracheal intubation and mechanical ventilation, and administering drug therapy to relieve bronchospasm, reduce airway inflammation, and alleviate severe anxiety and restlessness.

ESSENTIAL DOCUMENTATION

Record the date and time of your entry. Record your assessment findings of respiratory distress, such as dyspnea, use of accessory breathing muscles, abnormal breath sounds, cyanosis, restlessness, confusion, anxiety, delirium, tachypnea, tachycardia, hypertension, and arrhythmias. Note the name of the doctor notified, the time of notification, and the orders given, such as oxygen and drug administration. Record your interventions, such as inserting I.V. lines, administering oxygen and drugs, monitoring pulse oximetry and arterial blood gas (ABG) studies, assisting with the insertion of hemodynamic monitoring lines, assisting with endotracheal intubation, maintaining mechanical ventilation, and suctioning. Chart your patient's responses to these interventions. Use flow sheets to record your frequent assessments, vital signs, hemodynamic measurements, intake and output, I.V. therapy, and laboratory and ABG values. Document the instructions and explanations given to the patient, such as for coughing and deep-breathing exercises. Describe emotional support given to the patient.

11/3/05	1500	At 1430 while receiving mechlorethamine via implanted port, pt. c/o chills and reported, "I have tightness in my chest. It feels like my throat is closing up." Drug infusion stopped and NSS infusing at 20 ml/hr. Pt. dyspneic, diaphoretic, and restless. P 122 and regular, BP 169/90, RR 34. O_2 sat. by pulse oximetry 88%. Expiratory wheezes noted bilaterally on posterior and anterior chest auscultation. Accessory muscle use observed. Dr. Jones stat paged at 1437 and told of assessment findings. Orders given. Non-rebreather mask applied at 12 L/minute. Pt. placed in tripod position to facilitate breathing. Stat ABGs drawn by Dr. Jones. I.V. aminophylline and methylprednisolone given. See MAR. At 1450 P 104, BP 140/84, RR 30. Pulse oximetry 95%. Pt. states her breathing is easier, no further chills. Breath sounds clear, no longer using accessory muscles. See flow sheets for documentation of frequent VS, I/O, and lab values. Reassured pt. that she will be closely monitored. ———————— Rita Clarke, RN

RESTRAINTS

Restraints are defined as any method of physically restricting a person's freedom of movement, physical activity, or normal access to his body. Restraints can cause numerous problems, including limited mobility, skin breakdown, impaired circulation, incontinence, psychological distress, and strangulation.

Effective January 1, 2001, the Joint Commission on Accreditation of Healthcare Organizations (JCAHO) issued revised standards that were intended to reduce the use of restraints. According to the revised standards regarding the use of restraints on the medical-surgical unit, restraint use is to be limited to emergencies in which the patient is at risk for harming himself or others. However, because restraints are used only in emergencies, your facility may authorize qualified registered nurses to initiate their use. The revised standards also emphasize staff education. It's important to know and follow your facility's policy on the use of restraints.

Time limitations have also been set on the use of restraints. Within 12 hours of placing a patient in restraints, a licensed independent practitioner must give an order for restraints; however, if the need for restraints is due to a significant change in the patient's condition, the licensed independent practitioner must examine the patient immediately. This order must be renewed every 24 hours. If a patient requires the use of restraints for at least two separate episodes in a 24-hour time period, JCAHO requires notification of the chief medical officer or chief executive officer.

The revised JCAHO standards require continuous monitoring to ensure patient safety, including monitoring the patient's vital signs, nutrition and hydration needs, circulation, and hygiene and toileting needs. The patient's family members must also be notified of the use of restraints if the patient consented to have them informed of his care. Moreover, the patient must be informed of the conditions necessary for his release from restraints.

ESSENTIAL DOCUMENTATION

Document each episode of the use of restraints, including the date and time they were initiated. Your facility may have a special form or flow sheet for this purpose. Record the circumstances resulting in the use of restraints and nonphysical interventions considered or used first. Describe the rationale for the specific type of restraints used. Chart the name of the licensed independent practitioner who ordered the restraints. Include the conditions or behaviors necessary for discontinuing the restraints and that these conditions were communicated to the patient. Document each in-person evaluation by the licensed independent practitioner. Record 15-minute assessments of the patient, including signs of injury, nutrition, hydration, circulation, range of motion, vital signs, hygiene, elimination, comfort, physical and psychological status, and readiness for removing the restraints. Record your interventions to help the patient meet the conditions for removing the restraints. Note that the patient was continuously monitored. Document any injuries or complications that occurred, the time they occurred, the name of the doctor notified, and the results of your interventions or actions.

8/28/05	1400	Pt. extremely confused and pulled I.V. out at 1345.
		Attempted to calm patient through nonthreatening
		verbal communication. No I.V. access available. Dr. Miller
		notified at 1350 and came to see pt. at 1353. Ativan
		2 mg I.M. given per Dr. Miller's order. After evalu-
		ation, Dr. Miller ordered 2-point restraints applied to
		prevent harm to patient. Pt. informed that restraints
		would be removed when he could remain calm and refrain
		from trying to remove I.V. Pt. doesn't want his family to
		be notified of restraint application. See restraint moni-
		toring sheet for frequent assessments and intervention
		notations. ———————————— Carol Sacks, RN

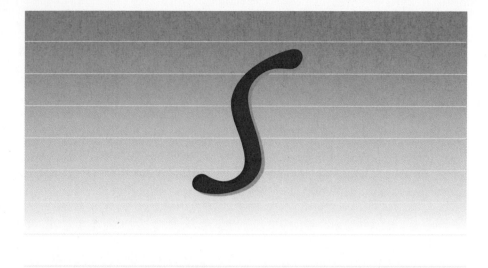

SECLUSION

During seclusion, a patient is separated from others in a safe, secure, and contained environment with close nursing supervision to protect himself, other patients, and staff members from imminent harm. Seclusion is used when nonphysical interventions are ineffective. Follow your facility's policy when placing a patient in seclusion, and familiarize yourself with the Joint Commission on Accreditation of Healthcare Organizations' standards on the use of seclusion for behavioral health care reasons in nonbehavioral health care settings, which became effective January 1, 2001.

Seclusion is based on three principles: containment, isolation, and decreased sensory input. In containment, the patient is restricted to an area in which he can be protected from harm. Moreover, others are protected from impulsive acts by the patient. Isolation permits the patient to withdraw from situations that are too intense for him to handle at that point. Decreased sensory input reduces external stimulation and sensory overload, allowing the patient to regroup and reorganize coping skills.

ESSENTIAL DOCUMENTATION

Record the date and time of each episode as well as the rationale for, and circumstances leading up to, the use of seclusion. Describe the nonphysical interventions that were tried first. In your note, chart the time that you notified the family members and their names. Document that you notified the doctor and obtained a verbal or written order. Write the verbal order in the doctor's orders, according to your facility's policy. Record each time the order for seclusion is renewed. Record the doctor's visit and his evaluation of the patient. Criteria for ending seclusion should be charted. Document what the patient was told about seclusion, including the behavior criteria for stopping seclusion. Chart your frequent assessments of the patient, such as nutrition, hydration, circulation, range of motion, mobility, hygiene, elimination, comfort, and psychological status. Record your interventions to help the patient meet these needs. Describe your interventions to help the patient reduce his need for seclusion and his responses to these interventions. Document that the patient is receiving continuous monitoring while in seclusion and by whom.

10/26/05	2000	Approached by pt. at 1930, crying and saying loudly, "I
		can't stand it, they will get me." Repeated this statement
		several times. Unable to say who "they" were. Pt. asked
		to sit in a seclusion room saying, "it's quiet and safe
		there. That's what I do at the psych. hospital." Called
		Dr. Wright at 1935 and told him of pt. request. Verbal
		order given for seclusion as requested by pt. Dr. Wright
		will be in to evaluate pt. at 2030. Pt. placed in empty
		pt. room on unit in close proximity to nurses' station.
		Told her that since seclusion was voluntary, she was
		free to leave seclusion when she felt ready. Rita
		Summers, CNA, assigned to continuously observe pt.
		P 82, BP 132/82, RR 18, oral T 98.7° F. Family notified
		of pt.'s request for seclusion, that pt. is free to leave
		seclusion on her own, will be continuously observed by
		CNA and assessed frequently by RN, and that doctor
		will be by to see her at 2030. Family stated they were
		comfortable with this decision. ———— Donna Blau, RN

SEIZURE MANAGEMENT

Seizures are paroxysmal events associated with abnormal electrical discharges of neurons in the brain. Partial seizures are usually unilateral, involving a localized or focal area of the brain. Generalized seizures involve the entire brain.

When your patient has a generalized seizure, observe the seizure characteristics to help determine the area of the brain involved; administer anticonvulsants as ordered; protect him from injury; and prevent serious complications, such as aspiration and airway obstruction. When caring for a patient at risk for seizures, take precautions to prevent injury and complications in the event of a seizure.

PREVENTING SEIZURES

Teach the patient the following measures to help him control and decrease the occurrence of seizures:

- Take the exact dose of medication at the times prescribed. Missing doses, doubling doses, or taking extra doses can cause a seizure.
- Eat balanced, regular meals. Low blood glucose levels (hypoglycemia) and inadequate vitamin intake can lead to seizures.
- Be alert for odors that may trigger an attack. Advise the patient and his family to inform the doctor of any strong odors they notice at the time of a seizure.
- Limit alcohol intake. The patient should check with the doctor to find out whether he can drink alcoholic beverages at all.
- Get enough sleep. Excessive fatigue can precipitate a seizure.
- Treat a fever early during an illness. If the patient can't reduce a fever, he should notify the doctor.
- Learn to control stress. If appropriate, suggest learning relaxation techniques such as deep-breathing exercises.
- Avoid trigger factors, such as flashing lights, hyperventilation, loud noises, heavy musical beats, video games, and television.

ESSENTIAL DOCUMENTATION

If a patient is at risk for seizures, document all precautions taken, such as padding the side rails, headboard, and footboard of the bed; keeping the bed in low position; raising side rails while the patient is in bed; placing an airway at the bedside; and having suction equipment nearby. Record that seizure precautions have been explained to the patient.

If your patient has a seizure, record the date and time it began as well as its duration and any precipitating factors. Identify any sensation that may be considered an aura. Describe involuntary behavior occurring at the onset, such as lip smacking, chewing movements, or hand and eye movements. Record any incontinence, vomiting, or salivation during the seizure. Describe where the movement began and the parts of the body involved. Note any progression or pattern to the activity. Document whether the patient's eyes deviated to one side and whether the pupils changed in size, shape, equality, or reaction to light. Note if the patient's teeth were clenched or open.

Document the patient's response to the seizure, drugs given, complications, and interventions. Record the name of the doctor that you notified, the time of notification, and any orders given. Finally, record your assessment of the patient's postictal mental and physical status every 15 minutes for 1 hour, every 30 minutes for 1 hour, and then hourly as long as there are no further complications, or according to your facility's policy.

Document patient teaching that you provide for the patient or his family, including instructions you give about preventing and managing seizures. (See *Preventing seizures.*)

| 11/19/05 | 1730 | At 1712, pt. had whole body stiffening, followed by alternating muscle spasm and relaxation, teeth clenched. Seizure lasted 2½ min. Breathing was labored during seizure, no cyanosis noted. Pt. sleeping at time of onset. Pt. incontinent during seizure, but no vomiting or salivation noted. Padded side rails, headboard, and footboard in place prior to seizure; bed in low position; suction and airway in room but not needed. Pt. placed on Ⓛ side, airway patent, breath sounds clear bilaterally. Dr. Gordon notified of seizure at 1716 and came to see pt. at 1720. Diazepam 10 mg given I.V. as ordered. Pt. currently sleeping, confused when aroused, not oriented to time or place. P 94, BP 142/88, RR 18 and regular, tympanic T 97.7° F. See flow sheets for frequent VS and neurologic assessments, per policy. Wife in to visit at 1725. Explained that pt. had a seizure and measures taken to treat it. Reviewed with wife how to prevent seizures and gave her copy of written material, "Preventing Seizures." Wife verbalized understanding. ——— Gale Hartman, RN |

SEXUAL ADVANCE BY COLLEAGUE

The Equal Employment Opportunity Commission defines sexual harassment as an unwelcome sexual advance, a request for sexual favors, and other verbal, nonverbal, or physical conduct of a sexual nature. However, such behavior as sexual activity between consenting adults or asking someone for a date isn't sexual harassment. Sexual harassment is a subtle but real form of sexual abuse. (See *Myths about sexual harassment,* page 370.)

An unwanted sexual advance by a colleague should be addressed immediately. Decline the advance in a direct and honest manner. However, if your colleague persists, or if the initial advance consists of sexually charged, degrading, or vulgar words or makes you a target of sexual jokes, touching, or pinching, tell the colleague making the advance that this behavior is harassment and that it won't be tolerated.

MYTHS ABOUT SEXUAL HARASSMENT

Common myths about sexual harassment include:
- If women would just say "No," it would stop.
- Harassment will stop if a person just ignores it.
- If women watched the way they dress, there wouldn't be a problem with sexual harassment.
- Only women can be sexually harassed.
- Sexual harassment is no big deal — it's the natural way men and women express affection and friendship.
- Most people enjoy sexual attention at work. Teasing and flirting make work fun.
- Sexual harassment is harmless. Persons who object have no sense of humor or don't know how to accept a compliment.
- Sexual harassment policies will negatively affect friendly relationships.
- Nice people couldn't possibly be harassers.

Most facilities have a policy for filing a complaint. If your facility doesn't have a policy, inform your immediate supervisor or the human resources department that the behavior you experienced constitutes sexual harassment, and ask how to proceed with a complaint.

The human resources department will contact the accused employee and inform him that a complaint has been filed against him. They'll advise the employee that this behavior must cease immediately. After you've reported the harassment, it's the responsibility of your employer to follow through according to local and federal guidelines. Confidentiality is important, and the privacy of individuals reporting or accused of sexual harassment must be protected as much as possible. A complaint may also be filed with the state Human Rights Commission or with the federal Equal Employment Opportunity Commission.

ESSENTIAL DOCUMENTATION

States vary in the way that sexual harassment issues are addressed and resolved. The human resources department in your facility can help you with documentation that complies with local and federal law and facility policy. In general, documentation should include:
- description of the incident, including the date, time, and location
- statements made by both parties (in quotes)
- names of individuals that you informed about the incident, such as the nursing supervisor and human resources manager, and their responses

- date, time, and location where the information was shared as well as any counseling or referral offered to you
- names of witnesses, if any
- names of anyone who supports your charge (other victims or witnesses).

Document each instance of harassment. Keep a copy of all the documentation at home. This will be useful if legal action is taken.

To: Tom Cooke, RN, Nursing Supervisor
    Martin Hillman, Director of Human Resources
From: Martha Clark, RN
    MICU
Date: 8/22/05
Time: 1320
At 1240, Dr. Parker asked me to go with him to a movie. I refused, saying I was busy. He said, "You don't have to be such a snob." I responded by repeating that I had other plans. He then began to follow me down the hall saying loudly, "Why won't you go out with me? Come on answer me. What's the matter? Are you frigid?" I requested that he stop speaking to me in this manner and, when he persisted, I called Tom Cooke, RN, nursing supervisor, at 1245 and asked him to address the situation. J. Smith, K. Brown, P. Green, and M. Carter were in the hallway and heard this exchange. The nursing supervisor arrived on the unit at 1310 and after speaking with me, instructed Dr. Parker to stop speaking loudly to me and advised me that I should report the incident to the human resources dept. He also asked that I put the event in writing. Dr. Parker did stop his behavior and apologized to me. He said, "I'm sorry I bothered you. I won't bother you again."

SEXUAL ADVANCE BY PATIENT

Several recent studies show that more than 50% of nurses have experienced sexual harassment on the job and more than 25% reported being victimized while on the job. Patients were the most frequent sources of sexual harassment and physical assault. Nursing, by its very nature of having to care for a patient's bodily needs, transgresses normal social rules regarding physical contact. A patient who relies on a nurse's caring attitude may exploit this. In addition, the intimacy of the nurse-patient relationship can mislead a patient into believing that a nurse might be receptive to such an advance.

The patient's motivation for making a sexual advance may be a need for friendliness or attention, a demonstration of anger, or a plea for reassurance about sexual attractiveness. In many cases, when a sexual advance by a patient occurs, the nurse will typically ignore it, pretend she hasn't heard it, or withdraw from contact with the patient. However, a better way to handle this type of behavior is to address it immediately and to be honest and direct with the patient, making a comment such as "I'm uncomfortable when you speak to me like that. Let's talk about something else" or "I don't want you to touch me that way."

If a verbal warning isn't effective in changing the patient's behavior, inform your nursing supervisor immediately and have a colleague present when care is delivered. In addition, speak with the patient's doctor about the patient's behavior. Consultation with psychiatric staff may help the patient control inappropriate behavior. Also, the psychiatric clinical nurse specialist can help the nursing staff plan this patient's care. Be sure to maintain the patient's privacy and confidentiality, discussing his behavior only with caregivers who need to know.

ESSENTIAL DOCUMENTATION

Follow your facility's policy for documenting a sexual advance by a patient. In addition to documenting the incident in the medical record, you may be required to fill out an incident report.

Record the date and time that the sexual behavior took place. Carefully document the care that the patient received as well as the inappropriate behavior. Record what the patient said to you, using his words (in quotes). List staff members who witnessed the behavior. Leave your emotions or feelings out of your charting. Document your response to the patient's behavior, putting your exact statements in quotes. Record the time that you notified the doctor and nursing supervisor, their names, and their responses.

10/14/05	0900	While taking the pt.'s VS at 0830, he touched my breast
		and asked me to "get in here and cuddle." I stepped
		back from the bed and told the pt., "I'm not comfortable
		when you touch me like that or speak in that way. I
		prefer that you not do it." Pt. stated, "You nurses are
		all alike. Come on over here." I stated, "Those remarks
		make me uncomfortable. Let's talk about something else."
		Pt. persisted in his remarks, and I left the room and
		returned at 0835 with Jan Smith, RN. Pt. stated, "Oh,
		you can't handle things on your own, you need help" and
		made no further comments or sexual approaches. VS
		completed at 0840. Dr. Hope and K. Smith, RN, nursing
		supervisor, informed at 0845 of pt.'s persistent sexual
		approach when I was alone with him and that he ceased
		his comments when a colleague accompanied me. K. Smith
		and Dr. Hope addressed inappropriate behaviors with
		pt. at 0855. Caregiver team meeting scheduled with all
		staff who will participate in care of the pt. to work out
		a care plan. ————————— Monica Smith, RN

SEXUAL ADVANCE BY VISITOR

The Equal Employment Opportunity Commission defines sexual harassment as unwelcome sexual advances, requests for sexual favors, and other verbal, nonverbal, or physical conduct of a sexual nature. Unwelcome sexual advances may come from anyone, including a person visiting a patient.

Address an unwanted sexual advance by a family member or visitor immediately. Tell the family member or visitor to stop the behavior; that it's inappropriate and won't be tolerated. If you don't feel comfortable confronting the family member or visitor, your facility should have a policy in place designating who will address this behavior. Your employer is responsible for ensuring that you're supported and protected from reprisals.

Immediately report the incident to the nursing supervisor and the human resources department. Most facilities have a policy for filing a complaint. If a policy doesn't exist, ask the nursing supervisor or human resources department how to proceed with a complaint.

ESSENTIAL DOCUMENTATION

Document sexual advances by a family member or visitor according to your facility's policy. Record the date, time, and location of the incident as well as the name of the family member or visitor. Describe the person's behaviors and record what was said, using his words (in quotes). Document the names of any witnesses, and note whether sexual advances were made to other staff members. Record the name of the nursing supervisor and the time of notification. Write a separate report for each instance of harassment.

To: *Karen Weber, RN, Nursing Supervisor*
    Sally Reising, Director, Human Resources
From: *Pam Thomas, RN*
Date: *10/24/05*
Time: *1750*
At *1730, pt.'s nephew, Conrad Minsk, stopped me outside Room 200 and invited me for a drink after work. I responded that I had other plans. Mr. Minsk continued to invite me to join him for drinks and dinner after work. He asked where I lived and put his hand on my arm. I removed his hand from my arm, and told him, "This behavior isn't appropriate. Please stop it now." The visitor got angry and stated, "I thought you nurses wanted to be picked up." The visitor left the facility shortly after. Nursing supervisor, Karen Weber, RN, notified of event at 1745 and directed me to file this report. There were no witnesses to this event.*

SHOCK

Shock is a systemic pathologic event characterized by diffuse cellular ischemia that can lead to cell, tissue, and organ death if not promptly recognized and treated. Shock is classified as hypovolemic (hemorrhage), cardiogenic (myocardial infarction), or distributive. Distributive type is further divided into septic (gram-negative bacterial infection), neurogenic (spinal cord injury), and anaphylactic (hypersensitivity such as bee sting) shock. (See *Classifying shock*.)

Because shock either causes or results from multisystem failure, it's typically treated in an intensive care unit. Nursing responsibilities related to shock center on prevention, early detection, emergent treatment, and support during recovery and rehabilitation.

ESSENTIAL DOCUMENTATION

Record the date and time of your entry. Document your assessment findings of shock, such as declining level of consciousness, hypotension, tachycardia in early shock and bradycardia in later shock, ECG changes, weakened pulses, dyspnea, tachypnea, declining arterial oxygen saturation and partial pressure of arterial oxygen, rising partial pressure of arterial carbon dioxide, respiratory and metabolic acidosis, oliguria, rising blood urea nitrogen and creatinine, diminished or absent bowel sounds, and pale, cool skin. Note the time that you notified the doctor, his name, and orders given, such as drug, fluid, blood, and oxygen administration. Record your in-

CLASSIFYING SHOCK

Type	Description
Hypovolemic	Results from a decrease in central vascular volume. Total body fluids may or may not be decreased. Causes include hemorrhage, dehydration, and fluid shifts (trauma, burns, anaphylaxis).
Cardiogenic	Results from a direct or indirect pump failure with decreasing cardiac output. Total body fluid isn't decreased. Causes include valvular stenosis or insufficiency, myocardial infarction, cardiomyopathy, arrhythmias, cardiac arrest, cardiac tamponade, pericarditis, pulmonary hypertension, and pulmonary emboli.
Distributive	Results from inadequate vascular tone that leads to massive vasodilation. Vascular volume remains normal and heart pumps adequately, but size of vascular space increases, causing maldistribution of blood within the circulatory system. It includes the following subtypes: ■ Septic shock—A form of severe sepsis characterized by hypotension and altered tissue perfusion. Vascular tone is lost and cardiac output may be decreased. ■ Neurogenic shock—Characterized by massive vasodilation from loss or suppression of sympathetic tone. Causes include head trauma, spinal cord injuries, anesthesia, and stress. ■ Anaphylactic shock—Characterized by massive vasodilation and increased capillary permeability secondary to a hypersensitivity reaction to an antigen.

terventions, such as assisting with the insertion of hemodynamic monitoring lines, inserting I.V. lines, administering drugs, continuous ECG monitoring, providing supplemental oxygen, inserting an indwelling urinary catheter, airway management, and pulse oximetry monitoring. Chart your patient's responses to these interventions. Use flow sheets to record your frequent assessments, vital signs, hemodynamic measurements, intake and output, I.V. therapy, and laboratory test and arterial blood gas values. Also, record patient teaching and emotional care given.

7/17/05	1930	At 1905 noted bloody abdominal dressing and abdominal
		distention. No bowel sounds auscultated. Pt. slow to
		respond to verbal stimulation, not oriented to time and
		place, and not readily following commands. Pupil response
		sluggish. Cardiac monitor reveals HR of 128, no arrhyth-
		mias noted. Peripheral pulses weak. Skin pale and cool;
		capillary refill 4-5 sec, BP 88/52. Breath sounds clear.
		Normal heart sounds. Breathing regular and deep,
		RR 24. O₂ sat. 88% on room air. Dr. Garcia notified of
		changes at 1910 and orders given. 100% nonrebreather
		mask applied, O₂ sat. increased to 92%. Foley catheter
		placed with initial 70 ml urine output. Stat ABG, hemo-
		globin, hematocrit, serum electrolytes and renal panel
		ordered. I.V. inserted in Ⓛ antecubital space with 18G
		catheter on first attempt. 1,000 ml I.V. dextrose 5%
		in 0.45% NSS infusing at 100 ml/hr. Explained all pro-
		cedures and drugs to pt. and wife. Wife verbalized
		understanding and fears. Reassured wife that pt. is
		being closely monitored. See flow sheets for documen-
		tation of frequent VS, I/O, I.V. fluids, neuro. checks,
		and lab values. ——————— Brian Wilcox, RN

SICKLE CELL CRISIS

Sickle cell anemia is a genetic disorder that occurs primarily, but not exclusively, in African Americans. It results from a defective hemoglobin molecule (hemoglobin S) that causes red blood cells to roughen and become sickle-shaped. Such cells impair circulation, resulting in chronic ill health (characterized by fatigue, dyspnea on exertion, and swollen joints), periodic crises, long-term complications, and premature death.

Although sickle cell anemia is a chronic disorder, acute exacerbations or crises periodically occur. If you suspect your patient with sickle cell anemia is in a crisis, notify the doctor immediately and anticipate oxygen and I.V. fluid administration and pain control.

ESSENTIAL DOCUMENTATION

Record the date and time of your entry. Document your assessment findings of a sickle cell crisis, such as severe abdominal, thoracic, muscular, and joint pain; jaundice; fever; dyspnea; pallor; and lethargy. Note the time that you notified the doctor, his name, and orders given, such as oxygen administration, analgesics, antipyretics, fluid administration, and blood transfusions. Record your interventions, such as initiating I.V. therapy using a large-bore catheter for blood and fluid administration, encouraging bed rest, placing warm compresses over painful joints, and administering drugs and oxygen. Chart your patient's responses to these interventions. Use flow sheets to record your frequent assessments as well as the patient's vital signs, intake and output, I.V. therapy, and laboratory test values. Document any patient teaching performed (crisis prevention, genetic screening) and emotional support given.

11/8/05	0900	19 y.o. male with history of sickle cell disease admitted to
		ED at 0825 with weakness and severe abdominal and joint
		pain. He reports nausea, vomiting, and poor oral intake X
		3 days. Skin and mucous membranes pale and dry. Joints
		warm, red, swollen and painful to touch. Pt. is dyspneic
		with clear breath sounds. Heart sounds normal. Pt. is
		alert and oriented to time, place, and person. Abdomen
		is painful to touch; auscultated bowel sounds in all 4
		quadrants. P 96 and regular, BP 120/74, RR 22 and
		labored, oral T 100.2° F. Pt. rates abdominal and joint
		pain at 7 on a 0 to 10 scale, w/10 being the worst pain
		imaginable. Dr. McBride in to evaluate pt at 0833. Electro-
		lytes, bilirubin, CBC, ABGs drawn and sent to lab. Placed on
		O_2 at 4 L/min by NC. I.V. line started in ® forearm on
		first attempt with #18G catheter. 1,000 ml of $D_5/0.45$
		NSS at 125 ml/hr. Tylenol 650 mg P.O. given for fever.
		Morphine 2 mg given I.V. over 4 min for pain at 0843.
		Pt. positioned with joints supported by pillows. Warm com-
		presses placed on elbow and knee joints. Voided 400 ml
		clear yellow urine. Urinalysis sent to lab. Explained all
		procedures and drugs to pt. Reinforced need for good
		hydration and encouraged oral fluids at 0853. Pt. rated
		pain as 3 out of 10, with 10 being the worst pain imagin-
		able. See flow sheets for documentation of frequent VS,
		I/O, I.V. fluids, and lab values. To be admitted to 6 West
		for pain control and I.V. hydration. Report called to Pat
		Stoner, RN. ———————— Helene Mumford, RN

SKIN CARE

In addition to helping shape a patient's self-image, the skin performs many physiologic functions. It protects internal body structures from the environment and potential pathogens, regulates body temperature and homeostasis, and serves as an organ of sensation and excretion. As a result, meticulous skin care is essential to overall health.

ESSENTIAL DOCUMENTATION

Record the date and time of your entry. Assess your patient's skin and describe its condition, noting changes in color, temperature, texture, tone, turgor, thickness, moisture, and integrity. Describe your interventions related to skin care and the patient's response. Note the time that you notified the doctor of any changes, his name, the orders given, your actions, and the patient's response. Describe patient teaching given, such as proper hygiene and the importance of turning and positioning every 2 hours.

12/22/05	1000	During a.m. care, noted pt.'s skin to be dry and flaking, especially the hands, feet, and lower legs. Pt. states skin feels itchy in these areas. Skin rough, intact, warm to touch. Skin tents when pinched. After bath, blotted skin dry and applied emollient. Explained the importance of drinking more fluids and using emollients. Encouraged pt. not to scratch skin and to report intense itching to nurse. Care plan amended to include use of superfatted soap with baths and application of emollients t.i.d. Dr. Johnson notified at 0945 and order given for Benadryl 0.25 mg P.O. q 6hr prn for intense itching. Pt. states, "The itching is not that bad right now after the emollient was applied." ——————————— Jason Dickson, RN

SKIN GRAFT CARE

A skin graft consists of healthy skin taken from either the patient (autograft) or a donor (allograft) that is then applied to a part of the patient's body. The graft resurfaces an area damaged by burns, traumatic injury, or surgery. Care procedures for an autograft or allograft are essentially the same. However, an autograft requires care for two sites: the graft site and the donor site.

Successful grafting depends on various factors, including clean wound granulation with adequate vascularization, complete contact of the graft with the wound bed, aseptic technique to prevent infection, adequate graft immobilization, and skilled care. Depending on your facility's policy, a doctor or specially trained nurse may change graft dressings.

ESSENTIAL DOCUMENTATION

Record the date and time of each dressing change. Note the location, size, and appearance of the graft site. Document all drugs used, and note the patient's response to these drugs. Describe the condition of the graft, and note any signs of infection or rejection. Chart the name of the doctor that you notified, the time of notification, and any concerns or complications discussed. Record the specific care given to the graft site, including how it was covered and dressed. Document any patient and family teaching that you provide and evidence of their understanding. Note the patient's reaction to the graft.

9/17/05	1300	Dressings carefully removed from ® anterior thigh skin graft site. Site is 4 cm X 4 cm, pink, moist, and without edema or drainage. Area gently cleaned by irrigating with NSS. Xeroflo placed over site and covered with burn gauze and a roller bandage. Pt. instructed not to touch dressing, to report if dressing becomes loose, and to avoid placing any weight on the site. Pt. verbalized understanding of the instructions. Pt. stated, "The site doesn't look as bad as I thought it would." ————————————————— Brian Wilcox, RN.

SMOKING

It's a well-known fact that smoking has adverse effects on health. Yet people continue to smoke – even in the hospital. Smoking in the hospital poses special risks beyond the usual health risks: secondhand smoke can aggravate many illnesses, fire and explosion may occur when a person smokes in an area where oxygen is being used, and a smoldering cigarette dropped in a wastebasket or on bed linens can start a fire.

Explain your facility's smoking policy to the patient on admission, and provide him with a written set of facility rules, if available. If you find your patient smoking in a nonsmoking area, remind him of the facility's smoking policy. Ask him to extinguish his smoking materials and to move to a designated smoking area, if possible. Alert the doctor if your patient is smoking against medical advice.

Talk to your patient about smoking cessation. If the patient is interested in quitting, discuss strategies for smoking cessation, including smoking cessation programs and nicotine replacement therapy. Alert the doctor about your patient's smoking habits. If a patient is unwilling to stop smoking, make plans for him to go to a smoking area at certain times of the day. If necessary, arrange for an escort.

ESSENTIAL DOCUMENTATION

Document that the patient received facility policies regarding smoking on admission. Record the patient's statement about his smoking, including the number of years he has smoked and the number of cigarettes he smokes per day. Describe his feelings about quitting and his experience with smoking cessation programs. Record patient teaching, such as discussing the hazards of smoking, the use of nicotine replacement therapy, and available information on smoking cessation programs and support groups. Describe the patient's response to teaching and any smoking cessation plans. Include any written materials given to the patient.

If your patient is smoking against facility policy, chart the date and time of the incident and where he was found smoking. Record what you told the patient and his response. Document any education that took place regarding smoking cessation and the patient's response. If the doctor was notified, record that you notified him, the time, his name, and any orders given. Describe any arrangements made for the patient to smoke. Some facilities may require you to complete an incident report.

8/18/05	1400	Upon entering room, found pt. smoking while sitting
		up in his chair. Pt. complied when asked to extinguish
		cigarette. Reinforced the facility's no smoking policy.
		Discussed health risks of smoking to pt. Explained that
		if pt. wished to smoke, he would need his dr.'s order
		to be escorted outdoors to a designated area. Pt.
		stated that he was aware of health risks and would like
		to try to quit. Pt. stated, "I've been smoking since my
		teens, I know it's bad and I want to quit but I can't."
		Pt. reports 2-pack/day, 30-year history of smoking. Pt.
		asked about the use of a nicotine patch. Dr. Pasad
		notified of pt.'s smoking habit and interest in the use
		of a nicotine patch. Order given for nicotine patch,
		see MAR. Use of nicotine patch, frequency, dosage,
		adverse effects, dangers of smoking while wearing
		patch, and s/s to report to dr. explained to pt. Pt.
		information dispensed with patch given to pt. to read.
		Pt. agrees to follow-up with Dr. Pasad after discharge
		for monitoring of smoking cessation. Gave pt. names
		and contact numbers for community support groups
		and cessation programs. ———— Bruce Mailor, RN

SPINAL CORD INJURY

In addition to spinal cord damage, spinal injuries include fractures, contusions, and compressions of the vertebral column (usually a result of trauma to the head or neck). The real danger lies in possible spinal cord damage. Spinal fractures most commonly occur in the 5th, 6th, and 7th cervical; 12th thoracic; and 1st lumbar vertebrae.

Most serious spinal injuries result from motor vehicle accidents, falls, diving into shallow water, and gunshot wounds; less serious injuries result from lifting heavy objects and minor falls. Spinal dysfunction may also result from hyperparathyroidism and neoplastic lesions.

If your patient has a spinal cord injury, limit the extent of the injury with immobilization, administer steroids as ordered, and take actions to prevent complications.

ESSENTIAL DOCUMENTATION

Record the date and time of your entry. Document measures taken to immobilize the patient's spine as well as measures taken to maintain airway patency and respirations. Document a baseline neurologic assessment, and chart the results of your cardiopulmonary, GI, and renal assessments. Note the time that you notified the doctor, his name, and orders given, such as spinal immobilization and administration of steroids, analgesics, or muscle relaxants. Record your interventions, such as administering drugs, maintaining spinal immobilization, preparing the patient for neurosurgery, positioning and logrolling the patient, assisting with rehabilitation, and providing skin and respiratory care. Chart your patient's responses to these interventions. Use flow sheets to record your frequent assessments and the patient's vital signs, intake and output, I.V. therapy, and laboratory test values. Include patient teaching and emotional care given.

9/17/05	0930	Pt. alert and oriented to time, place, and person. Speech clear and coherent. No facial drooping or ptosis, tongue midline, swallows without difficulty. Readily follows commands. PERRLA. Pt. reports "mild tenderness" in lower back and states, "It's better than yesterday." Can perform active ROM of upper extremities with 5/5 muscle strength bilaterally in arms and hands. No voluntary muscle movement inferior to the iliac crests and pt. reports no sensation to touch, pressure, or temperature. Lower body muscles flaccid, patellar and Achilles reflexes absent. P 82 and regular, BP 126/72, RR 12 and regular, oral T 98.2° F. Breath sounds clear, normal heart sounds. Indwelling catheter in place and draining clear, yellow urine. See I/O sheet. Active bowel sounds are present in all 4 quadrants. Had brown, formed mod. size BM this a.m. Skin warm, dry, and intact with no tenting when pinched. Body alignment maintained while pt. logrolled with assist of 2 into ® side-lying position. Skin intact, no areas of redness noted. Reinforced importance of using incentive spirometer q/hr while awake. Pt. gave proper demo of its use. Pt. instructed to report any pain or changes in sensations. Discussed plan to begin bladder training today and remove indwelling catheter early tomorrow. Pt. expressed understanding of teaching and plans. ——— ———————————————————————— Brian Wilcox, RN

SPLINT APPLICATION

By immobilizing the site of an injury, a splint alleviates pain and allows the injury to heal in proper alignment. It also minimizes possible complications, such as excessive bleeding into the tissues, restricted blood flow caused by bone pressing against vessels, and possible paralysis from an unstable spinal cord injury. In cases of multiple serious injuries, a splint or spine board allows caretakers to move the patient without risking further damage to bones, muscles, nerves, blood vessels, and skin.

ESSENTIAL DOCUMENTATION

Record the date and time of splint application. Document the circumstances and cause of the injury. Record the patient's complaints, noting whether symptoms are localized. Chart your assessment of the splinted region, noting swelling, deformity, and tissue and skin discoloration. Also, record neurovascular status before and after splint application. (See *Assessing neurovascular status.*)

ASSESSING NEUROVASCULAR STATUS

When assessing an injured extremity, always include the following steps and compare your findings bilaterally.

- Inspect the color of fingers or toes.
- Note the size of the digits to detect edema.
- Simultaneously touch the digits of the affected and unaffected extremities and compare temperature.
- Check capillary refill by pressing on the distal tip of one digit until it's white. Then release the pressure and note how soon the normal color returns. It should return quickly in the affected and unaffected extremities.
- Check sensation by touching the fingers or toes and asking the patient how they feel. Note reports of any numbness or tingling.
- Tell the patient to close his eyes; then move one digit and ask him which position it's in to check proprioception.
- Tell the patient to wiggle his toes or move his fingers to test movement.
- Palpate the distal pulses to assess vascular patency.

Record your findings for the affected and unaffected extremities, using standard terminology to avoid ambiguity. Warmth, free movement, rapid capillary refill, and normal color, sensation, and proprioception indicate sound neurovascular status.

Note the patient's level of discomfort, using a 0-to-10 pain scale, with 0 representing no pain and 10 representing the worst pain imaginable. Describe the type of wound, if any, noting the amount of bleeding and the amount and type of any drainage. Document the type of splint being used, and describe where it has been placed. If the bone end should slip into surrounding tissue or if transportation causes any change in the degree of dislocation, be sure to note it. Record the time that you notified the doctor, his name, and any orders given. Record all patient education, noting whether written instructions were given. Note that the patient received instruction for follow-up care.

10/5/05	0900	Pt. fell off bicycle and landed on Ⓛ arm. Ⓛ wrist swollen, no deformity or discoloration noted. 6 cm X 1 cm abrasion noted along Ⓛ medial forearm. Pt. reports "throbbing" of Ⓛ wrist, rates pain as 6 on a scale of 0 to 10, w/10 being the worst pain imaginable. Pt. denies pain in Ⓛ hand or fingers, Ⓛ radial pulse strong, Ⓛ hand warm, capillary refill less than 3 sec., able to wriggle fingers of Ⓛ hand and feel light touch. No c/o numbness or tingling in Ⓛ hand. Abrasion cleaned with NSS and covered with sterile gauze dressing. Rigid splint applied to Ⓛ forearm, extending from palm of Ⓛ hand to just below Ⓛ elbow. Mother and son given discharge instructions. Mother verbalized understanding and says she will take pt. to pediatrician for follow-up care. Report called to pediatrician, Dr. Feng. No orders or instructions given to this nurse. —— Steven Bobeck, RN

STATUS ASTHMATICUS

An acute, life-threatening obstructive lung disorder, status asthmaticus doesn't respond to conventional asthma therapy and requires more aggressive treatment. Uncontrolled, status asthmaticus can lead to respiratory arrest or heart failure. Status asthmaticus may be triggered by allergens, occupational and environmental irritants, infections such as pneumonia, cold weather, and exercise.

If your patient's asthma continues to worsen despite medical treatment, suspect status asthmaticus and call the doctor immediately. Anticipate administration of inhaled beta$_2$-adrenergic or anticholinergic drugs, subcutaneous (subQ) epinephrine, I.V. aminophylline, corticosteroids, and fluids; oxygen administration; or intubation and mechanical ventilation.

ESSENTIAL DOCUMENTATION

Record the date and time of your entry. Document your assessment findings of status asthmaticus, such as severe dyspnea, tachypnea, tachycardia, air hunger, chest tightness, labored breathing, use of accessory muscles of breathing, nasal flaring, restlessness, extreme anxiety, frequent position changes, skin color changes, feelings of suffocation, wheezes (wheezing may not be heard with severe airway obstruction), low arterial oxygen saturation, or stridor.

Note the time that you notified the doctor, his name, and orders given, such as drug and fluid administration or oxygen therapy. Also, chart the time that you notified the respiratory therapist, her name, her actions, and the patient's response. Record your interventions, such as administering inhaled, I.V., and subQ drugs; administering oxygen; providing I.V. fluids; placing the patient in an upright position; calming the patient; and assisting with endotracheal intubation and mechanical ventilation. Chart your patient's responses to these interventions. Use flow sheets to record your frequent assessments and the patient's vital signs, intake and output, I.V. therapy, and laboratory test and arterial blood gas values. Include patient teaching and emotional care given.

| 12/13/05 | 0955 | Called to room at 0930 and found pt. severely dyspneic stating, "I'm . . . suffocating . . ." Unable to speak more than 1 word at a time. Anxious facial expression, using nasal flaring and accessory muscles to breathe, restless and moving around in bed, skin pale. P 112 and regular, BP 142/88, RR 32 and labored. Wheezes audible without stethoscope, heard in all lung fields on auscultation. O_2 sat. 87%. Pt. placed in high Fowler's position and 35% oxygen by facemask applied. Called Dr. Dillon at 0937 and reported assessment findings. Orders given by Dr. Dillon. Stat ABG drawn at 0945 by Mike Traynor, RRT. I.V. line started on first attempt with #22G angiocath in ® hand. 1,000 ml NSS infusing at 100 ml/hr. Methylprednisolone 150 mg given I.V.P. Nebulized albuterol administered by Mr. Traynor, RRT. Stayed with pt. throughout event, explaining all procedures and offering reassurances. See flow sheets for documentation of frequent VS, I/O, I.V., and ABG values. —————————————Tom Gardner, RN |
| | 1010 | ABG results: pH 7.33, PaO_2 75 mm Hg, $PaCO_2$ 50 mm Hg, O_2 sat. 89%. Wheezes still heard in all lung fields but not as loud. Wheezing no longer audible without stethoscope. Pt. still dyspneic but states breathing has eased. Can speak several words at a time. Skin still pale, use of accessory muscles not as prominent. RR 24 and less labored. P 104, BP 138/86. Dr. Dillon notified at 1000 of ABG results and assessment findings. No new orders. Repeat nebulized albuterol treatment ordered and given by Mr. Traynor. ————————————— Tom Gardner, RN |

STATUS EPILEPTICUS

Status epilepticus is a state of continuous seizure activity or the occurrence of two or more sequential seizures without full recovery of consciousness in between. It can result from abrupt withdrawal of anticonvulsant drugs, hypoxic encephalopathy, acute head trauma, metabolic encephalopathy, or septicemia secondary to encephalitis or meningitis.

Status epilepticus is a life-threatening event that requires immediate treatment to avoid or reduce the risk of brain damage. If your patient develops status epilepticus, notify the doctor right away, maintain a patent airway, protect the patient from harm, and administer anticonvulsant drugs, as ordered.

ESSENTIAL DOCUMENTATION

Record the date and time that the seizure activity started, its duration, and precipitating factors. Note whether the patient reported warning signs (such as an aura). Document the characteristics of the seizure and related patient behaviors, such as pupil characteristics, level of consciousness, breathing, skin color, bowel and bladder continence, and body movements. Record the time that you notified the doctor, his name, and orders given, such as I.V. administration of anticonvulsants. Document your nursing actions, such as maintaining a patent airway, suctioning, patient positioning, loosening of clothing, monitoring vital signs, and neurologic assessment. Record the patient's response to treatment and document ongoing assessments. Note that you stayed with the patient throughout the seizure and record any emotional support given to family members. Finally, record your assessment of the patient's postictal and physical status. Chart frequent assessments, vital signs, and neurologic assessments on the appropriate flow sheets.

9/17/05	1730	While eating dinner at 1655, housekeeper Mary Smith
		noticed pt. lost consciousness and called for help. Pt.
		had full body stiffness, followed by alternating episodes
		of muscle spasm and relaxation. Breathing was labored
		and sonorous. Pt. was incontinent of bowel and bladder.
		Skin ashen color. Seizure lasted approx. 2 min. Clothing
		loosened and pt. placed on Ⓛ side. Pt. unconscious after
		seizure, not responding to verbal stimuli. Airway patent,
		pt. breathing on own. P 92, BP 128/62, RR 18 and un-
		even. Approx. 1 min later seizure recurred and was
		continuous. Dr. Maddox notified of assessment findings
		at 1703; diazepam 5 mg I.V. X 1 dose ordered and given
		STAT and phenytoin 1 gram I.V. X 1 dose ordered and
		given STAT. Started 35% O₂ via facemask. Seizure
		stopped at 1710. Stayed with pt. throughout seizures. Pt.
		breathing on own, RR 20 and regular, O₂ sat. 95%. P 88
		and regular, BP 132/74, tympanic T 98.2° F. Pt. sleeping
		and not responding to verbal stimuli. O₂ mask removed.
		Incontinence care provided. Will maintain on Ⓛ side and
		monitor closely during recovery. See flow sheets for
		documentation of frequent VS, I/O, and neuro. signs.
		—————————————— Mary Stafford, RN

STROKE

A stroke is a sudden impairment of cerebral circulation in one or more of the blood vessels supplying the brain. A stroke interrupts or diminishes oxygen supply and commonly causes serious damage or necrosis in brain tissues. Clinical features of a stroke vary with the artery affected and, consequently, the portion of the brain it supplies, the severity of damage, and the extent of collateral circulation. A stroke may be caused by thrombosis, embolus, or intracerebral hemorrhage and may be confirmed by computed tomography or magnetic resonance imaging. Treatment options vary, depending on the cause of the stroke.

The sooner you detect signs and symptoms of a stroke, the sooner your patient can receive treatment and the better his prognosis will be.

If you suspect a stroke in your patient, ensure a patent airway, breathing, and circulation. Perform a neurologic examination, and alert the doctor of your findings.

ESSENTIAL DOCUMENTATION

Record the date and time of your nurse's note. Record the events leading up to the suspected stroke and the signs you noted. If the patient can communicate, record symptoms using his own words. Evaluate the patient's airway, breathing, and circulation. Document your findings, actions taken, and the patient's response. Record your neurologic and cardiovascular assessments, actions taken, and the patient's response. Document the name of the doctor notified, the time of notification, and whether orders were given.

Assess your patient frequently, and record the specific time and results of your assessments. Avoid using block charting. Use a frequent vital signs assessment sheet to document vital signs. (See "Vital signs, frequent," page 442.) A neurologic flow sheet such as the NIH Stroke Scale may be used to record your frequent neurologic assessments. (See *Using the NIH Stroke Scale,* pages 388 and 389.)

11/10/05	2030	When giving pt. her medication at 2015, noted drooping
		of Ⓛ eyelid and Ⓛ side of mouth. Pt. was in bed breath-
		ing comfortably with RR 24, P 112, BP 142/72, axillary
		T 97.2° F. Breath sounds clear. Normal heart sounds.
		PEARLA, awake and aware of her surroundings, answer-
		ing yes and no by shake of head, speech slurred with
		some words inappropriate. Follows simple commands. Ⓛ
		hand grasp weaker than Ⓡ hand grasp. Ⓛ foot slightly
		dropped and weaker than Ⓡ. Glasgow Coma score of
		13. See Glasgow Coma Scale flow sheet for frequent
		assessments. Skin cool, dry. Peripheral pulses palpable.
		Capillary refill less than 3 sec. Called Dr. Lee at 2020.
		Stat CT scan ordered. Administered O_2 at 2 L/min by
		NC. I.V. infusion of NSS at 30 ml/hr started in Ⓡ
		forearm with 18G catheter. Continuous pulse oximetry
		started with O_2-sat. of 96% on 2 L O_2. Dr. Lee in to see
		pt. at 2025. Pt. being prepared for transfer to ICU.
		Dr. Lee will notify family of transfer. — Luke Newell, RN

(Text continues on page 390.)

AccuChart

USING THE NIH STROKE SCALE

The National Institutes of Health (NIH) Stroke Scale is widely used in conjunction with a neurologic examination to assess neurologic status and detect deficits in the patient suspected of having a stroke. For each item, choose the score that reflects what the patient can actually do at the time of assessment. Add the scores for each item and record the total. The higher the score, the more severe the neurologic deficits.

CATEGORY	DESCRIPTION	SCORE	BASELINE DATE/TIME	DATE/TIME
1a. Level of consciousness (LOC)	Alert Drowsy Stuporous Coma	0 1 2 3	7/15/05 1100 1	
1b. LOC questions (Month, age)	Answers both correctly Answers one correctly Incorrect	0 1 2	0	
1c. LOC commands (Open/close eyes, make fist, let go)	Obeys both correctly Obeys one correctly Incorrect	0 1 2	1	
2. Best gaze (Eyes open — patient follows examiner's finger or face.)	Normal Partial gaze palsy Forced deviation	0 1 2	0	
3. Visual (Introduce visual stimulus/threat to patient's visual field quadrants.)	No visual loss Partial hemianopia Complete hemianopia Bilateral hemianopia	0 1 2 3	1	
4. Facial palsy (Show teeth, raise eyebrows, and squeeze eyes shut.)	Normal Minor Partial Complete	0 1 2 3	2	
5a. Motor arm — left (Elevate extremity to 90 degrees and score drift/movement.)	No drift Drift Can't resist gravity No effort against gravity No movement Amputation, joint fusion (explain)	0 1 2 3 4 9	4	
5b. Motor arm — right (Elevate extremity to 90 degrees and score drift/movement.)	No drift Drift Can't resist gravity No effort against gravity No movement Amputation, joint fusion (explain)	0 1 2 3 4 9	0	

USING THE NIH STROKE SCALE *(continued)*

CATEGORY	DESCRIPTION	SCORE	BASELINE DATE/TIME	DATE/ TIME
6a. Motor leg — left (Elevate extremity to 30 degrees and score drift/movement.)	No drift Drift Can't resist gravity No effort against gravity No movement Amputation, joint fusion (explain)	0 1 2 3 4 9	4	
6b. Motor leg — right (Elevate extremity to 30 degrees and score drift/movement.)	No drift Drift Can't resist gravity No effort against gravity No movement Amputation, joint fusion (explain)	0 1 2 3 4 9	0	
7. Limb ataxia (Finger-nose, heel-down shin testing)	Absent Present in one limb Present in two limbs	0 1 2		
8. Sensory (Pinprick to face, arm, trunk, and leg — compare side to side.)	Normal Partial loss Severe loss	0 1 2	R L 0 2	R L
9. Best language (Name items; describe a picture and read sentences.)	No aphasia Mild to moderate aphasia Severe aphasia Mute	0 1 2 3	1	
10. Dysarthria (Evaluate speech clarity by patient repeating listed words.)	Normal articulation Mild to moderate dysarthria Near to unintelligible or worse Intubated or other physical barrier	0 1 2 9	1	
11. Extinction and inattention (Use information from prior testing to identify neglect or double simultaneous stimuli testing.)	No neglect Partial neglect Complete neglect	0 1 2	0	
		Total	17	

Individual administering scale: *Helen Hareson, RN*

STUMP CARE

Patient care directly after limb amputation includes monitoring drainage from the stump, positioning the affected limb, assisting with exercises prescribed by a physical therapist, and wrapping and conditioning the stump. Postoperative care of the stump will vary slightly, depending on the amputation site (arm or leg) and the type of dressing applied to the stump (elastic bandage or plaster cast).

After the stump heals, it requires only routine daily care, such as proper hygiene and continued muscle-strengthening exercises. The prosthesis – when in use – also requires daily care. Typically, a plastic prosthesis (the most common type) must be cleaned, lubricated, and checked for proper fit. As the patient recovers from the physical and psychological trauma of amputation, he'll need to learn correct procedures for routine daily care of the stump and prosthesis.

ESSENTIAL DOCUMENTATION

Record the date, time, and specific procedures of all postoperative care. Chart your assessment of the stump, such as appearance, type of drain and character and amount of drainage, appearance of suture line and surrounding tissue, and type of wound stabilizers (such as adhesive strips or sutures). Record the time that you notified the doctor of any concerns or abnormal findings, such as irritation or signs of infection; his name; and orders given. Document the specific care given to the stump, such as cleaning; application of drugs, lotion, or ointments; massage; and dressing, bandaging, and wrapping. Chart the patient's tolerance of exercises and his psychological reaction to the amputation. Record patient teaching about stump care. This may be charted on a patient-teaching flow sheet.

7/17/05	0830	ⓛ BKA incision well-approximated, sutures intact. Slight redness and swelling along suture line. No drainage noted. Pt. reports stump pain of 2 on scale of 0 to 10, w/10 being the worst pain imaginable. Incision cleaned with NSS, blotted dry, dressed with dry sterile gauze, and covered with snug fitting stump stocking. Foot of bed slightly elevated. Pt. instructed to keep knee extended to prevent flexion contractures, lie in prone position at least 4 hr/day, and report stump discomfort. Pt. looked at stump during care and asked many questions related to stump care and rehabilitation. —————————————— Nick Heninger, RN

SUBARACHNOID HEMORRHAGE

Subarachnoid hemorrhage occurs when there is bleeding in the space between the arachnoid membrane and the pia mater. The most common cause of subarachnoid hemorrhage is trauma, but the condition may also develop as a result of severe hypertension, aneurysm, or an arteriovenous malformation rupture. Subarachnoid hemorrhage is fatal in 40% of cases. Of those who survive, half have permanent neurologic deficits.

If you suspect subarachnoid hemorrhage in your patient, alert the doctor immediately. Perform frequent neurologic assessments, observe for central nervous system changes, prevent complications (such as hydrocephalus, hyponatremia, seizures, and increased intracranial pressure [ICP]), and maintain a patent airway and adequate ventilation. Anticipate administering drugs to reduce inflammation, prevent seizures, control pain, and reduce inflammation as well as transferring your patient to an intensive care unit (ICU).

ESSENTIAL DOCUMENTATION

Record the date and time of your entry. Document your assessment findings of subarachnoid hemorrhage, such as a sudden and severe headache, nausea, vomiting, nuchal rigidity, tachycardia, hypertension, blurry vision, dilated pupils, positive Kernig's or Brudzinski's sign, photophobia, focal motor or sensory deficits, decreased level of consciousness, or seizures. Note the time that you notified the doctor, his name, and orders given, such as transferring the patient to the ICU, diagnostic testing, supplemental oxygen, calcium channel blockers to reduce cerebral vasospasm, anticonvulsants, and analgesics.

Record your interventions, such as administering drugs, establishing I.V. access, administering oxygen, maintaining the head of the bed at 30 degrees, dimming the lights, inserting an indwelling urinary catheter, maintaining a patent airway, maintaining mechanical ventilation, monitoring pulse oximetry values, maintaining seizure precautions, continuous cardiac monitoring, and preparing the patient for diagnostic tests and transfer to the ICU. Chart your patient's responses to these interventions.

If the patient has an ICP monitor, follow the documentation guidelines outlined in "Intracranial pressure monitoring," page 238. Record your frequent neurologic, cardiopulmonary, and renal assessments. A neurologic flow sheet such as the Glasgow Coma Scale may be used to record your frequent neurologic assessments. (See *Using the Glasgow Coma Scale,* page 251.) Use flow sheets to record your frequent assessments, vital signs, hemodynamic monitoring, intake and output, and I.V. therapy. If the patient undergoes an invasive procedure such as a craniotomy, document postprocedural observations and care as well as the patient's tolerance of the procedure. Record patient and family teaching and emotional support provided.

12/30/05	1400	Called to pt.'s room at 1325 by wife saying that pt. has "a sudden, excruciating headache." Speech is sluggish with occasional inappropriate words. Pt. follows commands slowly. Oriented to person but not time and place. PERRLA. Opens eyes to verbal stimuli. Moving all extremities. Glasgow Coma score 12. See Glasgow Coma flow sheet. Pt. c/o nausea, blurry vision, and photophobia. P 104 and regular, BP 148/88, RR 25, tympanic T 98.8° F. ① facial drooping and ① hand weakness noted. Negative Kernig's and Brudzinski's signs. Head of bed placed at 30 degrees. Lights dimmed. Initiated seizure precautions, bed in low position, side rails padded, airway taped to head of bed. Dr. Eastman notified of pt.'s s/s and assessment findings at 1330 and came to see pt. at 1335. Orders given to transfer pt. to neuro. ICU. Report called to Courtney Sturmberg, RN at 1340. Pt. given O₂ at 4 L/min by NC. Pulse oximetry on O₂ at 4 L/min is 92%. Intermittent infusion device patent in ① forearm. Nimodipine 60 mg given orally after assessing at gag reflex. Morphine sulfate 4 mg I.V. given for HA. Phenergan 12.5 mg I.V. given for nausea. See MAR. CT scan scheduled for 1430. Pt. to be transferred to ICU from CT scan. Explained all procedures and drugs to pt. and wife. Wife understands seriousness of pt.'s condition and the need for close monitoring in ICU. Emotional support given to wife. Assured her that pt. will be closely monitored in ICU. See flow sheets for documentation of frequent VS, I/O, I.V. fluids, and neuro. checks. ———————— Brian Wilcox, RN

SUBDURAL HEMATOMA

A potentially life-threatening condition, a subdural hematoma is the collection of blood in the space between the dura mater and the arachnoid membrane in the brain. Bleeding may be due to tears in the veins or a rupture of the arteries crossing the subdural space. Typically, subdural hematoma is caused by severe blunt trauma to the head. Venous bleeding accumulates gradually over days to weeks but arterial bleeding may develop within 48 hours.

If you suspect a subdural hematoma in your patient, alert the doctor immediately. Perform frequent neurologic assessments, monitor and take measures to prevent increased intracranial pressure (ICP), and maintain a patent airway and adequate ventilation. Anticipate surgery to evacuate the hematoma.

ESSENTIAL DOCUMENTATION

Record the date and time of your entry. Record your assessment findings of subdural hematoma, such as a decline in the level of consciousness, seizures, headache, altered respiratory patterns, ipsilateral pupil fixed and dilated, hemiparesis, and hemiplegia. Monitor and record signs of increased ICP, such as increased systolic blood pressure, widened pulse pressure, and bradycardia. Note the time that you notified the doctor, his name, and orders given, such as transferring the patient to the intensive care unit, surgical intervention, osmotic diuretics, or endotracheal intubation and mechanical ventilation. Record your interventions, such as administering drugs, establishing I.V. access, administering oxygen, proper positioning, inserting an indwelling urinary catheter, maintaining a patent airway, following seizure precautions, maintaining mechanical ventilation, monitoring pulse oximetry values, and preparing the patient for diagnostic tests and surgery. Chart your patient's responses to these interventions.

If the patient has an ICP monitor, follow the documentation guidelines outlined in "Intracranial pressure monitoring," page 238. Record your frequent neurologic, cardiopulmonary, and renal assessments. A neurologic flow sheet such as the Glasgow Coma Scale may be used to record your frequent neurologic assessments. Use flow sheets to record your frequent assessments, vital signs, hemodynamic monitoring, intake and output, I.V. therapy, and laboratory values. If the patient undergoes surgery, document postprocedural observations and care as well as the patient's tolerance of the procedure. Record patient and family teaching and emotional support given.

11/17/05	2000	Pt.'s wife reports that pt. fell off a ladder 2 days ago
		and hit his head. States he didn't see a doctor at that
		time because he "felt fine." Wife states pt. is becoming
		confused and c/o headache. Pt. is drowsy and oriented
		to person but not time and place. ® pupil 5 mm with
		sluggish response to light, Ⓛ pupil 3 mm with brisk re-
		sponse to light. Pt. opens eyes to verbal stimuli, answers
		questions inappropriately, and pushes away noxious stim-
		uli. Glascow Coma score 12. Moving all extremities, hand
		grasps equal. P 58 and and regular, BP 130/62, RR 24
		and regular, tympanic T 97.4° F. Breath sounds clear, no
		dyspnea noted, normal heart sounds. Skin warm and dry,
		peripheral pulses palpable. Pulse oximetry on room air
		95%. Dr. Kay notified of assessment findings at 1930,
		came to see pt. at 1935, and orders given for stat skull
		X-ray and CT scan. I.V. line started in ® antecubital on
		first attempt with #18G angiocath. 1,000 ml of D₅W in-
		fusing at 30 ml/hr. Pt. left for radiology at 1945 on
		stretcher, accompanied by this RN. Explained need for
		X-ray and CT scan to pt. and wife. Wife understands
		seriousness of pt.'s condition and the need for X-ray
		and CT scan to detect bleeding. See flow sheets for doc-
		umentation of frequent VS, Glasgow Coma scores, I/O,
		I.V. fluids. ———————————— Peter Mallory, RN

SUBSTANCE ABUSE BY COLLEAGUE, SUSPICION OF

An estimated 7% of the 1.9 million nurses in the United States are addicted to alcohol or drugs. This addiction may be a result of the high stress levels in nursing today or other personal problems. The suspicion of substance abuse may not be limited to nursing colleagues but may include other members of the health care team, such as doctors, assistive personnel, or multidisciplinary team members. (See *Reporting a colleague's substance abuse: Your obligations.*)

LEGAL CASEBOOK

REPORTING A COLLEAGUE'S SUBSTANCE ABUSE: YOUR OBLIGATIONS

Although the decision to report a coworker is never easy, you have an ethical obligation to intervene if you suspect that a colleague is abusing drugs or alcohol. Intervening enables you to fulfill your moral obligation to your colleague: By reporting abuse, you compel her to take the first step toward regaining control over her life and undergoing rehabilitation. You also fulfill your obligation to patients by protecting them from a nurse whose judgment and care don't meet professional standards.

SIGNS OF DRUG OR ALCOHOL ABUSE IN A COLLEAGUE

Signs of drug or alcohol abuse may include:
- rapid mood swings, usually from irritability or depression
- frequent absences, lateness, and use of private quarters such as bathrooms
- frequent volunteering to administer drugs
- excessive errors or problems with controlled substances, such as reports of broken vials or spilled drugs
- illogical or sloppy charting
- inability to meet deadlines or minimum job requirements
- increased errors in treatment
- poor personal hygiene
- inability to concentrate or remember details
- odor of alcohol on the breath
- discrepancies in opioid supplies
- slurred speech, unsteady gait, flushed face, or red eyes
- patient complaints of no relief from opioids supposedly administered when the nurse is on duty
- social withdrawal.

If you detect signs of substance abuse, make sure that your suspicions are as accurate as possible. (See *Signs of drug or alcohol abuse in a colleague.*) Be aware that allegations of substance abuse are serious and potentially damaging. Follow your facility's policy for reporting suspicions of substance abuse. Use the appropriate channels for your facility and report your suspicions to your nursing supervisor. You'll be asked to document your suspicion on the appropriate form for your facility, possibly an incident or variance report.

ESSENTIAL DOCUMENTATION

Record the date, time, and location of the incident. Include a description of what you observed and what was said, using direct quotes. Write down the names of any witnesses. Record only objective facts, and make sure to leave out opinions and judgments. Document the name of the nursing supervisor that you notified of the incident, and record any instructions given.

To: *Theresa Stiller, RN*
     Nursing supervisor
From: *Pamela Stevens, RN*
Date: *12/3/05*
Time: *2245*
At about 2100 on 12/1/05, Janet Fox in room 501 told me "Your injections of
morphine are much better than those the other nurse gives." I asked her what she
meant. She told me, "Nurse Barrett's injections never do much for me, but yours
always do." Two nights later, at 2215, I went to the restroom. When I opened the
door, I saw Ms. Barrett injecting some solution into her thigh using a syringe.
She told me to get out and I did. We didn't talk about the incident afterward.
I immediately notified Theresa Stiller, RN, nursing supervisor, who advised me to
write out this incident report so she could assess the situation. Ms. Stiller came to
the unit at 2220 and met privately with Ms. Barrett. At 2230 Ms. Barrett and Ms.
Stiller left the unit together, after which Ms. Stiller asked the other RNs and myself
to assume Ms. Barrett's assignments.

SUBSTANCE WITHDRAWAL

Substance withdrawal occurs when a person who's addicted to a substance (alcohol or drugs) suddenly stops taking that substance. Withdrawal symptoms may include tremors, nausea, insomnia, and seizures.
Substance withdrawal can result in death.

If your patient is at risk for substance withdrawal or shows signs of
withdrawal, contact the doctor immediately and anticipate a program of
detoxification, followed by long-term therapy to combat drug dependence.

ESSENTIAL DOCUMENTATION

Document the patient's substance abuse and addiction history, noting the
substance, the amount and frequency of use, the date and time when last
used, and any history of withdrawal. Note specific manifestations that the
patient had during previous withdrawals. If available, use a flow sheet that
lists the signs and symptoms associated with withdrawal from specific substances. Document current blood, urine, and Breathalyzer results. Frequently monitor the patient for signs and symptoms of withdrawal, and
document the findings. Record your nursing interventions and the patient's
response. Document the names of individuals notified regarding the patient, such as the doctor, substance abuse counselor, and social worker, and
the date, time, and reason of notification. Document orders or instructions
given and your nursing actions. Chart any patient education regarding

withdrawal, such as manifestations that the patient should anticipate, nursing care you'll provide, and evidence of the patient's understanding.

9/17/05	1000	Pt. admitted to Chemical Dependency Unit for withdrawal
		from ethanol. Has a 30-year history of alcohol dependence
		and states, "I can't keep this up anymore. I need to get off
		the booze." Reports drinking a fifth of vodka per day for
		the last 2 months and that her last drink was today shortly
		before admission. Her blood alcohol level is 0.15%. She
		reports having gone through the withdrawal process 4 times
		before but has never completed rehabilitation. Reports the
		following symptoms during previous withdrawals: anxiety,
		nausea, vomiting, irritability, and tremulousness. Currently
		demonstrates no manifestations of ethanol withdrawal. Dr.
		Jones notified of pt.'s admission and blood alcohol level
		results. Orders given. Lorazepam 2 mg P.O. given at 0930.
		Pt. instructed regarding s/s of ethanol withdrawal and
		associated nursing care. She expressed full understanding
		of the information. Will reinforce teaching when blood
		tests reveal no alcohol in blood. ———— Brian Winters, RN

SUICIDAL INTENT

People with suicidal intent not only have thoughts about committing suicide, but they also have a concrete plan. People contemplating suicide commonly give evidence of their intent either by self-destructive behaviors or comments about suicide. Take all self-destructive behaviors and comments about suicide seriously. Follow your facility's policy on caring for a patient with suicidal intent. If you suspect a patient is at risk for self-destructive behavior or a suicide attempt, immediately notify the doctor and assess the patient for suicide clues. (See *Legal responsibilities when caring for a suicidal patient,* page 398.)

ESSENTIAL DOCUMENTATION

Record your patient's statements or behaviors and any circumstances that led you to suspect suicidal intent. Use the patient's own words, in quotes. Document the patient's response to your inquiry about his thoughts of harming or killing himself and the presence and nature of a specific suicide plan. Document the patient's suicide history and the presence of suicide clues such as:

LEGAL RESPONSIBILITIES
WHEN CARING FOR A SUICIDAL PATIENT

Whether you work on a psychiatric unit or a medical unit, you'll be held responsible for the decisions you make about a suicidal patient's care. If you're sued because your patient has harmed himself while in your care, the court will judge you on the basis of:
- whether you knew (or should have known) that the patient was likely to harm himself
- whether, knowing he was likely to harm himself, you exercised reasonable care in helping him avoid injury or death.

- characteristics of depression (sad countenance, poor eye contact, declining self-care, isolation, lack of communication, poor appetite, and unkempt appearance)
- expressed or displayed feelings of hopelessness, unworthiness, futility, or lack of control over life
- suspicious questions such as "How long does it take to bleed to death?"
- statements about the benefits of death such as "My family won't have to worry about me anymore."
- giving away personal belongings and demonstration of an unusual amount of interest in death preparation, such as getting affairs in order and making funeral arrangements
- hearing voices, especially those telling the patient to harm himself
- history of significant personal loss
- withdrawal from those close to him
- loss of interest in persons, property, and pursuits previously important
- insomnia or hypersomnia
- substance abuse history.

Record the results of your mental status examination of the patient, including the patient's appearance, orientation, cognition, speech, mood, affect, thought processes, and judgment. Record the time that you notified the doctor of the patient's suicidal intent, the doctor's name, and orders given. Include your nursing interventions and the patient's response. (Also see "Suicide precautions.") Update the nursing care plan to reflect the patient's suicidal intent.

10/17/05	1100	Pt. reports that she lost her job yesterday. 3 months
		ago she had a miscarriage. She states, "I don't think I'm
		supposed to be here." Speaks with a low-toned voice,
		appears sad, avoids eye contact, and has an unkempt
		appearance. Reports getting no more than 3 hours of
		sleep per night for several weeks and states, "That's
		why I lost my job — I couldn't stay awake at work." Pt.
		reports having thoughts about suicide but declares, "I
		would never kill myself." She denies having a suicide
		plan. Has no history of previous suicide attempts. Pt.
		lives alone with no family nearby. Doesn't belong to
		a church and denies having any close friends. Denies
		having a history of drug or alcohol abuse or psychiatric
		illness. Pt. alert and oriented to person, place, and
		time. Speech clear and coherent. Answers questions
		appropriately. Dr. Patterson called at 1045 and told of
		this conversation with pt. She will see pt. for further
		evaluation at 1130. Will maintain constant observation
		of pt. until evaluated by dr. —— Roger C. Trapley, RN

SUICIDE PRECAUTIONS

Patients who have been identified as at risk for self-harm or suicide are placed on some form of suicide precautions based on the gravity of the suicidal intent. If your patient has suicidal ideations or makes a suicidal threat, gesture, or attempt, contact the doctor immediately and institute suicide precautions. Follow your facility's policy when caring for a potentially suicidal patient. Notify the nursing supervisor, other members of the health care team, and the risk manager, and update the patient's care plan.

ESSENTIAL DOCUMENTATION

Record the date and time that suicide precautions were initiated and the reasons for the precautions. Chart the time that you notified the doctor, his name, and orders given. Also, include the names of other people involved in making this decision. Document the measures taken to reduce the patient's risk of self-harm; for example, removing potentially dangerous items from the patient's environment, accompanying the patient to the bathroom, and placing him in a room by the nurses' station with sealed windows. Record the level of observation, such as close or constant observation, and who's performing the observation. Chart that the patient was instructed about the suicide precautions and his response. Throughout the period of suicide precautions, maintain a suicide precautions flow sheet that includes mood, behavior, and location as well as nursing interventions and patient responses.

10/17/05	1600	Pt. stated, "Every year about this time, I think about offing myself." History of self-harm 1 year ago when he lacerated both wrists on the 3rd anniversary of his father's suicide. States that he has been thinking about cutting his wrists again. Dr. Gordon notified and pt. placed on suicide precautions. Leah Halloran, RN, nursing supervisor, and Michael Stone, risk manager, also notified. Pt. placed in room closest to nurses' station, verified that the sealed window can't be opened. With pt. present, personal items inventoried and those potentially injurious were placed in the locked patient belongings cabinet. Instructed pt. that he must remain in sight of the assigned staff member at all times, including being accompanied to the bathroom and on walks on the unit. Betsy Richter is assigned to constantly observe pt. this shift. Pt. contracted for safety stating, "I won't do anything to hurt myself." See flow sheet for q15min assessments of mood, behavior, and location. ———————————————————— Sandy Peres, RN

SUICIDE PREVENTION CONTRACT

Nurses and other mental health practitioners often develop a contract for safety, also known as a *no-harm* or *no-suicide contract,* when a patient verbalizes suicidal thoughts or has plans to injure or kill himself. Although a no-suicide contract isn't a legally binding document and doesn't guarantee against suicidal behavior, it's one tool that the nurse can use to help prevent suicide. A no-suicide contract is an agreement or pact between the patient and nurse outlining the actions that the patient will take if he becomes suicidal. By agreeing to the contract, the patient understands that the nurse will offer support and concern and remain available to help the patient address his feelings of hopelessness and depression. (Untreated depression is a major cause of suicide.)

Typically, a no-suicide contract is written with the patient and stated in simple, easily understood language. (See *Sample no-suicide contract.*) Some points to emphasize when drafting a no-suicide contract include:
- the patient will agree not to die by suicide

SAMPLE NO-SUICIDE CONTRACT

A no-suicide contract such as the one below can be used as part of the treatment plan for a patient who verbalizes suicidal thoughts or a plan to commit suicide.

NO-SUICIDE CONTRACT

I, *James Kelly* _____, agree not to kill myself, attempt to kill myself, or injure myself.

I agree to come to my next appointment on ___*September 7*___ at ___*9:00 am*___ .

I agree to get rid of the things that I have thought about using to kill myself.

I agree to call 911 if I feel that I am in immediate danger of harming or killing myself.

I agree to call any and all of the people listed below at the following phone numbers if I am not in immediate danger of harming myself but am having suicidal thoughts.

John Kelly _____ *123-456-7890* _____
Name   Phone #
123 Broad Street
Address
Patty Williams _____ *123-456-5555* _____
Name   Phone #
123 Main Street
Address

I will call the 1-800-SUICIDE phone number, the 24-hour suicide prevention line, if I cannot reach any of the people listed above. I know this suicide prevention line can be called from anywhere in the United States at any time.

James Kelly _____
Signature of Client

Barbara Johnson _____
Signature of Nurse

John Kelly _____
Signature of family member/friend

- the patient will contact an appropriate family member, supportive friend, or a local suicide hotline service to obtain help instead of committing suicide.

Including these points in the contract reinforces the idea that suicide is never an acceptable action and that the patient needs to seek immediate assistance whenever he feels suicidal. It's important to remember that a patient who is thinking about or planning suicide is in severe distress and emotional pain, feels hopeless, and is desperate to obtain relief from his suffering. Having essential information written down about what to do when feeling suicidal allows the patient to reach out to others for help when he is in an emotionally charged state and incapable of figuring out what to do on his own.

ESSENTIAL DOCUMENTATION

Document that the patient and nurse have an unequivocal agreement that, under no circumstances, will the patient die by suicide and that it's never acceptable to die by suicidal means. Record the patient's negative life experiences that are contributing to his depression, such as any serious losses, breakup of a relationship, physical or sexual abuse, or feeling of being trapped. Also, document any signs and symptoms of mental illness that the patient may be experiencing.

If the patient's family or friends witnessed the agreement, have them sign it, and document their names and participation. Indicate that the patient has verbalized understanding of the contract, what it means, and what he will do if he feels suicidal. Document that you instructed the patient where to keep the no-suicide contract for easy access, such as in a wallet or near the phone. Indicate that the no-suicide contract is one strategy used in the patient's care plan, making sure to document all relevant assessment data and the treatment plan. (See "Suicide precautions," page 399, for common procedures and documentation.) Make sure that you and the patient sign, date, and time the contract. If the patient doesn't want to sign the contract, document that he declined to sign the agreement and the specific actions you are taking to ensure his safety. Include a copy of the no-suicide contract in the care plan and the patient's chart.

| 7/17/05 | 0830 | Pt.'s hx states that he recently lost his mother and father in a MVC. He states that he has been thinking about ending his life recently. No-suicide agreement signed by pt. and me and witnessed by pt.'s brother, John Kelly. Pt. verbally expressed understanding of the contract. Pt. instructed to keep the contract where he can easily access it. Copy of contract placed in pt.'s chart. —————————————— Barbara Johnson, RN |

SURGICAL INCISION CARE

In addition to documenting vital signs and level of consciousness when the patient returns from surgery, pay particular attention to maintaining records pertaining to the surgical incision and drains and the care that you provide. Also, read the records that travel with the patient from the postanesthesia care unit. Look for a doctor's order indicating who will perform the first dressing change.

ESSENTIAL DOCUMENTATION

Chart the date, time, and type of wound care performed. Describe the wound's appearance (size, condition of margins, and necrotic tissue, if any), odor (if any), location of any drains, drainage characteristics (type, color, consistency, and amount), and the condition of the skin around the incision. Record the type of dressing and tape applied. Document additional wound care procedures provided, such as drain management, irrigation, packing, or application of a topical medication. Record the patient's tolerance of the procedure. Chart the time that you notified the doctor of any abnormalities or concerns, his name, and orders given. Note explanations or instructions given to the patient.

Record special or detailed wound care instructions and pain management measures on the nursing care plan. Document the color and amount of measurable drainage on an intake and output form. (See *Intake and output*, page 231.)

If the patient will need wound care after discharge, provide and document appropriate instructions. Record that you explained aseptic technique, described how to examine the wound for signs of infection and other complications, demonstrated how to change the dressing, and provided written instructions for home care. Include the patient's understanding of your instructions.

12/10/05	0830	Dressing removed from 8-cm midline abdominal incision; no drainage noted on dressing. Incision well-approximated and intact with staples. Margin ecchymotic. Skin around incision without redness, warmth, or irritation. Small amt. of serosanguineous drainage cleaned from lower end of incision with NSS and blotted dry with sterile gauze. 3 dry sterile 4" X 4" gauze pads applied and held in place with paper tape. Jackson Pratt drain intact in LLQ draining serosanguineous fluid, emptied 40 ml. See I/O sheet for drainage records. Jackson Pratt insertion site without redness or drainage. Split 4" X 4" gauze applied around Jackson Pratt drain and taped with paper tape. Pt. stated he had only minor discomfort before and after discharge and that he didn't need any pain meds. Pt. instructed to call nurse if dressing becomes loose or soiled and for incision pain. Pt. demonstrated how to splint incision with pillow during C&DB exercises. ———————— Grace Fedor, RN

SURGICAL SITE IDENTIFICATION

To prevent wrong-site surgery and improve the overall safety of patients undergoing surgery, the Joint Commission on Accreditation of Healthcare Organizations launched the Universal Protocol for Preventing Wrong Site, Wrong Procedure, Wrong Person Surgery in 2004. This protocol encompasses three important steps:

■ A *preoperative verification process* to ascertain that all important documents and tests are on hand before surgery and that these materials are evaluated and consistent with one another as well as with the patient's expectations and the surgical team's understanding of the patient, surgical procedure, surgical site, and any implants that may be used. All missing information and inconsistencies must be resolved before starting surgery.

■ *Marking the operative site,* by the surgeon performing the surgery and with the involvement of the awake and aware patient, if possible. The mark should be the surgeon's initials or YES.

■ Taking a *"time out"* immediately before surgery is started, in the location where the surgery is to be performed, so that the entire surgical team can confirm the correct patient, surgical procedure, surgical site, patient position, and any implants or special equipment requirements.

ESSENTIAL DOCUMENTATION

Most facilities use a detailed checklist to ensure that all steps of the verification process have been completed. Each member of the intraoperative team should document the checks that they performed to ensure proper surgical site identification. All documentation on the checklist should include the date, time, and initials of the team member providing the check. When using initials on a checklist, be sure that you sign your full name and initials in the signature space provided. Any discrepancies in the verification process should be noted on the checklist with a description of actions taken to rectify the discrepancy. Include the names of any people notified and their actions. (See *Preoperative surgical identification checklist,* page 406.)

Preoperatively, document that you identified the patient using two identifiers. Confirm that the patient understands the procedure and that he can correctly describe the surgery being performed and identify the surgical site. Check that the consent form has been signed and that it includes the name of the surgery and the surgical site. The preoperative verification checklist also includes checking the medical record for the physical examination, medication record, laboratory studies, radiology and ECG reports, and anesthesia and surgical records and confirmation that the medical record is consistent with the type of surgery planned and the identified surgical site.

In the intraoperative area, the checklist includes documenting that the patient was identified by staff as well as by the patient or his family. Documentation also includes confirmation of the surgical procedure by the staff as well as the patient or family member. The surgical site should be clearly marked and the patient or family member should verify that the marked surgical site is correct. Ideally, site marking should be completed by the surgeon performing the surgery. The checklist should also indicate that the medical record is consistent with the planned surgery and surgical site. The availability of implants and special equipment, if relevant, should also be noted.

Documentation of "time out" occurs in the operating room, before the surgical procedure starts, and includes verbal consensus by the entire surgical team of identification of the patient, surgical site, and surgical procedure and the availability of implants and special equipment, if needed. Document any discrepancies in verification during "time out" and interventions taken to correct the discrepancy.

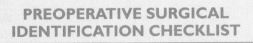

PREOPERATIVE SURGICAL IDENTIFICATION CHECKLIST

A preoperative surgical identification checklist such as the one below is commonly used to ensure the safety of patients undergoing surgery.

PREOPERATIVE SURGICAL IDENTIFICATION CHECKLIST

Patient's name *Thomas Smith*   Date *1/6/06*   Time *1032*

Medical record number *123456*   Initials *MC*

	HEALTH TEAM MEMBER INITIALS	DATE	TIME
Preoperative verification			
Patient identified using two identifiers	MC	1/6/06	1032
Informed consent with surgical procedure and site (side/level) signed and in chart	MC	1/6/06	1045
History and physical complete and in chart	MC	1/6/06	1045
Laboratory studies reviewed and in chart	MC	1/6/06	1045
Radiology and ECG reports reviewed and in chart	MC	1/6/06	1045
Medications listed in chart	MC	1/6/06	1045
Patient/family member/guardian verbalizes surgical procedure and points to surgical site	MC	1/6/06	1055
Surgical site marked	HD	1/6/06	1100
Patient, surgery, and marked site verified by patient/family/guardian	MC	1/6/06	1100
Surgical procedure and site, medical record, and tests are consistent	MC	1/6/06	1100
Proper equipment and implants available	MC	1/6/06	1100
Describe any discrepancies and actions taken:	N/A		
"Time out" verification			
Patient verification with two identifiers	BT	1/6/06	1135
Surgical site verified	BT	1/6/06	1135
Surgical procedure verified	BT	1/6/06	1135
Implants and equipment available	N/A		
Verbal verification of team obtained	BT	1/6/06	1135
Describe any discrepancies and actions taken:	N/A		

Signature *Mary Cooke, RN*   **Initials** *MC*   **Signature** *Beverly Thomas, RN* **Initials** *BT*

Signature *Howard Dunn, MD*   **Initials** *HD*   **Signature** _____ **Initials** _____

SUTURE REMOVAL

The goal of suture removal is to remove skin sutures from a healed wound without damaging newly formed tissue. The timing of suture removal depends on the shape, size, and location of the sutured incision; the absence of inflammation, drainage, and infection; and the patient's general condition. Usually, for a sufficiently healed wound, sutures are removed 7 to 10 days after they were inserted. Techniques for removal depend on the method of suturing; however, all techniques require sterile procedure to prevent contamination. Although sutures are usually removed by a doctor, a nurse may remove them in some facilities on the doctor's order.

ESSENTIAL DOCUMENTATION

Record the date and time of suture removal, and note that you explained the procedure to the patient. Include the type and number of sutures, appearance of the suture line, and whether a dressing or butterfly strips were applied. Document signs of wound complications, the name of the doctor that you notified, the time you of notification, and orders given. Record the patient's tolerance of the procedure.

12/14/05	1030	Order written by Dr. Feng for nurse to remove sutures from Ⓡ index finger. Suture line well-approximated and healed, site clean and dry, no redness or drainage noted. Procedure for suture removal explained to pt. All 3 sutures removed without difficulty. Dry bandage applied to finger, according to dr.'s order. No c/o pain or discomfort following removal. Explained incision care to pt. and gave written instructions. Pt. verbalized understanding of instructions. ———————— Amy Prima, RN

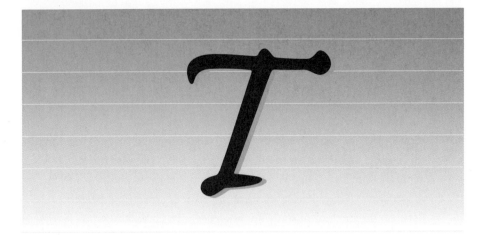

TERMINATION OF LIFE SUPPORT

According to the right-to-die laws of most states, a patient has the right to refuse extraordinary life-supporting measures if he has no hope of recovery. If the patient can't make this decision, the patient's next of kin is usually permitted to decide if life support should continue. A written statement of the patient's wishes is always preferable. Because of the Patient Self-Determination Act, each health care facility is required to ask the patient upon admission if he has an advance directive. (See "Advance directive," page 9.) An advance directive is a statement of the patient's wishes that becomes valid if he's unable to make decisions for himself. An advance directive may include a living will, which goes into effect when the patient can't make decisions for himself, as well as a durable power of attorney for health care, which names a designated person to make health care decisions when the patient can't. The Patient Self-Determination Act also states that the patient must receive written information concerning his right to make decisions about his medical care.

If life support is to be terminated, read the patient's advance directive to ensure that the present situation matches the patient's wishes, and verify that the risk manager has reviewed the document. Check that the appropriate consent forms have been signed. Ask the patient's family whether they would like to see the chaplain and whether they would like to be with the patient before, during, and after life-support termination.

ESSENTIAL DOCUMENTATION

Document whether an advance directive is present and whether it matches your patient's present situation and life support wishes. Note that your facility's risk manager has reviewed the advance directive. Document that a consent form has been signed to terminate life support, according to facility policy. Document the names of persons who were notified of the decision to terminate life support and their responses. Describe physical care for the patient before and after life-support termination. Note whether the family was with the patient before, during, and after termination of life support. Record whether a chaplain was present. Document the time of termination, name of the doctor who turned off the equipment, and names of people present. Record vital signs after extubation as well as the time the patient stopped breathing, the time he was pronounced dead, and who made the pronouncement. Document the family's response, your interventions for them, and postmortem care for the patient.

10/02/05	1800	Advance directive provided by pt.'s wife. Document
		reviewed by risk manager, Michael Stone, who verified
		that it matched the pt.'s present situation. Wife signed
		consent form to terminate life support. Wife spent
		approx. 10 min. alone with pt. before termination of
		life support. Declined to have anyone with her during
		this time. Life support terminated at 1730 by Dr. Brown,
		with myself, Chaplain Greene, and pt.'s wife present.
		VS after extubation: P 50, BP 50/20, no respiratory
		effort noted. Pronounced dead at 1737. Pt.'s wife
		tearful. Chaplain Greene and myself stayed with her
		and listened to her talk about her 35 years with her
		husband. Pt. bathed and dressed in pajamas for family
		visitation. ———————————— Lucy Danios, RN

THORACENTESIS

Thoracentesis involves the aspiration of fluid or air from the pleural space. It relieves pulmonary compression and respiratory distress by removing accumulated air or fluid that results from injury or such conditions as tuberculosis and cancer. It also provides a specimen of pleural fluid or tissue for analysis and allows the instillation of chemotherapeutic agents or other drugs into the pleural space.

ESSENTIAL DOCUMENTATION

Note that the procedure, its risks and advantages, alternative treatments, and the consequences of no treatment have been explained to the patient and that a consent form has been signed. Record the date and time of the thoracentesis and the name of the person performing the procedure. Document the location of the puncture site, the volume and description (color, viscosity, and odor) of the fluid withdrawn, and specimens sent to the laboratory. Chart your patient's vital signs and respiratory assessment before, during, and after the procedure. Record any postprocedural tests such as a chest X-ray. Note any complications (such as pneumothorax, hemothorax, or subcutaneous hematoma), the name of the doctor notified and the time of notification, orders given, your interventions, and the patient's response. Also, record the patient's reaction to the procedure.

After the procedure, record the patient's vital signs every 15 minutes for 1 hour. Then continue to record the patient's vital signs and respiratory status as indicated by his condition. These frequent assessments may be charted on a frequent vital signs flow sheet.

11/10/05	1100	Procedure risks and benefits, alternatives, and conse-
		quences of no treatment explained to pt. and written
		consent obtained by Dr. McCall. Breath sounds decreased
		in RLL and pt. SOB. Pulse oximetry 88% on 4 L O₂ by NC.
		P 102, BP 148/84, RR 32 and labored. Pt. positioned over
		secured bedside table. RLL thoracentesis performed by
		dr. without incident. Sterile 4" X 4" dressing applied to
		site. Site clean and dry, no redness or drainage present.
		900 ml of blood-tinged serosanguineous fluid aspirated.
		Specimen sent to lab as ordered. During procedure P 108,
		BP 144/82, RR 30, pt. SOB, pulse oximetry 90%. Post-
		procedure P 98, BP 138/80, RR 24, breath sounds clear
		bilaterally, no dyspnea noted. Pt. denies SOB. Pulse oxim-
		etry 96% on 4 L O₂ by NC. No c/o pain or discomfort
		at puncture site. CXR done at 1045, results pending. See
		frequent VS sheet for q15min VS and respiratory assess-
		ments. ———————————— Ellen Pritchett, RN

THROMBOLYTIC THERAPY

Thrombolytic drugs are used to dissolve a preexisting clot or thrombus, commonly in an acute or emergency situation. Some of the thrombolytic drugs currently used include alteplase, reteplase, anistreplase, and streptokinase. Thrombolytic drugs are used to treat acute myocardial infarction, pulmonary embolism, acute ischemic stroke, deep vein thrombosis, arterial thrombosis, arterial embolism, and to clear occluded arteriovenous and I.V. cannulas. Patients receiving these drugs must be closely monitored for bleeding and allergic reactions.

ESSENTIAL DOCUMENTATION

Record the date and time of your note. Chart the name, dosage, frequency, route, and intended purpose of the thrombolytic drug. Note whether the desired response is observed, such as cessation of chest pain, return of ECG changes to baseline, clearing of a catheter, or improved blood flow to a limb. Document your cardiopulmonary, renal, and neurologic assessments. Chart vital signs frequently, according to your facility's policy. Record partial thromboplastin time and other coagulation studies. Frequently assess and document signs and symptoms of complications, such as bleeding, allergic reaction, or hypotension. Note the time that you notified the doctor of complications and abnormal laboratory test values, his name, orders given, your interventions, and the patient's response. Document other nursing interventions related to thrombolytic therapy such as measures to avoid trauma. Use flow sheets to record your frequent assessments, vital signs, hemodynamic measurements, intake and output, I.V. therapy, and laboratory test values. Include any patient teaching and emotional care provided.

9/18/05	1010	Pt. receiving streptokinase 100,000 International Units/
		hr by I.V. infusion for Ⓛ femoral artery thrombosis.
		Ⓛ leg and foot cool, dorsalis pedis pulse now faintly
		palpable, 2 sec capillary refill in Ⓛ foot, able to wiggle
		Ⓛ toes. P 82 and regular, BP 138/72, RR 18 unlabored,
		oral T 97.2° F. Breath sounds clear, no dyspnea. Normal
		heart sounds, skin warm and pink (except for Ⓛ leg), no
		edema. Alert and oriented to time, place, and person.
		No c/o headache, hand grasps strong and equally bilater-
		ally, PERRLA. Speech clear and coherent. Voiding on own,
		urine output remains greater than 75 ml/hour. Urine
		and stool negative for blood, no flank pain. No bruising,
		bleeding, or hematomas noted. No c/o itching, nausea,
		chills. No rash noted. Maintaining pt. on bed rest. Avoid-
		ing I.M. injections. See flow sheets for documentation of
		frequent assessments, VS, I/O, and lab values. Reinforced
		the purpose of thrombolytic therapy in dissolving clot
		and the need to observe for bleeding. Pt. verbalized un-
		derstanding that he's to report blood in urine or stool,
		headache, and flank pain. —————— Cindy Trent, RN

TRACHEOSTOMY CARE

Tracheostomy care is performed to ensure airway patency of the tracheostomy tube by keeping it free from mucus buildup, maintain mucous membrane and skin integrity, prevent infection, and provide psychological support. The patient may have one of three types of tracheostomy tubes: uncuffed, cuffed, or fenestrated. An uncuffed tracheostomy tube, which may be plastic or metal, allows air to flow freely around the tube and through the larynx, reducing the risk of tracheal damage. A cuffed tube, made of plastic, is disposable. The cuff and the tube won't separate accidently because they're bonded. A cuffed tube also doesn't require periodic deflating to lower pressures, and it reduces the risk of tracheal damage. A fenestrated tube, also made of plastic, permits speech through the upper airway when the external opening is capped and the cuff is deflated. It also allows easy removal of the inner cannula for cleaning. However, a fenestrated tracheostomy tube may become occluded. When using any one of these tubes, use aseptic technique to prevent infection until the stoma has healed. When caring for a recently performed tracheotomy, use sterile gloves at all times. After the stoma has healed, clean gloves may be used.

ESSENTIAL DOCUMENTATION

Record the date and time of tracheostomy care. Document the type of care performed. Describe the amount, color, consistency, and odor of secretions. Chart the condition of the stoma and the surrounding skin. Note the patient's respiratory status. Record the duration of any cuff deflation, amount of any cuff inflation, and cuff pressure readings and specific body position. Note any complications, the time that you notified the doctor, his name, and orders given. Record your interventions and the patient's response. Document the patient's tolerance of the procedure. Be sure to report any patient or family teaching and their level of comprehension. Depending on your facility's policy, patient teaching may be recorded on a patient-teaching record.

11/19/05	2200	Trach. care performed using sterile technique. Wiped skin around stoma and outer cannula with sterile gauze soaked in NSS. Dried area with sterile gauze and applied sterile trach. dressing. Skin around stoma intact, no redness. Inner cannula cleaned with hydrogen peroxide and wire brush. Small amount creamy-white, thick, odorless secretions noted. Trach. ties clean and secure. Before procedure RR 18 and regular, unlabored. Breath sounds clear. After trach. care, RR 16 and regular, with clear breath sounds. Pt. verbalized no discomfort or respiratory distress. Pt.'s wife verbalized desire to assist with procedure when next scheduled to be performed. ———————————— Laurie Wilkes, RN

TRACHEOSTOMY OCCLUSION

On occasion, mucus may obstruct a tracheostomy tube, causing occlusion. When suctioning or withdrawing the inner cannula doesn't clear an occluded tube, follow your facility's policy. Stay with the patient while someone else calls the doctor or appropriate code. Continue to try to ventilate the patient using whichever method works; for example, a handheld resuscitation bag. Don't remove the tracheostomy tube entirely because doing so may close the airway completely.

ESSENTIAL DOCUMENTATION

Record the date and time of the tracheostomy occlusion. Describe your efforts to clear the tube and the results. Note the time that you notified the doctor, his name, his interventions, and any orders given. If appropriate, record the time that a code was called. Use a code sheet to document the events of the code. (See *The code record,* page 54.) Record the patient's respiratory status during the time of occlusion and after resolution of the occlusion. Note the patient's response to the event.

9/12/05	2045	Pt. noted to be cyanotic, with labored breathing at 2025. Diminished breath sounds in all lobes bilaterally. P 108, BP 102/64, RR 32 and shallow. Breathing not eased by suctioning or withdrawing inner cannula. Stayed with pt. and manually ventilated him with handheld resuscitation bag, meeting much resistance. Mary French, RN, called code at 2030. Code team arrived at 2032. Dr. Brown inserted new #18 Fr. trach. tube. Pt. immediately began taking deep breaths, skin color pink, breath sounds heard in all lobes bilaterally. After 5 min. on room air, O_2 sat. 96%, P 84, BP 138/68, RR 24. Explained all procedures to pt. and offered emotional support. See code flow sheet for code record. ———————————— Darcy Taylor, RN

TRACHEOSTOMY SUCTIONING

Tracheostomy suctioning involves the removal of secretions from the trachea or bronchi by means of a catheter inserted through the tracheostomy tube. In addition to removing secretions, tracheostomy suctioning also stimulates the cough reflex. This procedure helps maintain a patent airway to promote the optimal exchange of oxygen and carbon dioxide and to prevent pneumonia that results from pooling of secretions. Requiring strict aseptic technique, tracheostomy suctioning should be performed as frequently as the patient's condition warrants.

ESSENTIAL DOCUMENTATION

Record the date and time that you performed tracheostomy suctioning as well as the reason for suctioning. Document the amount, color, consistency, and odor of the secretions. Note any complications as well as nursing actions taken and the patient's response to them. Record any pertinent data regarding the patient's response to the procedure.

11/19/05	2145	Pt. coughing but unable to raise secretions. Skin dusky P 98,
		BP 110/78, RR 30 noisy and labored. Explained suction pro-
		cedure to pt. Using sterile technique, suctioned moderate
		amount of creamy, thick, odorless secretions from trache-
		ostomy tube. After suctioning, skin pink, respirations quiet.
		P 88, BP 112/74, RR 24. Breath sounds clear. Pt. resting
		comfortably in bed; states he needs to cough and deep-
		breathe more frequently. —————— Ken Wallings, RN

TRACHEOSTOMY TUBE REPLACEMENT

Because a tracheostomy tube may be expelled accidentally, make sure that a sterile tracheostomy tube and obturator of the same size and one size smaller than the one used (in case the trachea starts to close after the tube is expelled) are always kept at the patient's bedside. If your patient's tracheostomy tube is expelled, stay with the patient and send a colleague to call the doctor or a code, if necessary. Use extreme caution when attempting to reinsert an expelled tracheostomy tube because of the risk of tracheal trauma, perforation, compression, and asphyxiation. Be sure to follow your facility's policy when a tracheostomy tube is expelled. Reassure the patient until the doctor arrives.

ESSENTIAL DOCUMENTATION

Record the date and time that the tracheostomy tube was expelled and how it happened. Document your immediate interventions and the patient's response. Chart the time that you notified the doctor, his name, the time of his arrival on the unit, his actions, and any orders given. Note whether a code was called, and document the events of the code on a code flow sheet. (See *The code record,* page 54.) Record your patient's respiratory status while the tube was out and after replacement. Document your patient's response to the procedure.

11/18/05	1835	Answered pt.'s call light at 1810 and found pt. cough-
		ing vigorously and trach. tube lying on the blanket.
		Attempted to reinsert same size (#25) trach. tube
		but stopped when resistance was met. Pt. gasping for
		breath, skin turning ashen color. Stayed with pt. and
		sent Martha Gray, RN, to call code at 1812. Pt. had
		labored breathing, skin pale. Code team arrived at 1814.
		#25 trach. tube inserted by Dr. Brown and fastened
		with trach. ties. Pt. breathing easily, clear breath sounds
		bilaterally. P 88, BP 158/84, RR 22, skin pink. Pt.'s doc-
		tor, Dr. Buford, called at 1820 and notified of the
		event. Dextromethorphan 10 mg P.O. q4hr p.r.n. for
		coughing ordered and given. New #25 trach. tube
		and obdurator placed at bedside. Told pt. he may have
		cough medicine q4hr and to ask for it if coughing
		resumes. ———————————————— Tanya Holden, RN

TRACHEOTOMY

Tracheotomy is the surgical creation of an external opening — called a *tracheostomy* — into the trachea and the insertion of an indwelling tube to maintain the airway's patency. If all attempts to establish an airway have failed, an emergency tracheotomy may be performed at the bedside to correct an airway obstruction resulting from laryngeal edema, foreign body obstruction, or a tumor. An emergency tracheotomy may also be performed when endotracheal intubation is contraindicated. A nonemergency tracheotomy is typically performed during surgery.

Use of a cuffed tracheostomy tube provides and maintains a patent airway, prevents the unconscious or paralyzed patient from aspirating food or secretions, allows the removal of tracheobronchial secretions from a patient who's unable to cough, replaces an endotracheal tube when long-

ASSESSING FOR COMPLICATIONS OF TRACHEOTOMY

Complication	Prevention	Detection
Aspiration	■ Evaluate the patient's ability to swallow. ■ Elevate his head and inflate the cuff during feeding and for 30 minutes afterward.	■ Assess for dyspnea, tachypnea, rhonchi, crackles, excessive secretions, and fever.
Bleeding at tracheotomy site	■ Don't pull on the tracheostomy tube; don't allow the ventilator tubing to do so either. ■ If dressing adheres to the wound, wet it with hydrogen peroxide and gently remove it.	■ Check the dressing regularly; slight bleeding is normal, especially if the patient has a bleeding disorder or if the tracheotomy was performed in the past 24 hours.
Infection at tracheotomy site	■ Always use strict aseptic technique. ■ Thoroughly clean all tubing. ■ Change the nebulizer or humidifier jar and all tubing daily. ■ Collect sputum and wound drainage specimens for culture.	■ Check for purulent, foul-smelling drainage from the stoma. ■ Be alert for other signs and symptoms of infection, such as fever, malaise, increased white blood cell count, and local pain.
Pneumothorax	■ Assess for subcutaneous emphysema, which may indicate pneumothorax. Notify the doctor if this occurs.	■ Auscultate for decreased or absent breath sounds. ■ Check for tachypnea, pain, and subcutaneous emphysema.
Subcutaneous emphysema	■ Make sure the cuffed tube is patent and properly inflated. ■ Avoid displacement by securing the ties and using lightweight ventilator tubing and swivel valves.	■ This complication is most common in mechanically ventilated patients. ■ Palpate the neck for crepitus. Listen for air leakage around the cuff, and check the tracheostomy site for unusual swelling.
Tracheal malacia	■ Avoid excessive cuff pressures. ■ Avoid suctioning beyond the end of the tube.	■ Assess for dry, hacking cough and blood-streaked sputum when tube is being manipulated.

term mechanical ventilation is required, and permits the use of positive-pressure ventilation.

ESSENTIAL DOCUMENTATION

Record the reason for the tracheotomy, the date and time that it took place, and who performed it. Document that the doctor explained the procedure to the patient. Describe the patient's respiratory status before and after the procedure. Include any complications that occurred during the procedure, the amount of cuff pressure (if applicable), and the respiratory therapy initiated after the procedure. Also, note the patient's response to respiratory therapy.

After insertion, assess the patient's vital signs and respiratory status every 15 minutes for 1 hour, every 30 minutes for 2 hours, and then every 2 hours until his condition is stable. These frequent assessments may be charted on a flow sheet. Also, monitor the patient frequently for any signs of complications, and document any pertinent findings. (See *Assessing for complications of tracheotomy.*)

7/22/05	1730	Need for emergency tracheotomy due to laryngeal
		edema explained briefly to pt. while setting up for the
		procedure. Pt. nodded his assent. Breath sounds dimin-
		ished bilaterally, using accesory muscles, anxious appear-
		ance, stridor audible on inspiration, skin pale and dia-
		phoretic. P 132, BP 148/88, RR 34 and labored. Pulse
		oximetry 83%. Assisted Dr. Jones with insertion of #18
		Fr. tracheostomy tube using sterile technique. Sterile
		trach. dressing applied and tube secured with ties. Post-
		procedure, P 102, BP 138/82, RR 26 and unlabored, skin
		pink, clear breath sounds bilaterally. Placed on 40% O₂
		by trach. collar. Pulse oximetry 95%. See frequent VS
		flow sheet for frequent post-procedure assessments.
		———————————————— David Kelly, RN

TRACTION CARE, SKELETAL

Mechanical traction exerts a pulling force on a part of the body – usually the spine, pelvis, or long bones of the arms and legs. It can be used to reduce fractures, treat dislocations, correct or prevent deformities, improve or correct contractures, or decrease muscle spasms. Skeletal traction immobilizes a body part for prolonged periods by attaching weighted equipment directly to the patient's bones. This may be accomplished with pins, screws, wires, or tongs.

ESSENTIAL DOCUMENTATION

Record the amount of traction weight used, noting the application of additional weights and the patient's tolerance. Document equipment inspections and patient care, including routine checks of neurovascular integrity, skin condition, respiratory status, and elimination patterns. Note the condition of the pin site and any care given. Also, document patient education.

8/3/05	0900	Skeletal traction to ℚ leg intact, with 5 lb of weight
		hanging freely without c/o discomfort. Pedal pulses
		strong bilaterally, no c/o numbness or tingling in legs
		or feet, skin of lower extremities warm and pink, able
		to move toes of both feet. Skin intact around pin sites;
		no redness, warmth, or drainage noted. Pin sites cleaned
		with peroxide, antibacterial ointment applied. Sterile
		gauze dressing applied. Traction connections tight, ropes
		and pulleys moving freely, no fraying noted, traction
		equipment in proper alignment. Breath sounds clear
		bilaterally. Moderate size, soft BM at 0830. Foley cathe-
		ter patent, drained 200 ml in 2 hr. See I/O flow
		sheet. Assisted pt. with ROM exercises to unaffected
		extremities. Skin intact, no redness or open areas noted.
		Pt. using trapeze to shift weight in bed every 1 to 2
		hours. Instructed pt. to report any pain or pressure
		from traction equipment. ———————— Lily Evans, RN

TRACTION CARE, SKIN

Mechanical traction exerts a pulling force on a part of the body, such as the spine, pelvis, or long bones of the arms and legs. Skin traction immobilizes a body part intermittently over an extended period through direct application of a pulling force on the skin. The force may be applied using adhesive or nonadhesive traction tape or another skin traction device, such as a boot, belt, or halter. Adhesive attachment allows more continuous traction, whereas nonadhesive attachment allows easier removal for daily skin care.

ESSENTIAL DOCUMENTATION

Document the date, time, and amount of traction weight used. Note the application of additional weights and the patient's tolerance. Document equipment inspections and patient care, including routine checks of neurovascular integrity, skin condition, respiratory status, and elimination patterns. Also, document patient education provided.

12/28/05	1400	Skin traction to ® leg intact, with 5 lb of weight hanging
		freely without c/o discomfort. Adhesive traction tape
		applied to lower ® leg. Pedal pulses strong bilaterally,
		no c/o numbness or tingling in legs or feet, skin of
		lower extremities warm and pink, able to move toes of
		both feet. Traction connections tight, ropes and pulleys
		moving freely, no fraying noted, traction equipment in
		proper alignment. Breath sounds clear bilaterally. No
		BM today, last BM yesterday morning. Foley catheter
		patent, draining approx. 150 ml/hr. See I/O flow sheet.
		Assisted pt. with ROM exercises to unaffected extrem-
		ities. Skin intact, no redness or open areas noted. Pt.
		using trapeze to shift weight in bed every 1 to 2 hours.
		Instructed pt. to report any pain or pressure from
		traction equipment. ———————— Rachel Hardwick, RN

TRANSCUTANEOUS ELECTRICAL NERVE STIMULATION

Transcutaneous electrical nerve stimulation (TENS) involves a portable, battery-powered device that transmits a painless electrical current to peripheral nerves or directly to a painful area over large nerve fibers. By blocking painful stimuli traveling over smaller fibers, the patient's perception of pain is altered. TENS reduces the need for analgesic drugs when used after surgery or for chronic pain. A typical course of treatment is 3 to 5 days. (See *Current uses of TENS,* page 420.)

CURRENT USES OF TENS

Transcutaneous electrical nerve stimulation (TENS) must be prescribed by a doctor and is most successful if it's administered and taught to the patient by a therapist skilled in its use. TENS has been used for temporary relief of acute pain such as postoperative pain, and for ongoing relief of chronic pain such as sciatica. Among the types of pain that respond to TENS are:

- arthritis
- bone fracture pain
- bursitis
- cancer-related pain
- lower back pain
- musculoskeletal pain

- myofascial pain
- neuralgias and neuropathies
- phantom limb pain
- postoperative incision pain
- sciatica
- whiplash.

ESSENTIAL DOCUMENTATION

In the medical record and nursing care plan, record the electrode sites and control settings. Document the patient's tolerance to treatment. Also, during each shift, document your evaluation of pain control.

9/21/05	1730	TENS electrodes placed over ® and ① posterior superior iliac spines and ® and ① gluteal folds for lower back pain. Stimulation frequency set at 80 Hz. Pt. verbalizes discomfort as 3 on a scale of 0 to 10, w/10 being the worst pain imaginable. Pt. verbalizes satisfaction with level of pain control at this time. ————— ———————————————————— Lydia Vrubel, RN

TRANSFUSION REACTION, DELAYED

A delayed transfusion reaction may occur 4 to 8 days following a blood transfusion and even up to 1 month later. This type of transfusion reaction occurs in people who have developed antibodies from previous blood transfusions, which cause red blood cell hemolysis during subsequent transfusions. Delayed transfusion reactions are typically mild and don't require treatment. If you suspect that a patient is having a delayed transfusion reaction, notify the doctor and blood bank.

ESSENTIAL DOCUMENTATION

Record the date and time of the suspected delayed transfusion reaction. Note the signs of a delayed reaction, such as fever, elevated white blood cell count, and a falling hematocrit. Document the name of the doctor that you notified, the orders given, your interventions, the patient's reaction, and the time that the doctor came to see the patient. Record the time that you notified the blood bank, the name of the person with whom you spoke, and any orders given, such as obtaining blood or urine samples and sending them to the laboratory. Some facilities require you to complete a transfusion reaction report. (See *Transfusion reaction report*, pages 44 and 45.) Record any patient education provided and the patient's reaction.

3/8/05	1215	Oral T 102.4° F at 1200. Pt. states he has chills, but no
		itching, nausea, or vomiting. No flushing, facial edema,
		or urticaria noted. P 82 and regular, BP 128/72, RR 20
		and unlabored. Lungs clear bilaterally. Labs from 0600
		show hct 35%, hgb 12.4, WBC 15,000. Notified Dr. Small
		of elevated temp, assessment findings, and lab values
		at 1205. Dr. Small will see pt. at 1230. Notified Anna
		Cohen in blood bank of possible delayed transfusion
		reaction at 1210. Urine for UA and 2 red-top tubes of
		blood drawn and sent to lab. Explained to pt. that fever
		may be a possible delayed blood transfusion reaction
		and usually requires no treatment. —— Dave Burns, RN

TRANSIENT ISCHEMIC ATTACK

Transient ischemic attacks (TIAs) are sudden, brief episodes of neurologic deficit caused by focal cerebral ischemia. They usually last 5 to 20 minutes and are followed by rapid clearing of neurologic deficits (typically within 24 hours). TIAs may warn of an impending stroke. About 50% to 80% of patients who experience a thrombotic stroke have previously suffered a TIA.

If you suspect your patient has suffered a TIA, immediately contact the doctor and anticipate orders for antiplatelet or anticoagulant drugs. Surgery may be considered to treat carotid artery obstruction. To reduce risk factors, recommend lifestyle changes, including weight loss, smoking cessation, proper nutrition, hypertension and diabetes management, and daily exercise.

ESSENTIAL DOCUMENTATION

Record the date and time that the signs and symptoms of a TIA occurred and the duration of the attack. Document the findings of your assessment, such as dizziness, diplopia, dark or blurred vision, visual field deficits, ptosis, difficulty speaking or swallowing, unilateral or bilateral weakness, staggered gait, transient blindness in one eye, altered level of consciousness, bruits on auscultation of the carotid artery, hypertension, or numbness in the fingers, arms, or legs. A Glasgow Coma Scale may be used to track the level of consciousness. (See "Level of consciousness, changes in," page 251.)

Chart the time that you notified the doctor of your assessment findings, his name, and any orders given, such as antiplatelet or anticoagulant drug administration. Record your nursing interventions, such as preparing your patient for diagnostic tests, monitoring neurologic signs, tracking laboratory test values, giving drugs, and ensuring your patient's safety. Be sure to include the patient's response to these interventions. Document your patient teaching, such as lifestyle modification, signs and symptoms of stroke to report to the doctor, and the importance of keeping follow-up laboratory appointments. Depending on your facility's policy, patient teaching may be recorded on a patient-teaching record.

| 9/6/05 | 1015 | Pt. reports dizziness and numbness and tingling in Ⓡ arm and fingers lasting 5 min. P 84, BP 162/84, RR 18, oral T 97.1° F. Peripheral pulses palpable. Skin pink, warm and dry. Normal heart sounds, clear breath sounds bilaterally. Bruits auscultated over both carotid arteries. Alert, oriented to time, place, and person. Speech clear and understandable, follows all directions. Strong hand grasps bilaterally, strong dorsi and plantar flexion against resistance, normal gait. PERRLA, no diplopia reported. See flow sheets for VS and neuro. assessments. Dr. Luden notified of assessment findings and orders received for Carotid Doppler studies. ——————————————— Carol Allen, RN |
| | 1025 | Pt. states dizziness and numbness and tingling in Ⓡ arm and fingers has resolved. Explained s/s of TIA and stroke for pt. to report. Discussed reasons for Doppler study. Dietitian called and will be in today to discuss low-cholesterol, low-fat diet with pt. and wife. See pt. teaching record.——————————— Carol Allen, RN |

TUBE FEEDING

Tube feeding involves the delivery of a liquid feeding formula directly to the stomach (known as gastric gavage), duodenum, or jejunum. Gastric gavage is typically indicated for a patient who can't eat normally because of dysphagia or oral or esophageal obstruction or injury. Gastric feedings may also be given to an unconscious or intubated patient or to a patient recovering from GI tract surgery who can't ingest food orally.

Duodenal or jejunal feedings decrease the risk of aspiration because the formula bypasses the pylorus. Jejunal feedings reduce pancreatic stimulation; thus, the patient may require an elemental diet. Patients usually receive gastric feedings on an intermittent schedule. However, for duodenal or jejunal feedings, most patients tolerate a continuous slow drip.

Liquid nutrient solutions come in various formulas for administration through a nasogastric tube, small-bore feeding tube, gastrostomy or jejunostomy tube, percutaneous endoscopic gastrostomy or jejunostomy tube, or gastrostomy feeding button. Tube feedings are contraindicated in patients who have no bowel sounds or a suspected intestinal obstruction.

ESSENTIAL DOCUMENTATION

On the intake and output sheet, record the date, volume of formula, and volume of water. (See *Intake and output,* page 231.) In your note, document abdominal assessment findings (including tube exit site, if appropriate); amount of residual gastric contents; verification of tube placement; amount, type, strength, and time of feeding; and tube patency. Discuss the patient's tolerance of the feeding, including complications, such as nausea, vomiting, cramping, diarrhea, or distention.

Note the result of any laboratory tests, such as urine and serum glucose, serum electrolyte, and blood urea nitrogen levels as well as serum osmolality. Document the time that you notified the doctor of complications, such as hyperglycemia, glycosuria, and diarrhea, as well as the doctor's name. Be sure to include any orders given, your actions, and the patient's response. Record the patient's hydration status and any drugs given through the tube. Note any drugs or treatments to relieve constipation or diarrhea. Include the date and time of administration set changes and the results of specimen collections. Describe any oral and nasal hygiene and dressing changes provided.

11/25/05	0700	Full-strength Pulmocare infusing via Flexiflow pump
		through Dobhoff tube in Ⓡ nostril at 50 ml/hr. Tube
		placement confirmed by aspirated gastric contents with
		pH of 5 and grassy-green color. 5 ml residual noted.
		HOB maintained at 45-degree angle. Pt. denies N/V,
		abdominal cramping. Active bowel sounds auscultated in
		all 4 quadrants, no abdominal distention noted. Mucous
		membranes moist, no skin tenting when pinched. Nares
		cleaned with cotton-tipped applicator dipped in NSS.
		Water-soluble lubricant applied to nares and lips. Skin
		around nares intact, no redness around tape noted.
		Helped pt. to brush teeth. Diphenoxylate elixir 2.5 mg
		given via tube feed for continuous diarrhea. Tube
		flushed with 30 ml H₂O, as ordered. See I/O sheet
		for shift totals. Urine dipstick neg. for glucose. Blood
		drawn this a.m. for serum glucose, electrolytes, and
		osmolality. Instructed pt to tell nurse of any dis-
		comfort or distention. ———————— Sandra Mann, RN

TUBERCULOSIS

Tuberculosis (TB) is an acute or chronic infection caused by *Mycobacterium tuberculosis*. TB is characterized by pulmonary infiltrates, formation of granulomas with caseation, fibrosis, and cavitation. The disease spreads by inhalation of droplet nuclei when infected persons cough and sneeze. Sites of extrapulmonary TB include the pleura, meninges, joints, lymph nodes, peritoneum, genitourinary tract, and bowel.

After exposure to *M. tuberculosis,* roughly 5% of infected people develop active TB within 1 year; in the remainder, microorganisms cause a latent infection. The host's immunologic defense system usually destroys the bacillus or walls it up in a tubercle. However, the live, encapsulated bacilli may lie dormant within the tubercle for years, reactivating later to cause an active infection.

If you suspect your patient has TB, place him on isolation precautions; don't wait for diagnostic test results. Follow communicable disease reporting regulations. Anticipate administration of a multidrug regimen, such as isoniazid, rifampin, and pyrazinamide.

ESSENTIAL DOCUMENTATION

If TB is a new diagnosis for the patient, document the results of his tuberculin skin test, chest X-rays, and sputum cultures. Confirm and document that the case has been reported to local health authorities. Include

PREVENTING TUBERCULOSIS

Explain respiratory and standard precautions to the hospitalized patient with tuberculosis (TB). Before discharge, tell him that he must take precautions to prevent spreading the disease such as wearing a mask around others, until his doctor tells him he's no longer contagious. He should tell all his health care providers, including his dentist and eye doctor, that he has TB so that they can institute infection-control precautions.

Teach the patient other specific precautions to avoid spreading the infection. Tell him to cough and sneeze into tissues and to dispose of the tissues properly. Stress the importance of washing his hands thoroughly in hot, soapy water after handling his own secretions. Also, instruct him to wash his eating utensils separately in hot, soapy water.

the name of the person making the report and the name of the agency receiving it. Record your assessment findings of TB, such as fatigue, weakness, anorexia, weight loss, night sweats, low-grade fever, cough, mucopurulent sputum, and chest pain. Chart precautions taken to prevent transmission of the disease. Record all drugs given on the medication administration record, according to your facility's policy. Document your interventions, such as administering oxygen or suctioning, and the patient's response to them. Record the time that the doctor was notified of any concerns and complications, his name, orders given, your actions, and the patient's response. Document patient teaching given, including information on drugs, hygiene, preventing the spread of infection, the importance of proper nutrition, and the importance of proper follow-up and compliance with drugs. (See *Preventing tuberculosis*.)

| 11/24/05 | 1400 | Pt. admitted to r/o TB. PPD injected in Ⓛ forearm at 1340. CXR performed and sputum sent for culture. Pt. placed in private isolation room with negative-pressure ventilation. Pt. reports recent weight loss of 10 lb, productive cough, night sweats, and low-grade fever. P 84, BP 142/78, RR 28, tympanic T 100.1° F. Administering O₂ at 4 L/min via NC. Following standard and airborne precautions when interacting with pt. Explained isolation precautions to pt.'s family as well as the need for him to wear a mask when he leaves his room. Instructed pt. to throw all tissues in waxed bag taped to side of bed. Administered rifampin, isoniazid, and pyrazinamide, per orders. See MAR. All medications and procedures explained to pt. ———————————— Carla Marron, RN |

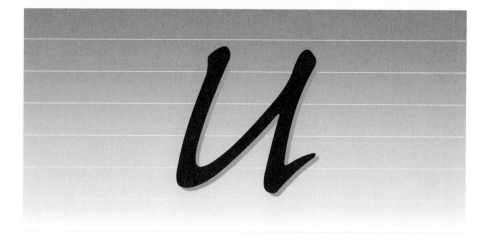

UNDERSTAFFING

Understaffing occurs when the facility administration fails to provide enough professionally trained personnel to meet the patient population's needs. Determining whether your unit has too few nurses or too few specially trained nurses may be difficult. The few guidelines that exist vary from state to state and are limited to specialty care units. The Joint Commission on the Accreditation of Healthcare Organizations' staffing standard sets no specific nurse-patient ratios. It states generally that the organization should provide an adequate number of staff whose qualifications are commensurate with defined job responsibilities and applicable licensure, laws and regulations, and certification.

If you find yourself assigned to more patients than you can reasonably care for or feel your unit is too understaffed to provide safe care, notify your nursing supervisor immediately. Be specific. Identify the type and amount of staff members you need. If the nursing supervisor can't or won't supply relief, notify the administration. If it doesn't offer a solution, write a memorandum detailing exactly what you did and said and what response you received. Don't walk off the job (you could be held liable for abandonment); instead, do the best you can.

Filing a written report isn't guaranteed to absolve you from liability if a patient is injured during your shift. You may still be found liable, especially if you could have foreseen and prevented the patient's injury; however, a written report will impress a jury as a sincere attempt to protect your patients. The report could also provide you with a defense if the al-

LEGAL CASEBOOK

COURT RULINGS RELATED TO UNDERSTAFFING

In the absence of well-defined staffing guidelines, the courts have had no reliable standard for ruling on cases of alleged understaffing. Each case has been decided on an individual basis.

The decision in the landmark case *Darling v. Charleston Community Memorial Hospital (1965)* was based partly on the issue of understaffing. A young man broke his leg while playing football and was taken to Charleston's emergency department where the on-call doctor set and cast his leg. The patient began to complain of pain almost immediately. Later, his toes grew swollen and dark, then cold and insensitive, and a stench pervaded his room. Nurses, who checked the leg only a few times per day, failed to report its worsening condition. When the cast was removed 3 days later, the necrotic condition of the leg was apparent. After making several surgical attempts to save the leg, the surgeon had to amputate below the knee.

After an out-of-court settlement with the doctor who applied the cast, the court found the hospital liable for failing to have enough specially trained nurses available at all times to recognize the patient's serious condition and alert the medical staff.

Since the *Darling* case, several similar cases have been tried — for example, *Cline v. Lun (1973)*, *Sanchez v. Bay General Hospital (1981)*, and *Harrell v. Louis Smith Memorial Hospital (1990)*. Almost every case involved a nurse who failed to continuously monitor her patient's condition — especially his vital signs — and to report significant changes to the attending doctor. In each case the courts have emphasized the:

- need for sufficient numbers of nurses to continuously monitor a patient's condition
- need for nurses who are specially trained to recognize signs and symptoms that require a doctor's immediate intervention.

leged malpractice involves something you should have done but didn't because of understaffing. (See *Court rulings related to understaffing*.)

ESSENTIAL DOCUMENTATION

Take notes during your shift and write a memorandum as soon as possible after your shift is over. Never document a staffing issue in the patient's chart. Record the name of the nursing supervisor with whom you spoke, the time of the conversation, exactly what you told the nursing supervisor, and her response. Include the names of other administrators you notified, the times they were notified, and their responses. Record any significant events that happened during the shift, noting a lack of care because of understaffing. Keep a copy of the memorandum for yourself, and send the original to the director of nursing.

To: Anita Lane, RN
    Director of Nursing
From: Laurel Baxter, RN
Date: 9/12/05
Time: 0100
Upon arrival to 6 West on 9/11/05 for the 7 p.m. to 7 a.m. shift, the 7 a.m. to 7 p.m. charge nurse, Patty O'Brien, told me that two RNs called in sick and replacements couldn't be found. I called Marisa Newcomb, RN, nursing supervisor, and told her that two RNs called in sick "Leaving four RNs to care for 15 critically ill patients. Patient acuity in the CCU is high at this time with four patients on ventilators, three patients with hemodynamic monitoring, two patients who underwent cardiac catheterization today, and one patient on an IABP. I was assigned to care for three critically ill patients, one was ventilator-dependent, one had acute heart failure, and the third patient was two days status post MI." Mrs. Newcomb reinforced that no nurses were available from other ICUs or from the p.r.n. pool and that we were to "do the best you can." I called you at 1900, but you had already left. I paged you but didn't get a response. My patient with heart failure developed acute pulmonary edema and respiratory distress, and I was unable to be in the other two patient's rooms from 2030 until 0030. The other nurses on the unit covered for me and assisted in delivering care to my patients. There were no patient injuries or complications during this time. However, I strongly feel the need to ensure adequate staffing in our unit to avoid future assignments such as the ones the other nurses and I had today and to avoid possible patient injuries and complications that could occur in this population of critically ill patients.
    I thank you for your time and consideration in this manner. I would like to set up a meeting with you and the unit director so the three of us can discuss possible options to prevent understaffing.

UNLICENSED ASSISTIVE PERSONNEL, CARE GIVEN BY

The American Nurses Association has defined unlicensed assistive personnel (UAP) as individuals trained to function in an assistive role to the registered professional nurse in the provision of patient care activities, as delegated by and under the supervision of that nurse. The nurse should only delegate care that the UAP is competent to perform. Even then, the nurse must evaluate the outcome and assure that the task and outcome are accurately documented in the medical record. Remember, responsibility for the task can be delegated but accountability can't. (See *Supervising unlicensed assistive personnel,* page 429.)

If your facility doesn't allow UAPs to document in the patient record, determine what care was provided, assess the patient and the task performed (for example, a dressing change), and document your findings. If your facility allows UAPs to chart, you may have to countersign their notes. If your facility's policy states that the UAP must provide care in your presence, don't countersign unless you actually witness her actions.

SUPERVISING UNLICENSED ASSISTIVE PERSONNEL

If you supervise unlicensed assistive personnel (UAP), you're responsible and liable for their performance. Limit your liability by educating yourself and advocating that your employer establish policies that clearly delineate the responsibilities of registered nurses, licensed practical nurses, and UAPs.

- Attend all educational programs your employer sponsors with respect to supervising UAPs.
- Encourage your supervisors to establish a written policy that defines the actions UAPs may take.
- Work cooperatively with UAPs in your clinical setting. If your employer decides to use UAPs, it's in your patients' best interest to establish a solid working relationship.
- Educate your patients about what UAPs can and can't do for them during your assigned work time. This will help them ask the appropriate individuals to assist them with their needs.
- If problems or disagreements arise over the appropriate functions for UAPs, report to your nursing-supervisor for immediate resolution.
- Review your state nurse practice act for provisions regarding delegation to UAPs. Follow all criteria for proper delegation set forth in the act.
- Stay current with your state nursing board's recommendations on the use of UAPs.

If the policy states that your presence isn't required, your countersignature indicates the note describes care that the UAP had the authority and competence to perform. It also indicates that you verified the procedure was performed. Unless your facility authorizes or requires you to witness someone else's notes, your signature will make you responsible for anything put in the notes above it.

ESSENTIAL DOCUMENTATION

If UAPs aren't allowed to chart, be sure to record the full name of the UAP who provided care (not just her initials). Describe the care that the UAP performed as well as your assessment of the patient.

12/12/05	0930	Morning care provided by UAP Terry Lien, who stated
		that pt. was unsteady on feet walking to bathroom to
		wash up. Went to see pt. who states that "Ms. Lien gave
		me a thorough sponge bath today." Explained to pt. that
		she was to call for assistance if she needed to get out
		of the chair. Pt. verbalized understanding. Call bell
		placed within pt.'s reach. Pt. demonstrated proper use
		of call bell. ———————— Katherine Landry, RN

UNRESPONSIVENESS BY PATIENT

Assessment of unresponsiveness is a crucial link in activating early life-saving techniques. Unresponsiveness is checked by calling the person's name and shaking his shoulder. If the patient remains unresponsive, call for help and take immediate measures to ensure airway, breathing, and circulation until the code team arrives.

Guidelines established by the American Heart Association direct you to keep a written, chronological account of a patient's condition while cardiopulmonary resuscitation (CPR) is being performed. This is usually charted on the code record, which documents detailed observations and interventions as well as drugs administered to the patient. (See *The code record,* page 54.) Remember to follow Advanced Cardiac Life Support guidelines when responding to a code.

Some facilities use a resuscitation critique form to identify actual or potential problems with the CPR process. This form tracks personnel responses and response times as well as the availability of appropriate drugs and functioning equipment.

ESSENTIAL DOCUMENTATION

Don't rely on your memory later; record the events as they occur. Writing "recorder" after your name indicates that you documented the code but didn't participate. Document the date and time that the code was called. Record the patient's name, the location of the code, the name of the person who discovered that the patient was unresponsive, the patient's condition, and whether the unresponsiveness was witnessed. Record the time that the doctor was notified, his name, and the name's of other members who participated in the code as well as the time that the family was notified. Note the exact time for each code intervention and include vital signs, heart rhythm, laboratory test results (arterial blood gas or electrolyte values), type of treatment (CPR, defibrillation, or cardioversion), drugs (name, dosage, and route), procedures (intubation, temporary or transvenous pacemaker, or central venous line insertion), and the patient's response. Indicate the time that the code ended and the patient's status. Some facilities require that the doctor leading the code and the nurse recording the code review the code record and sign it.

In your note, record the events leading up to the code, the assessment findings that prompted you to call a code, who initiated CPR, and any other interventions performed before the code team arrived. Include the patient's response to these interventions. Indicate in your note that a code sheet was used to document the events of the code.

8/9/05	1650	Summoned to pt.'s room at 1557 by a shout from
		roommate. Found pt. unresponsive in bed without
		respirations or pulse. Roommate stated, "He was
		watching TV; then all of a sudden he started gasping
		and holding his chest." Code called at 1559. Initiated
		CPR with Leslie Adams, RN. Code team arrived at 1600
		and continued resuscitative efforts. (See code record).
		Pt. moaned and opened eyes at approx. 1610. Notified
		Dr. Brower at home at 1615 and explained situation—
		will be in immediately. Report called to Tom Kennedy,
		RN, and pt. transferred to ICU at 1638. Family
		notified of pt.'s condition and transfer. ————
		—————————————— Michelle Robbins, RN

URINARY CATHETER INSERTION, INDWELLING

Also known as a Foley or retention catheter, an indwelling urinary catheter remains in the bladder to provide continuous urine drainage. A balloon inflated at the catheter's distal end prevents it from slipping out of the bladder after insertion.

An indwelling catheter is inserted using sterile technique and only when absolutely necessary. Insertion should be performed with extreme care to prevent injury to the patient and possible infection.

An indwelling catheter is most commonly used to relieve bladder distention caused by urine retention and allow continuous urine drainage when the urinary meatus is swollen from childbirth, surgery, or local trauma. Other indications for an indwelling catheter include urinary tract obstruction caused by a tumor or enlarged prostate, urine retention or infection from neurogenic bladder paralysis caused by spinal cord injury or disease, and any illness in which the patient's urine output must be closely monitored.

ESSENTIAL DOCUMENTATION

Record the date and time that the indwelling urinary catheter was inserted. Note the size and type of catheter used. Also, describe the amount, color, and other characteristics of the urine emptied from the bladder. Intake and output should be recorded on the patient's intake and output record. (See *Intake and output,* page 231.) If large volumes of urine have been emptied, describe the patient's tolerance for the procedure. Note whether a urine specimen was sent for laboratory analysis. Document any patient teaching performed.

12/12/05	1115	Explained reason for insertion of indwelling urinary catheter to pt. prior to hysterectomy. Pt. stated she understood the need but wasn't looking forward to its insertion. Reassured her that the insertion shouldn't be painful if she relaxes. Showed her how to do breathing exercises during insertion. #16 Fr. Foley catheter inserted at 1045. Emptied 450 ml from bladder. Urine dark amber, no odor, or sediment. Specimen sent to lab for U/A. Pt. states she has no discomfort and can't feel catheter in place. See I/O flow sheet. ————— Molly Malone, RN

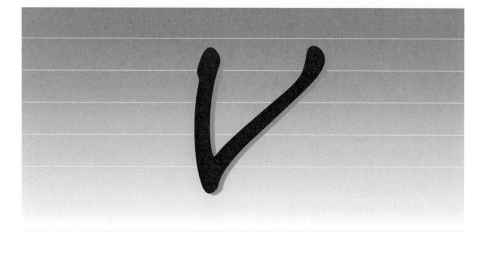

VAGAL MANEUVERS

When a patient suffers sinus, atrial, or junctional tachyarrhythmias, vagal maneuvers – Valsalva's maneuver and carotid sinus massage – can slow his heart rate. These maneuvers work by stimulating nerve endings, which respond as they would to an increase in blood pressure. They send this message to the brain stem, which in turn stimulates the autonomic nervous system to increase vagal tone and decrease the heart rate. Usually performed by a doctor, vagal maneuvers may also be performed by a specially trained nurse under a doctor's supervision.

In Valsalva's maneuver, the patient holds his breath and bears down, raising his intrathoracic pressure. When this pressure increase is transmitted to the heart and great vessels, venous return, stroke volume, and systolic blood pressure decrease. Within seconds, the baroreceptors respond to the changes by increasing the heart rate and causing peripheral vasoconstriction. When the patient exhales at the end of this maneuver, his blood pressure rises to its previous level. This increase, combined with the peripheral vasoconstriction caused by bearing down, stimulates the vagus nerve, decreasing the heart rate.

In carotid sinus massage, manual pressure applied to the left or right carotid sinus slows the patient's heart rate. The patient's response to carotid sinus massage depends on the type of arrhythmia. If he has sinus tachycardia, his heart rate will slow gradually during the procedure and speed up again after it. In atrial tachycardia, the arrhythmia may stop and the heart rate may remain slow. With atrial fibrillation or flutter, the ventricular rate may not change; atrioventricular block may even worsen.

Nonparoxysmal tachycardia and ventricular tachycardia won't respond to carotid sinus massage.

ESSENTIAL DOCUMENTATION

Record the date and time of the procedure, who performed it, and why it was necessary. Note the patient's response, any complications, and the interventions taken. If possible, obtain a rhythm strip before, during, and after the procedure.

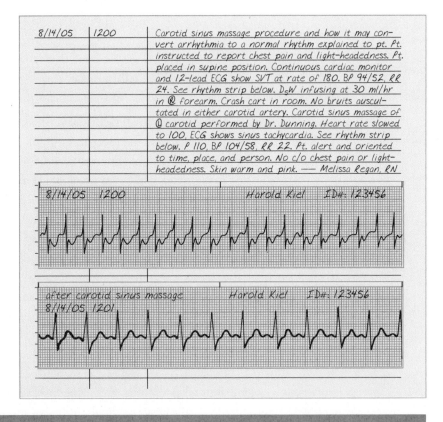

8/14/05	1200	Carotid sinus massage procedure and how it may con-
		vert arrhythmia to a normal rhythm explained to pt. Pt.
		instructed to report chest pain and light-headedness. Pt.
		placed in supine position. Continuous cardiac monitor
		and 12-lead ECG show SVT at rate of 180. BP 94/52, RR
		24. See rhythm strip below. D₅W infusing at 30 ml/hr
		in ® forearm. Crash cart in room. No bruits auscul-
		tated in either carotid artery. Carotid sinus massage of
		ℚ carotid performed by Dr. Dunning. Heart rate slowed
		to 100. ECG shows sinus tachycardia. See rhythm strip
		below. P 110, BP 104/58, RR 22. Pt. alert and oriented
		to time, place, and person. No c/o chest pain or light-
		headedness. Skin warm and pink. — Melissa Regan, RN

VASCULAR ACCESS DEVICE, ACCESSING

Surgically implanted under local anesthesia by a doctor, a vascular access device consists of a silicone catheter attached to a reservoir, which is covered with a self-sealing silicone rubber septum. It's used most commonly when an external central venous catheter isn't desirable for long-term I.V. therapy. The most common type of vascular access device is a vascular access port (VAP). Typically, VAPs deliver intermittent infusions. They're used to deliver chemotherapy and other drugs, I.V. fluids, and blood. They can also be used to obtain blood.

To access a VAP, a noncoring or Huber needle is inserted into the reservoir. An extension set is flushed with normal saline solution and then attached to the needle. After checking for blood return, the port is flushed with normal saline solution, according to your facility's policy.

While the patient is hospitalized, a luer-lock injection cap may be attached to the end of an extension set to provide ready access for intermittent infusions. In addition to saving time, a luer-lock cap reduces the discomfort of accessing the port and prolongs the life of the port septum by decreasing the number of needle punctures.

ESSENTIAL DOCUMENTATION

Record the date and time that the port was accessed. Note whether signs or symptoms of infection or skin breakdown are present. Describe any pain or discomfort that the patient experienced when the port was accessed. If you used ice or local anesthetic, make sure to chart it. Describe how the area was cleaned before accessing the port. Note whether resistance was met when inserting the needle and whether you obtained a blood return. Include the number of attempts made to access the port. Record any problems with the normal saline flush, such as swelling or pain. Chart the time that the doctor was notified of any problems, his name, any orders given, your interventions, and the patient's response. Also, document patient education performed.

10/20/05	1200	No breakdown, redness, warmth, or drainage noted at VAP
		access site in Ⓡ chest. Pt. states he doesn't use a local
		anesthetic to access the site since "It doesn't really hurt."
		Site cleaned with chlorhexidine, per protocol, and
		anchored by hand while noncoring needle was inserted
		perpendicular to port septum on first attempt. No
		resistance noted. Blood return observed and device
		flushed with NSS, per protocol. Antibiotic infusing with-
		out problem. Pt. has been using VAP at home for 3 months
		and verbalized understanding of its use. Pt. will access
		device with next drug infusion, with nurse watching to
		evaluate his technique. ———— Chelsea Burton, RN

VASCULAR ACCESS DEVICE, CARE OF

After implantation of a vascular access port (VAP), monitor the site for signs of hematoma and bleeding. Edema and tenderness may persist for about 72 hours. The incision site requires routine postoperative care for 7 to 10 days. You'll also need to assess the implantation site for signs of infection, device rotation, and skin erosion. No dressing is necessary except during infusions or to maintain an intermittent infusion device.

If your patient is receiving a continuous or prolonged infusion, change a transparent dressing and needle every 7 days. You'll also need to change the tubing and solution as you would for a long-term central venous infusion.

After a bolus injection or at the end of an infusion, flush the VAP with normal saline solution followed by heparin, according to your facility's policy. If your patient is receiving an intermittent infusion, flush the port periodically with heparin solution. When the VAP isn't being used, flush it every 4 weeks. During the course of therapy, you may need to clear a clotted VAP with a fibrinolytic drug, as ordered.

ESSENTIAL DOCUMENTATION

Record the date and time of your entry. Record the appearance of the site, indicating any bleeding, edema, or hematoma. Document any sign of skin infection or device rotation. Indicate the type of therapy that the patient is receiving, such as continuous infusion or intermittent therapy. Document normal saline solution and heparin flushes as well as measures taken to maintain a patent infusion. Record all dressing, needle, and tubing changes.

7/31/05	0930	VAP site clean, dry, and intact. No redness, warmth,
		drainage, bleeding, swelling, or discoloration noted.
		Noncoring needle, extension set, transparent dressing,
		tubing, and solution replaced. Port flushed with heparin
		solution, per protocol. ———————— Mae Robinson, RN

VASCULAR ACCESS DEVICE, WITHDRAWING ACCESS

When you care for a patient with a vascular access port (VAP), you'll need to remove the noncoring Huber needle every 7 days (according to your facility's policy) or at the end of therapy. After you remove the dressing, attach a 10-ml syringe containing normal saline solution, according to facility policy, and aspirate for blood; then flush the catheter. Follow this with a heparin flush in a 10-ml syringe, according to facility policy. As you inject the last 0.5 ml, reclamp the extension tubing to maintain positive forward flow. Stabilize the port with your nondominant thumb and forefinger while you gently pull the needle upward. Protective devices are available to prevent a rebound needle stick. Discard the needle in the appropriate container. Apply an adhesive dressing over the site for 30 to 60 minutes.

ESSENTIAL DOCUMENTATION

Record the date and time that access is withdrawn from the VAP, and note that you've explained the procedure to the patient. Document the solutions, amounts, and size of the syringes used to flush the extension tubing. Depending on your facility's policy, these solutions may need to be documented on the medication administration record as well. Note whether you aspirated blood or met resistance. Record that the needle was removed, noting any clots on the needle tip. Describe the condition of the site and the type of dressing applied.

12/19/05	1930	Explained procedure for deaccessing VAP to pt. Pt. was
		concerned about pain. Reassured her that removing
		needle shouldn't cause her any pain. Blood easily
		aspirated from extension tubing. Flushed tubing with
		5 ml NSS, followed by 5 ml of 100 unit/ml heparin,
		using 10-ml syringes. While stabilizing VAP, needle was
		easily withdrawn. Except for needle puncture wound,
		skin at access site is intact and without redness,
		drainage, swelling, bleeding, or hematoma. Adhesive
		bandage placed over site. Told pt. bandage may be
		removed in 30 to 60 minutes. —— Danielle Ford, RN

VENTRICULAR ASSIST DEVICE

A temporary life-sustaining treatment for the failing heart, the ventricular assist device (VAD) diverts systemic blood flow from a diseased ventricle into a centrifugal pump; thus temporarily reducing ventricular work, which allows the myocardium to rest and contractility to improve. The VAD functions somewhat like an artificial heart. The major difference is that the VAD assists the heart, whereas the artificial heart replaces it.

The permanent VAD is implanted in the patient's chest cavity, although it still provides only temporary support. The device receives power through the skin by a belt of electrical transformer coils (worn externally as a portable battery pack). It can also be operated by an implanted, rechargeable battery for short periods of time.

Candidates for the VAD include patients with massive myocardial infarction, irreversible cardiomyopathy, acute myocarditis, an inability to be weaned from cardiopulmonary bypass, valvular disease, bacterial endocarditis, or heart transplant rejection. The device may also be used in patients awaiting a heart transplant.

ESSENTIAL DOCUMENTATION

Record the date and time of your entry. Note the patient's condition after the insertion of the VAD. Record the results of your cardiopulmonary findings (including hemodynamic measurements) as well as neurologic and renal assessments. Document pump adjustments and the patient's response. Chart signs and symptoms of poor perfusion and ineffective pumping (such as arrhythmias, hypotension, slow capillary refill, cool skin, oliguria or anuria, or anxiety and restlessness), pulmonary embolism (such as dyspnea, chest pain, tachycardia, productive cough, or low-grade fever), and stroke or neurologic deficits.

Record the time that the doctor was notified of complications, his name, orders given, your interventions, and the patient's response. Document any drugs given (such as heparin); the dosage, frequency, and route; and the patient's response. Record the appearance of the cannula insertion site, site care, and dressing changes. Document all patient teaching and emotional support provided. Patient teaching may be recorded on a patient-teaching flow sheet. Use flow sheets to record your frequent assessments, including vital signs, intake and output, I.V. therapy, hemodynamic parameters, and laboratory test values (such as complete blood count and coagulation studies).

| 7/31/05 | 1030 | VAD continues to function without problems. No pump adjustments made. Pt. states he feels much better since VAD insertion 3 days ago. Pt. is alert and oriented to time, place, and person. Moving all extremities, strong hand grasps. Skin warm, pink, and dry. Breath sounds clear. Urine output remains greater than 60 ml/hr. Peripheral pulses palpable, 3 sec capillary refill. P 70 and regular, BP 110/68, RR 18, oral T 98.8° F. Cardiac monitor shows NSR, no arrhythmias noted. CO 5.6 L/min. PAP 25/16, PAWP 15 mm Hg, CVP 8 cm H₂O, MAP 36.6, and LAP 10 mm Hg. Cannula site without redness, warmth, drainage, or bleeding. Site cleaned and dressed according to policy. CBC w/diff, electrolytes, BUN, creatinine, PT–PTT drawn this a.m. Results pending. See flow sheets for documentation of frequent VS, I.V. therapy, I/O, hemodynamic parameters, and lab values. Transplant coordinator in to talk with pt. about transplant process. —— ———————————————— Carol Allen, RN |

VIOLENT PATIENT

When a patient demonstrates violent behavior, quick action is needed to protect him, other patients, and the staff from harm. Follow your facility's policy for dealing with a violent patient. Call for help immediately and contact security. The doctor, nursing supervisor, and risk manager should also be informed of the patient's violence. Stay with the patient, without crowding him.

If your own safety is threatened, have another coworker stay with you. Remove dangerous objects from the area. Never block your exit or the patient's exit from a room. Use your communication skills to try to calm the patient. Don't challenge him or argue with him. Use a calm and non-threatening tone of voice and stance. Listen to the patient and acknowledge his anger.

Depending on their policies, some institutions prepare to handle violent individuals by mobilizing personnel. You may be required to call a specific code through the paging operator such as "code orange room 462B." Specific staff members would respond to the call, such as security personnel, male staff members, and individuals trained to handle volatile situations. The patient would then be approached and physically subdued and restrained enough to ensure safety without harming the patient, staff, or other patients. When the patient is restrained, he'll need to be closely monitored and assessed, and the cause of the episode will need to be determined. He may also require continued chemical or physical restraints if his behavior persists and no physical cause is determined.

ESSENTIAL DOCUMENTATION

Record the date and time of your note. Chart the location of the incident. Describe the patient's violent behaviors and record exactly what the patient said in quotes. Record your immediate interventions and the patient's response. Chart the names of the people you notified, such as the doctor, the nursing supervisor, security, and the risk manager, when you notified them, and their responses. Note any injuries that occurred as a result of the violence. Complete an incident report, according to facility policy, repeating the exact information in your nurse's note. Include the names, addresses, and telephone numbers of witnesses.

7/29/05	1715	Heard shouts and a crash from pt.'s room at 1645. Upon
		entering room, saw dinner tray and broken dishes on
		floor. Pt. was standing, red-faced, with fist in air yelling,
		"My dog gets better food than this." Called for help and
		maintained a distance of approx. 5' from pt. When Ann
		Stilson, RN, and Jason Black, RN, arrived, I told them to
		wait in hall. Pt. was throwing books and other items from
		nightstand to floor. Firmly told pt. to stop throwing
		things and that I wanted to help him. I stated, "I can
		see you're angry. How can I help you?" Pt. responded,
		"Try getting me some decent food." Asked a nurse in the
		hall to call dietary office to see what other choices were
		on menu for tonight. Told pt. I would try to get him
		other food choices. Asked pt. to sit down with me to talk.
		Pt. sat on edge of his bed and I sat on chair approx. 4'
		from pt. Pt. started to cry and said, "I'm so scared. I
		don't want to die." Listened to pt. verbalize his fears
		for several minutes. When asked, pt. stated he would like
		to speak with chaplain and would agree to talk with a
		counselor. He apologized for his behavior and stated he
		was embarrassed. Contacted Dr. Hartwell at 1705 and told
		him of pt.'s behavior. Doctor approved of psych. consult
		and gave verbal order. On-call psychiatrist paged at 1708.
		Hasn't yet returned call. Nursing supervisor, Jack Fox,
		RN, also notified of incident. Pt. has no visible injuries.
		Will further assess pt. when calmer. —Kristen Burger, RN

VISION IMPAIRMENT

A visual impairment in your patient may range from only a minor loss of vision to total blindness. If your patient has a visual impairment, determine what he can see and whether he uses any assistive devices to enhance his vision. Perform a safety assessment, orient him to his room and the unit, and remove possible hazards (such as wastebaskets, electric cords, and other obstructions). Assess his ability to maneuver around his environment. A patient with a recent loss of vision, such as the patient wearing an eye patch after eye surgery, may require more assistance than a patient who has had a gradual decline in vision or long-term visual loss.

ESSENTIAL DOCUMENTATION

Record the length of time that your patient has had a visual impairment. Describe the degree of his vision loss; for example, whether he can see faces, shapes, and objects; read large print; or has a loss of peripheral vision or depth perception. Document whether assistive devices are being used, such as glasses, contact lenses, or a pocket magnifying glass. Describe his ability to move around the environment safely. Record your interventions, such as obtaining a brighter light for the room and arranging personal objects within reach. Chart that you've notified other departments of the patient's visual impairment. Document your patient teaching, such as orienting the patient to his room, the unit, and the use of the call bell. Include other instructions such as calling for help when getting out of bed.

8/9/05	1900	Pt. admitted for ® hip replacement in a.m. Has had a gradual decline in vision over last 5 years due to macular degeneration. Pt. states she can see shapes and objects but has difficulty identifying faces from a distance. She uses a handheld magnifying glass to read large print books and also enjoys listening to books on tape. Pt. was able to safely maneuver around her room and unit; however, wastebasket and foot stool were moved against the wall. Showed pt. location of call bell attached to side rail of bed and emergency pull-cord in bathroom. Dietary office notified and will send an aide to read food choices to pt. Visual impairment marked in medical record, recorded on preop. checklist. ———————————— Marcy Phillips, RN

VITAL SIGNS, FREQUENT

A patient may require frequent monitoring of vital signs after surgery or certain procedures and diagnostic tests or during a critical illness. A frequent vital signs flow sheet allows you to quickly document vital signs the moment you take them without having to take the time to write a progress note. A flow sheet also allows you to readily detect changes in the patient's condition.

Sometimes, recording only vital signs isn't sufficient to give a complete picture of the patient's status. In such a case, you'll also need to write a progress note. Make sure the data on the vital signs flow sheet are consistent with the data in your progress note.

Essential documentation

Record the date on the flow sheet. Chart the specific time each set of vital signs is taken. If there's a significant change in vital signs, write a progress note documenting the change, the time the doctor was notified, his name, any orders given, your actions, and the patient's response. (See *Frequent vital signs flow sheet*.)

ACCUCHART

FREQUENT VITAL SIGNS FLOW SHEET

When the patient requires frequent vital sign assessments, a flow sheet such as this may help facilitate documentation by eliminating the need to continually make entries in the notation section of the chart. In the example below, blood pressure is monitored every 15 minutes.

FREQUENT VITAL SIGNS FLOW SHEET

DATE	TIME	KEY	BP	P	RR	T	CVP	PAP			COMMENTS	TITRATED I.V.'S	MEDS STAT AND PRN	INITIALS
								S/D	M	W				
11/13/05	0900	S	122/84	98	18	98⁶								MC
	0915	S	124/82	94	18									MC
	0930	S	122/78	92	20									MC
	0945	S	120/80	94	18									MC
	1000	S	128/78	94	20									MC

Key: S = Stethoscope   D = Doppler   P = Palpation   T = Transducer

W X Y

WALKER USE

A walker consists of a metal frame with handgrips and four legs buttressing the patient on three sides. One side remains open. Because this device provides greater stability and security than do other ambulatory aids, it's recommended that the patient with insufficient strength and balance use crutches or a cane.

ESSENTIAL DOCUMENTATION

Record the date and time of your entry. Record the type of walker used, such as a standard, stair, or reciprocal walker. Note whether any attachments are used, including platform attachments or wheels. Describe the degree of guarding that the patient requires. Chart the distance walked and the patient's tolerance. Document all teaching related to the use of the walker.

11/20/05	1200	Pt. ambulated with reciprocal walker without assistance
		from own room to day room using 2-point gait, approx.
		50'. Required only occasional verbal cues. Pt. was slightly
		SOB at end of walk. VS before walk P 82, BP 130/78,
		RR 18. After walk P 94, BP 138/82, RR 26. Reinforced
		sitting and standing using the walker. Pt. gave proper
		demo.————————————— Carole Parker, RN

WOUND ASSESSMENT

When caring for a patient with a wound, complete a thorough assessment so that you'll have a clear baseline from which to evaluate healing and the appropriateness of therapy. Care may need to be altered if the wound doesn't respond to therapy. Many facilities have a specific wound care protocol that specifies different treatment plans based on wound assessment. A wound should be assessed with each dressing change.

ESSENTIAL DOCUMENTATION

Record the date and time of your entry. Be sure to include the following points when documenting wound assessment:
- wound size, including length, width, and depth in centimeters
- wound shape
- wound site, drawn on a body plan to document exact location
- wound stage
- characteristics of drainage, if any, including amount, color, and presence of odor
- characteristics of the wound bed, including description of tissue type, such as granulation tissue, slough, or epithelial tissue, and percentage of each tissue type
- character of the surrounding tissue
- presence or absence of eschar
- presence or absence of pain
- presence or absence of undermining or tunneling (in centimeters).

Many facilities also have a special form or flow sheet on which to document wounds. (See *Wound and skin assessment tool,* pages 446 and 447.)

| 12/14/05 | 1330 | Pt. admitted to unit for fem-pop bypass tomorrow. Pt. has open wound at tip of 2nd ℚ toe, approx. 0.5 cm X I cm X 0.5 cm deep. Wound is round with even edges. Wound bed is pale with little granulation tissue. No drainage, odor, eschar, or tunneling noted. Pt. reports pain at wound site, rates pain as 4 on scale of 0 to 10, w/10 being the worst pain imaginable. Surrounding skin cool to touch, pale, and intact. Pt. understands not to cross legs or wear tight garments. ——— Mark Silver, RN |

ACCUCHART

WOUND AND SKIN ASSESSMENT TOOL

When performing a thorough wound and skin assessment, a pictorial demonstration is often helpful to identify the wound site or sites. Using the wound and skin assessment tool below, the nurse identified the left second toe as a partial-thickness wound, vascular ulcer, that's red in color using the classification of terms that follow.

PATIENT'S NAME (LAST, MIDDLE, FIRST)	ATTENDING PHYSICIAN	ROOM NUMBER	ID NUMBER
Brown, Ann	Dr. A. Dennis	123-2	01726

WOUND ASSESSMENT:

NUMBER	1	2	3	4	5	6
DATE	11/03/05					
TIME	1215					
LOCATION	Ⓛ second toe					
STAGE	II					
APPEARANCE	G					
SIZE-LENGTH	0.5 cm					
SIZE-WIDTH	1 cm					
COLOR/FLR.	RD					
DRAINAGE	0					
ODOR	0					
VOLUME	0					
INFLAMMATION	0					
SIZE INFLAM.	0					

KEY

Stage:
  I. Red or discolored
  II. Skin break/blister
  III. Sub 'Q' tissue
  IV. Muscle and/or bone

Appearance:
  D = Depth
  E = Eschar
  G = Granulation
  IN = Inflammation
  NEC = Necrotic
  PK = Pink
  SL = Slough
  TN = Tunneling
  UND = Undermining
  MX = Mixed (specify)

Color of Wound
Floor:
  RD = Red
  Y = Yellow
  BLK = Black
  MX = Mixed (specify)

Drainage:
  0 = None
  SR = Serous
  SS = Serosanguineous
  BL = Blood
  PR = Purulent

Odor:
  0 = None
  MLD = Mild
  FL = Foul

Volume:
  0 = None
  SC = Scant
  MOD = Moderate
  LG = Large

Inflammation:
  0 = None
  PK = Pink
  RD = Red

WOUND AND SKIN ASSESSMENT TOOL
(continued)

WOUND ANATOMIC LOCATION:

(circle affected area)

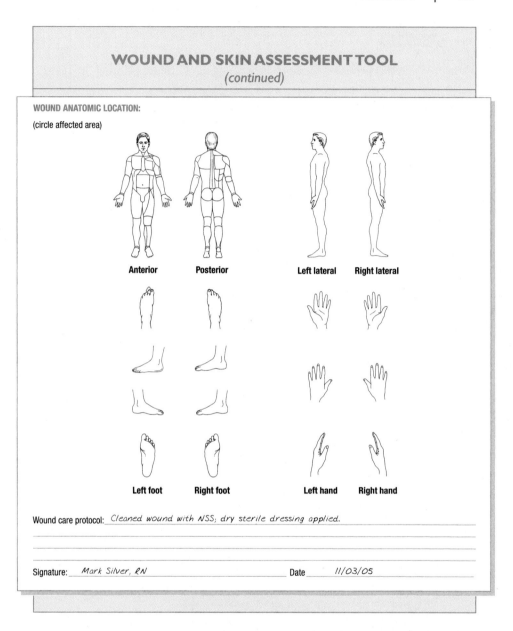

Anterior   Posterior   Left lateral   Right lateral

Left foot   Right foot   Left hand   Right hand

Wound care protocol: *Cleaned wound with NSS; dry sterile dressing applied.*

Signature: *Mark Silver, RN*   Date   *11/03/05*

WOUND CARE

When caring for a surgical wound, your intent is to help prevent infection by stopping pathogens from entering the wound. In addition to promoting patient comfort, such procedures protect the skin surface from maceration and excoriation caused by contact with irritating drainage. They also allow you to measure wound drainage to monitor fluid and electrolyte balance.

The two principal methods for managing a draining wound are dressing and pouching. Dressing is the best choice when skin integrity isn't compromised by caustic or excessive drainage. Lightly seeping wounds with drains as well as wounds with minimal purulent drainage can usually be managed with packing and gauze dressings. Copious, excoriating drainage calls for pouching to protect the skin.

ESSENTIAL DOCUMENTATION

Document the date and time of the procedure as well as the type of wound management. Record the amount of soiled dressing and packing removed. Describe wound appearance (size, condition of margins, and presence of necrotic tissue) and odor (if present). Chart the type, color, consistency, and amount of drainage for each wound. Indicate the presence and location of drains. Note any additional procedures, such as irrigation, packing, or application of a topical medication. Record the type and amount of new dressing or pouch applied. Note the patient's tolerance of the procedure and any instructions given.

Document special or detailed wound care instructions and pain management steps on the care plan. Record the color and amount of drainage on the intake and output sheet.

11/17/05	1030	Dressing removed from ® mastectomy incision. 1.5 cm
		round area of serosanguineous drainage noted on
		dressing. No odor noted. 11-cm incision well-approximated,
		staples intact. Skin around incision intact, no redness. Site
		cleaned with sterile NSS. Six sterile 4" X 4" gauze pads
		applied. Jackson Pratt drain at lateral edge of incision
		emptied for 10 ml serosanguineous fluid, no odor noted.
		See I/O flow sheet for shift totals. Explained dressing
		change and signs and symptoms of infection to report. Pt.
		verbalized understanding. Pt. states incision is tender but
		doesn't require pain medication. ———— Deborah Liu, RN

WOUND DEHISCENCE

Although surgical wounds typically heal without incident, occasionally the edges of a wound may fail to join or may separate even after they seem to be healing normally. This complication, called *dehiscence,* may be partial and superficial or complete with disruption of all layers. It commonly occurs from 3 to 11 days after surgery.

Dehiscence occurs most commonly in abdominal wounds after a sudden strain, such as a sneeze or cough, vomiting, or sitting up in bed. Obese patients are at higher risk due to constant strain placed on the wound and slow healing of fatty tissue. Other factors that may contribute to dehiscence include poor nutrition (either from inadequate intake or diabetes mellitus), chronic pulmonary or cardiac disease, and localized wound infection.

If wound dehiscence occurs, stay with the patient while someone immediately contacts the doctor. Place the patient in a reclining position, with knees flexed. Cover the wound with sterile gauze pads soaked in sterile normal saline solution; then cover the wound with dry sterile gauze pads and tape them in place. Stay with the patient until the doctor provides further instructions. Depending on the degree of dehiscence, the patient may need sutures or adhesive strips to close the wound.

ESSENTIAL DOCUMENTATION

Note the date and time that the problem occurred, the patient's activity preceding dehiscence, his condition, the name of the doctor, and the time of notification. Note any orders given. Document the actions you took and the patient's response. Describe the appearance of the wound and the amount, color, consistency, and odor of any drainage. Record the patient's vital signs. Frequent vital signs may be recorded on a frequent vital signs flow sheet. (See "Vital signs, frequent," page 442). Document all patient teaching and emotional support provided.

| 8/24/05 | 0945 | During dressing change at 0925, noted dehiscence of distal 2" of midline abdominal incision. Superficial layers of tissue observed, no evisceration noted. Pt. placed in reclined position with knees flexed. Pt. states, "I felt something give when I coughed." Wound covered with sterile 4" X 4" gauze soaked in NSS, then covered with dry sterile dressing. P 100, BP 150/84, RR 18, T 98.6° F. Dr. McBride notified at 0930. Adhesive strips ordered and applied to wound. Pt. to be kept on bed rest until Dr. McBride visits pt. at 1030. Pt. instructed to stay in bed with knees flexed and to call nurse for assistance with moving in bed. Reviewed splinting incision with pillow if he has to cough or sneeze. Call bell placed within reach, and pt. demonstrated how to use it. ———————— Maureen Dunlop, RN |

WOUND EVISCERATION

A complication of wound dehiscence, evisceration occurs when a portion of the viscera (usually a bowel loop) protrudes through the incision. Evisceration can lead to peritonitis and septic shock, a potentially fatal condition.

Wound evisceration most commonly occurs 6 to 7 days after surgery and may be caused by poor nutrition, chronic pulmonary or cardiac disease, localized wound infection, or stress on the incision from coughing. A midline abdominal incision has a higher risk of wound evisceration.

If wound evisceration occurs, stay with the patient while someone immediately contacts the doctor. Place the patient in a reclining position, with knees flexed. Cover the exposed viscera with sterile gauze pads soaked in normal saline solution. Then place a sterile, waterproof drape over the dressings and keep the dressings moist. Anticipate preparing the patient for surgery.

ESSENTIAL DOCUMENTATION

Note when the evisceration occurred, the patient's activity preceding the problem, his overall condition, the name of the doctor, and the time of notification. Note any orders given. Document the actions that you took and the patient's response. Describe the appearance of the wound and eviscerated organ and the amount, color, consistency, and odor of any drainage. Record the patient's vital signs and his response to the incident.

Frequent vital signs may be recorded on a frequent vital signs flow sheet. (See "Vital signs, frequent," page 442.) Document your patient teaching and emotional support given to the patient.

10/18/05	1135	Called to room by pt. who stated, "I think I felt something pulling when I coughed." Pt. lying curled on side splinting abdomen with arms, moaning. Eviscerated bowel pink and moist, no drainage. Area covered with NSS-soaked gauze. Sterile, waterproof drape placed over dressing. Skin color pale, diaphoretic. P 112, BP 92/58, RR 28, tympanic T 98.2° F. Stayed with pt. while Karen Schultz, RN, called Dr. Brown who came by immediately, orders given. O₂ at 2 L/min by NC applied. I.V. line started in ® antecubital with 18G catheter on first attempt. 1,000 ml lactated Ringer's solution infusing at 100 ml/hr. Being kept NPO for probable surgery. Pt. fearful and weeping. Offering reassurance and explaining all procedures. See flow sheet for VS. —————— Carla Molino, RN

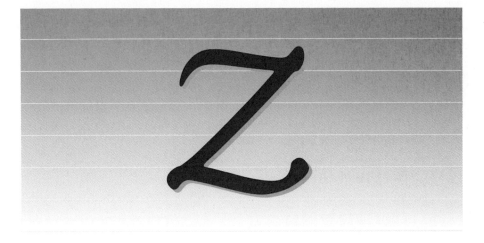

Z-TRACK INJECTION

The Z-track method of I.M. injection prevents leakage, or tracking, into the subcutaneous (subQ) tissue. It's typically used to administer drugs that irritate and discolor subQ tissue, primarily iron preparations such as iron dextran. It may also be used in an elderly patient who has a decreased muscle mass. Lateral displacement of the skin during the injection helps to seal the drug in the muscle.

Discomfort and tissue irritation may result from drug leakage into subQ tissue. Failure to rotate sites in patients who require repeated injections can interfere with the absorption of medication. Unabsorbed medications may build up in deposits that can reduce the desired pharmacologic effect and may lead to abscess formation or tissue fibrosis.

ESSENTIAL DOCUMENTATION

Record the medication and dosage as well as the date, time, and site of injection on the patient's medication record. Include the patient's response to the injected drug, if appropriate. (See *Z-track injection*, page 452.)

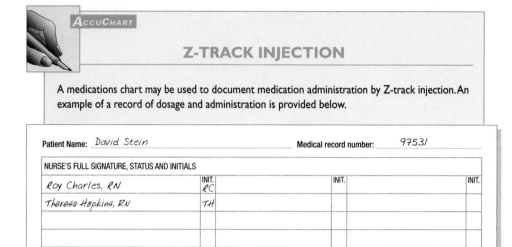

Z-TRACK INJECTION

A medications chart may be used to document medication administration by Z-track injection. An example of a record of dosage and administration is provided below.

Patient Name: _David Stein_   Medical record number: _97531_

NURSE'S FULL SIGNATURE, STATUS AND INITIALS

	INIT.		INIT.		INIT.
Roy Charles, RN	RC				
Theresa Hopkins, RN	TH				

DIAGNOSIS: Heart failure, atrial flutter, COPD

ALLERGIES: ASA   DIET: Cardiac

ROUTINE/DAILY ORDERS FINGERSTICKS/INSULIN COVERAGE		DATE: 6/10		DATE: 6/11		DATE: 6/12		DATE: 6/13		DATE: 6/14		DATE: 6/15		DATE: 6/16		DATE: 6/17		DATE: 6/18		DATE: 6/19	

ORDER DATE	MEDICATIONS DOSAGE, ROUTE, FREQUENCY	TIME	SITE	INT.	SITE	INT.	SITE	INT.	SITE	INT.	SITE	INT.	SITE	INT.	SITE	INT.	SITE	INT.	SITE	INT.	SITE	INT.
6/10/05	Iron dextran 50 mg I.M. daily by Z-track X 3 doses	0900	Ⓡ GM	RC	Ⓛ GM	TH	Ⓡ GM	TH														

Adapted with permission from Katz, S. et al. "Studies of Illness in the Aged: The Index of ADL-A Standardized Measure of Biological and Psychosocial Function," *JAMA* 185:914-19, ©1963.

Appendices

- Documentation systems

- Electronic health record

- JCAHO National Patient Safety Goals

- Abbreviations to avoid

- NANDA nursing diagnoses

Selected references

Index

Documentation systems

Depending on your health care facility's policies, you'll use one or more documentation systems to record your nursing interventions and evaluations and the patient's response.

Health care facilities may use traditional narrative charting or an alternative system, such as problem-oriented medical record (POMR), problem-intervention-evaluation (PIE), FOCUS, charting-by-exception (CBE), FACT, core, or outcome documentation systems. In addition, many health care facilities use computerized charting systems. (See "Electronic health record," page 470.)

TRADITIONAL NARRATIVE CHARTING

Narrative charting is a straightforward chronologic account of the patient's status, the nursing interventions performed, and the patient's response to those interventions. Documentation is usually included in the progress notes and is supplemented by flow sheets. The Joint Commission on Accreditation of Healthcare Organizations' (JCAHO) standards require all health care facilities to set policies on how frequently patients should be assessed. Document patient assessments as often as your institution requires and more frequently when you observe any of the following:

- change in the patient's condition
- patient's response to a treatment or medication
- lack of improvement in the patient's condition
- patient's or family member's response to teaching.

Document exactly what you hear, observe, inspect, do, or teach. Include as much specific, descriptive information as possible. Always document how your patient responds to care, treatments, and medications as well as his progress toward the desired outcome. Also, include notification to the doctor of changes that have occurred. Document this communication, the doctor's response, new orders that are followed, and the patient's response.

You can organize your notes by using a head-to-toe approach or by referring to the care plan and documenting the patient's progress in relation to the plan and unresolved problems. Regardless of the way you organize your narrative note, be specific and document chronologically, recording exact times.

11/26/05	2255	Patient 4 hr postop; awakens easily, oriented to time, place, and person but groggy, incision site in front of Ⓛ ear extending down and around the ear and into neck— approximately 15 cm in length—without dressing. No swelling or bleeding, bluish discoloration below Ⓛ ear noted, sutures intact. Jackson-Pratt drain in Ⓛ neck below ear with 20-ml bloody drainage measured. Drain remains secured with suture and anchored to Ⓛ anterior chest wall with tape. P 82, BP 132/88, RR 18, oral T 98.8° F. Pt. denied pain but stated she felt nauseated and promptly vomited 100 ml of clear fluid. Pt. attempted to get OOB to ambulate to bathroom with assistance, but felt dizzy upon standing. Assisted to lie down in bed. Voided 200 ml clear, yellow urine in bedpan. Pt. encouraged to deep-breathe and cough qhr, and turn frequently in bed. Lungs clear bilaterally. Antiembolism stockings applied to both lower extremities. Explanations given regarding these preventive measures. Pt. verbalized understanding. ———————— Bridget Smith, RN
	2300	Pt. continues to feel nauseated. Compazine 1 mg I.V. given. See MAR———————————— Bridget Smith, RN
	2335	Pt. states she's no longer nauseated. No further vomiting. Rating pain in incisional areas as 7 on a scale of 0 to 10, w/ 10 being worst pain imaginable. Medicated with morphine 2 mg I.V. See MAR——————— Bridget Smith, RN
	2355	Pt. rates pain as 1/10. Demonstrated taking deep breaths and coughing effectively. ——————— Bridget Smith, RN

PROBLEM-ORIENTED MEDICAL RECORD

The POMR system focuses on specific patient problems. Developed by doctors and later adapted by nurses, POMR has five components:

- Database: Subjective and objective data about the patient form the initial care plan. These data are collected during the initial patient assessment and include such information as the reason for hospitalization, medical history, allergies, medications, physical and psychosocial findings, self-care abilities, educational needs, and discharge planning concerns.

■ Problem list: A numbered list of the patient's current problems in chronologic order according to the date each was identified provides an overview of the patient's health status. You can refer to the problem by number when writing your notes. When a problem is resolved, note the date and time, and sign or initial it according to your facility's policy. Resolved problems shouldn't be highlighted with a felt-tip highlighter because highlighting often doesn't appear when medical records are copied, increasing the risk of errors.

■ Initial plan: This includes expected outcomes and plans for further data collection, patient care, and teaching. Involve the patient and significant others in planning and setting goals.

■ Progress notes: Typically, you must write a note for each current problem every 24 hours or when the patient's condition changes. SOAP, SOAPIE, or SOAPIER is used to structure progress notes. If you have nothing to record for a component, simply omit the letter from the note.

The components of SOAPIER include:

– **S**ubjective data: reason for seeking care or other information the patient or family members tell you

– **O**bjective data: factual, measurable data, such as observable signs and symptoms, vital signs, or test values

– **A**ssessment data: conclusions based on subjective and objective data and formulated as patient problems or nursing diagnoses

– **P**lan: strategy for relieving the patient's problems, including short-term and long-term actions

– **I**nterventions: measures you've taken to achieve expected outcomes

– **E**valuation: analysis of the effectiveness of your interventions

– **R**evision: changes from the original care plan.

■ Discharge summary: This covers each problem on the list and notes whether it was resolved. Discuss any unresolved problems and specify your plan for dealing with the problems after discharge. Also, record communications with other facilities, home health agencies, and the patient.

11/26/05	2400	#1 Nausea related to anesthetic. ————————
		S: Pt. states, "I feel nauseated." ————————
		O: Pt. vomited 100 ml of clear fluid at 2255. ———
		A: Pt. is nauseated. ————————————
		P: Monitor nausea and give antiemetic as necessary. ——
		I: Pt. given Compazine 1 mg. I.V. at 2300. ———
		E: Pt. states she's no longer nauseated at 2335. ———
		#2 Risk for infection related to incision sites. ———
		O: Incision site in front of Ⓛ ear extending down and
		around the ear and into neck — approximately 15 cm in
		length — without dressing. No swelling or bleeding, bluish
		discoloration below Ⓛ ear noted, sutures intact. Jackson-
		Pratt drain in Ⓛ neck below ear with 20-ml bloody
		drainage. Drain remains secured in place with suture.
		P 82, BP 132/88, RR 18, oral T 98.8° F. ————————
		A: No infection at present. ————————
		P: Monitor incision sites for redness, drainage, and
		swelling. Monitor JP drain output. Teach pt. S&S of
		infection prior to discharge. Monitor temperature.
		#3 Delayed surgical recovery. ————————
		O: Pt. oriented to time, place, and person, but groggy. Pt.
		attempted to get OOB at 2245 to ambulate to bathroom
		but felt dizzy upon standing. Lungs clear bilaterally. P 98,
		BP 110/68, RR 18 on return to bed.————————
		A: Pt. is dizzy when getting OOB. Pt. needs post-op edu-
		cation about mobility and coughing and deep-breathing
		exercises. ————————————
		P: Assisted pt. to use bedpan. Teach pt. to call for
		assistance and to get OOB by dangling legs on side of bed
		for a few minutes before attempting to stand. Monitor
		blood pressure. Teach coughing and deep breathing,
		turning, use of antiembolism stockings. ————————
		I: Allowed pt. to lie down in bed after feeling dizzy. Pt.
		used bedpan and voided 200 ml clear, yellow urine at
		2245. Assisted in coughing and deep-breathing exercises
		and taught about turning, use of antiembolism stockings.
		E: Lungs remain clear bilaterally. Pt. needs assistance with
		ambulation.————————
		#4 Acute pain related to surgical incision. ————————
		S: 2245 pt. states "No" when asked if she has pain. At
		2335 pt. states, "It hurts." ————————
		O: Pt. reports incisional pain as 7 on scale of 0 to 10, w/
		10 being worst pain imaginable. ————————
		A: Pt. is in pain and needs pain medication. ————————
		P: Give pain meds as ordered. ————————
		I: Pt. given morphine 2 mg I.V. at 2335. ————————
		E: Pt. states pain is 1/10 at 2340. —— Bridget Smith, RN

PROBLEM-INTERVENTION-EVALUATION SYSTEM

The PIE system organizes information according to the patients' problems. It requires you to keep a daily assessment flow sheet and progress notes. Integrating the care plan into the progress notes eliminates the need for a separate care plan and provides a record with a nursing – rather than medical – focus.

The daily assessment flow sheet includes areas for documenting assessment of major categories, such as respiration or pain, along with routine care and monitoring. It usually provides space to document the times that treatments are given and continued assessment of a specific area such as neurologic checks every hour. Progress notes are organized according to PIE:

■ **P**roblem: Use data collected from your initial assessment to identify pertinent nursing diagnoses. Use the list of nursing diagnoses accepted by your facility, which usually corresponds to the diagnoses approved by the North American Nursing Diagnosis Association (NANDA). (See "NANDA nursing diagnoses," page 480.) Some facilities use a separate problem list such as the POMR system. When documenting a problem, label it in the progress notes as *P* and number it; for example, P#1. This way you can refer to it later by its number without having to redocument the problem statement.

■ **I**ntervention: Document the nursing actions you take for each nursing diagnosis. Label each entry as *I* followed by *P* and the problem number; for example, IP#1.

■ **E**valuation: The patient's response to treatment makes up your evaluation. Use the label *E* followed by *P* and the problem number; for example, EP#1.

11/26/05	2400	P#1: Nausea related to anesthetic. ————————
		IP#1: Pt. given Compazine 1 mg I.V. at 2300. ———
		EP#1: Pt. vomited 100-ml clear fluid at 2255. Pt. now
		states no nausea after given Compazine. ————
		P#2: Risk for infection related to incision sites. ———
		IP#2: Drainage from Jackson-Pratt drain measured.
		Site monitored for redness, drainage, and swelling.
		Temperature monitored. ——————————
		EP#2: Incision site in front of ⓁŁ ear extending down
		and around the ear and into neck—approximately 15 cm
		in length—without dressing. No swelling or bleeding,
		bluish discoloration below Ⓛ ear noted, sutures intact.
		JP drain in Ⓛ neck below ear with 20 ml of bloody
		drainage. Drain remains secured in place with suture.
		P 82, BP 132/88, RR 18, oral T 98.8° F.————
		P#3: Delayed surgical recovery. —————————
		IP#3: At 2245, assisted patient getting back in bed and
		using bedpan after attempting to get up. Explained to
		pt. how to dangle legs and get OOB slowly. Voided 200
		ml clean, yellow urine. Assisted with and taught about
		coughing and deep-breathing exercises, turning, and use
		of antiembolism stockings. Assessed breath sounds. ———
		EP#3: Pt. reported feeling dizzy after first attempt to
		get OOB. Pt. did coughing and deep-breathing exercises
		effectively, and lungs clear bilaterally. P 98, BP 110/68,
		RR 18.———————————————————
		P#4: Acute pain related to surgical incision.————
		IP#4: Assessed pain as 7 on scale of 0 to 10, w/ 10
		being the worst pain imaginable. Gave pt. morphine 2
		mg I.V. at 2335. ———————————————
		EP#4: Prior to med. administration, pt. reported pain
		as 7/10. At 2340, pt. reports pain as 1/10. ————
		————————————— Bridget Smith, RN

FOCUS CHARTING

FOCUS charting is organized into patient-centered topics, or foci. It encourages you to use assessment data to evaluate these concerns.

Use a progress sheet with columns for the date, time, focus, and progress notes. In the focus column, write each focus as a nursing diagnosis, a sign or symptom, a patient behavior, a special need, an acute change in the patient's condition, or a significant event. In the progress notes column, organize information using three categories: data (D), action (A), and response (R). In the data category, include subjective and objective information that describes the focus. In the action category, include immediate and future nursing actions based on your assessment of the patient's

Date	Time	Focus	Progress notes
11/26/05	2400	Nausea related to anesthetic	D: Pt. states she's nauseated. Vomited 100-ml clear fluid at 2255. ————————————
			A: Given Compazine 1 mg I.V. at 2300. ———
			R: Pt. reports no further nausea at 2335. No further vomiting. ———————————
		Risk for infection related to incision sites	D: Incision site in front of Q ear extending down and around the ear and into neck— approximately 15 cm in length—without dressing. Jackson-Pratt drain in Q neck below ear secured in place with suture. P 82, BP 132/88, RR 18, oral T 98.8° F.————————————
			A: Assessed site and emptied drain. Taught patient S&S of infection. ———————
			R: No swelling or bleeding; bluish discoloration below Q ear noted. JP drained 20-ml bloody drainage. Pt. states understanding of teaching.—
		Delayed surgical recovery	D: Pt. reported dizziness after trying to get OOB to use the bathroom. P 98, BP 110/68, RR 18.——
			A: Assisted patient back in bed and with use of bedpan. Taught pt. how to dangle legs and get OOB slowly. Also taught coughing and deep-breathing exercises, turning in bed, and use of antiembolism stockings. ————————
			R: Pt. voided 200 ml in bedpan. Did coughing and deep breathing appropriately. Lungs clear bilaterally. Using antiembolism stockings. ———
		Acute pain related to surgical incision	D: Pt. reports pain as 7 on 0 to 10 scale, w/ 10 being worst pain imaginable. ———————
			A: Given morphine 2 mg I.V. at 2335. ———————
			R: Pt. reports pain as 1/10 at 2355. —————————
			———————————— Bridget Smith, RN

condition and any changes to the care plan you deem necessary based on your evaluation. In the response category, describe the patient's response to nursing or medical care. Using all three categories ensures concise documentation based on the nursing process. All other routine nursing tasks and assessment data can be documented on flow sheets and checklists.

CHARTING-BY-EXCEPTION

CBE radically departs from traditional systems by requiring documentation of only significant or abnormal findings in the narrative portion of the record. To use CBE documentation effectively, you must know and adhere to established guidelines for nursing assessments and interventions, and follow written standards of practice that identify the nurse's basic responsibilities. You document only deviations from the standards. Guidelines for interventions come from standardized care plans, patient care guidelines, doctor's orders, incidental orders, and standards of nursing practice. In addition, you may need to supplement your CBE documentation with progress notes.

The CBE format involves the use of a nursing diagnosis–based standardized care plan and several types of flow sheets:

■ Nursing diagnosis–based standardized care plans: These preprinted care plans are used when identifying a nursing diagnosis. Individualize your plan in the blank spaces provided.

■ Nursing care flow sheet: This form is used to document your assessments and interventions and is usually designed for a 24-hour period. After completing an assessment, compare your findings with the normal parameters defined in the printed guidelines on the form. Also, compare your assessment findings with the previous nurse's notes to see if the patient's condition has changed. If your findings are within normal parameters and haven't changed since the last nursing assessment, you can check-mark the category and add your initials. If your findings aren't within normal limits or don't match the previous assessment, put an asterisk in the box and document your findings in the comment section or other designated area such as the progress notes. (See *Nursing care flow sheet for charting-by-exception,* pages 462 and 463.)

■ Graphic record: This flow sheet is used to document trends in vital signs, weight, intake and output, and activity level. As with the nursing care flow sheet, use check marks and initials to indicate expected findings and asterisks to indicate abnormal findings. Record abnormalities in your progress notes.

■ Patient-teaching record: Use this form to track and document patient teaching and document outcomes. Include teaching resources, social and behavioral measures, dates when goals are met, and other pertinent observations.

(Text continues on page 464.)

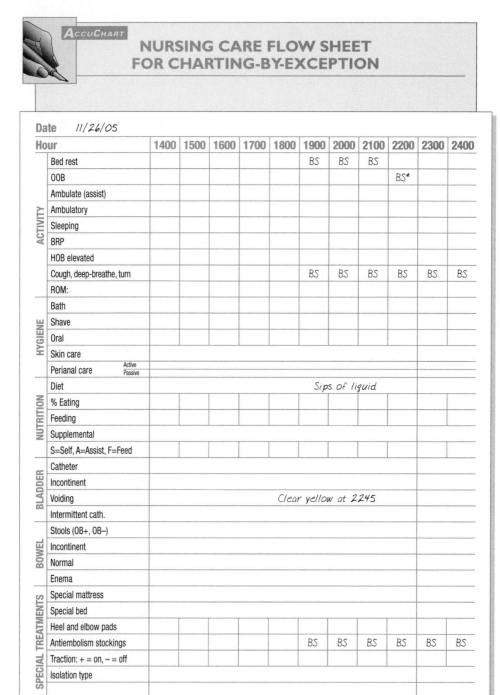

AccuChart

NURSING CARE FLOW SHEET
FOR CHARTING-BY-EXCEPTION

Date 11/26/05

Hour		1400	1500	1600	1700	1800	1900	2000	2100	2200	2300	2400
ACTIVITY	Bed rest						BS	BS	BS			
	OOB									BS*		
	Ambulate (assist)											
	Ambulatory											
	Sleeping											
	BRP											
	HOB elevated											
	Cough, deep-breathe, turn						BS	BS	BS	BS	BS	BS
	ROM:											
HYGIENE	Bath											
	Shave											
	Oral											
	Skin care											
	Perianal care Active Passive											
NUTRITION	Diet				Sips of liquid							
	% Eating											
	Feeding											
	Supplemental											
	S=Self, A=Assist, F=Feed											
BLADDER	Catheter											
	Incontinent											
	Voiding				Clear yellow at 2245							
	Intermittent cath.											
BOWEL	Stools (OB+, OB−)											
	Incontinent											
	Normal											
	Enema											
SPECIAL TREATMENTS	Special mattress											
	Special bed											
	Heel and elbow pads											
	Antiembolism stockings						BS	BS	BS	BS	BS	BS
	Traction: + = on, − = off											
	Isolation type											

NURSING CARE FLOW SHEET
FOR CHARTING-BY-EXCEPTION *(continued)*

ASSESSMENT FINDINGS

Key: ✓ = normal findings   ★ = significant finding

	Day	Evening	Night	
Neurologic	☐	✓ BS	☐	
Cardiovascular	☐	✓ BS	☐	
Pulmonary	☐	✓ BS	☐	
Gastrointestinal *Given Compazine 1 mg IV.*	☐	★ BS	☐	*vomited X 1 100 ml of clear fluid at 2255.* ̄c *relief.* ———
Genitourinary	☐	✓ BS	☐	
Surgical dressing and incision	☐	★ BS	☐	*Incision ⓛ ear around ear into neck 15 cm Jackson-Pratt drain, 20-ml bloody drainage.*
Skin integrity	☐	✓ BS	☐	
Psychosocial	☐	✓ BS	☐	
Educational	☐	★ BS	☐	*Taught C&DB, use of antiembolism stockings, and OOB slowly* ̄c *legs dangling first.* ———
Peripheral vascular	☐	✓ BS	☐	
Signatures	*Bridget Smith, RN*			

NORMAL ASSESSMENT FINDINGS

Neurologic
- Alert and oriented to time, place, and person
- Speech clear and understandable
- Memory intact
- Behavior appropriate to situation and accommodation
- Active range of motion (ROM) of all extremities; symmetrically equal strength
- No paresthesia

Cardiovascular
- Regular apical pulse
- Palpable bilateral peripheral pulses
- No peripheral edema
- No calf tenderness

Pulmonary
- Resting respirations 10 to 20 per minute, quiet and regular
- Clear sputum
- Pink nail beds and mucous membranes

Gastrointestinal
- Abdomen soft and nondistended
- Tolerates prescribed diet without nausea or vomiting
- Bowel movements within own normal pattern and consistency

Genitourinary
- No indwelling catheter in use
- Urinates without pain
- Undistended bladder after urination
- Urine clear yellow to amber color

Surgical dressing and incision
- Dressing dry and intact
- No evidence of redness, increased temperature, or tenderness in surrounding tissue
- Sutures, staples, adhesive strips intact
- Sound edges well approximated
- No drainage present

Skin integrity
- Skin color normal
- Skin warm, dry, and intact
- Moist mucous membranes

Psychosocial
- Interacts and communicates in an appropriate manner with others

Educational
- Patient or significant others communicate understanding of the patient's health status, care plan, and expected response
- Patient or significant others demonstrate ability to perform health-related procedures and behaviors as taught

Peripheral vascular
- Affected extremity pink, warm, and movable within average ROM
- Capillary refill time < 3 seconds
- Peripheral pulses palpable
- No edema: sensation intact without numbness or paresthesia
- No pain on passive stretch

■ Patient discharge note: This form may be used to document ongoing discharge planning. A typical discharge form includes places to document patient instructions, appointments for follow-up care, medication and diet instructions, signs and symptoms to report, level of activity, and patient education.

■ Progress notes: The progress notes are used to document revisions to the care plan and interventions that don't lend themselves to any of the flow sheets. Because most flow sheets should have areas in which to document abnormal findings, the progress notes typically contain little assessment and intervention data.

FACT DOCUMENTATION

The FACT system, which incorporates many CBE principles, has four key elements: **F**low sheets, **A**ssessments with baseline parameters, **C**oncise integrated progress notes and flow sheets documenting the patient's condition and responses, and **T**imely entries recorded when care is given. FACT requires that you document only exceptions to the norm or significant information about the patient. (See *Documenting with FACT.*)

FACT documentation begins with a complete initial baseline assessment on each patient using standardized parameters. This format involves an assessment-action flow sheet, a frequent assessment flow sheet, and progress notes. Flow sheets cover 24- to 72-hour periods. Always include the date and time, and sign all entries.

■ Assessment-action flow sheet: Use this form to document ongoing assessments and interventions. Normal assessment parameters for each body system are printed on the form along with planned interventions. Individualize the flow sheet according to patient need. In the appropriate place on the form (next to "normal"), check off assessments or interventions completed, or use the space provided to document abnormalities or completed interventions that are different than those printed on the form.

■ Frequent assessment flow sheet: Use this form to chart vital signs and frequent assessments. For example, on a surgical unit this form would include a postoperative assessment section.

AccuChart

DOCUMENTING WITH FACT

Developed in 1987 at Abbott Northwestern Hospital in Minneapolis, the FACT system records nursing assessment findings and interventions that are exceptions to the norm. This sample shows portions of a postoperative assessment flow sheet using the FACT format.

ASSESSMENT AND ACTION RECORD

	Date Time	11/26/05 2245	11/26/05 2335	11/26/05 2355
Neurologic Alert and oriented to time, place, and person. PEARL. Symmetry of strength in extremities. No difficulty with coordination. Behavior appropriate to situation. Sensation intact without numbness or paresthesia.		✓ groggy	✓	✓
Orient patient.				
Refer to neurologic flow sheet.				
Pain No report of pain. If present, include patient statements about intensity (0 to 10 scale), location, description, duration, radiation, precipitating and alleviating factors.		✓	7/10	1/10
Location			incision on left face	incision on left face
Relief measures			morphine 2 mg I.V.	
Pain relief: Y = Yes N = No				Y
Cardiovascular Apical pulse 60 to 100. S$_1$ and S$_2$ present. Regular rhythm. Peripheral (radial, pedal) pulses present. No edema or calf tenderness. Extremities pink, warm, movable within patient's range of motion (ROM).		✓	✓	✓
I.V. solution and rate				
Respiratory Respiratory rate 12 to 20 at rest, quiet, regular, and nonlabored. Lungs clear and aerated equally in all lobes. No abnormal breath sounds. Mucous membranes pink.		✓		✓
O$_2$ therapy				
TCDB/Incentive spirometer		✓		✓
Musculoskeletal Extremities pink, warm, and without edema; sensation and motion present. Normal joint ROM, no swelling or tenderness. Steady gait without aids. Pedal, radial pulses present. Rapid capillary refill.		OOB → dizzy → BR	✓	
Activity (describe)			BR	BR
Nurse's signature and title		Bridget Smith, RN	Bridget Smith, RN	Bridget Smith, RN

Key: ✓ = Meets assessment criteria

- Progress notes: This form includes an integrated progress record on which you'll use narrative notes to document the patient's progress and any significant incidents. As with FOCUS charting, write narrative notes using the data-action-response (DAR) method. Update progress notes related to patient outcomes every 48 hours or as required by your facility.

11/26/05	2400	D: Pt. states she's nauseated. Vomited 100 ml clear fluid at 2255.
		A: Given Compazine 1 mg I.V. at 2300.
		R: Pt. reports no further nausea at 2335. No further vomiting. ———————————— Bridget Smith, RN

CORE CHARTING

Core charting focuses on the nursing process — the core, or most important part of documentation. It consists of a database, care plan, flow sheets, progress notes, and discharge summary. Core charting requires you to assess and record a patient's functional and cognitive status within 8 hours of admission. The database and care plan are used as the initial assessment and focus on the patient's body systems and activities of daily living. They include a summary of the patient's problems and appropriate nursing diagnoses. Flow sheets are used to document the patient's activities and response to nursing interventions, diagnostic procedures, and patient teaching. Progress notes contain information for each problem organized in the data-action-response (DAR) format. Finally, the discharge summary includes information related to nursing diagnosis, patient teaching, and follow-up care.

11/26/05	2400	D: Pt. indicates being nauseated. Vomited 100-ml clear fluid at 2255.
		A: Given Compazine 1 mg I.V. at 2300.
		R: Pt. reports no further nausea at 2335. No further vomiting.
		D: Incision site in front of Ⓛ ear extending down and around the ear and into neck—approximately 15 cm in length—without dressing. Jackson-Pratt drain in Ⓛ neck below ear secured in place with suture. P 82, BP 132/88, RR 18, oral T 98.8° F.
		A: Assessed site and emptied drain. Taught patient S&S of infection.
		R: No swelling or bleeding; bluish discoloration below Ⓛ ear noted. JP drained 20-ml bloody drainage. Pt. states understanding of teaching.
		D: Pt. reported dizziness after trying to get OOB to use the bathroom. P 98, BP 110/68, RR 18.
		A: Assisted patient back in bed and with use of bedpan. Taught pt. how to dangle legs and get OOB slowly. Also taught coughing and deep-breathing exercises, turning in bed, and use of antiembolism stockings.
		R: Pt. voided 200 ml in bedpan. Did coughing and deep breathing appropriately. Lungs clear bilaterally. Using antiembolism stockings.
		D: Pt. reports pain as 7 on 0 to 10 scale, w/ 10 being worst pain imaginable.
		A: Given morphine 2 mg I.V. at 2335.
		R: Pt. reports pain as 1/10 at 2345. Bridget Smith, RN

OUTCOME DOCUMENTATION

Outcome documentation presents the patient's condition in relation to predetermined outcomes on the care plan, focusing on desired outcomes rather than problems. This system uses progress notes, flow sheets, and care plans. Some facilities use a separate teaching plan (see *Multidisciplinary patient-family education record,* page 468). Outcome documentation features these components:

■ Database: This includes subjective and objective data identifying the patient's problems and learning needs. The database is a foundation for ongoing evaluation.

■ Care plan: The care plan establishes priorities, identifies expected outcomes and nursing interventions, and documents the plan. Traditional handwritten plans, preprinted standardized plans, clinical pathways, and patient care guidelines can be used.

AccuChart

MULTIDISCIPLINARY
PATIENT-FAMILY EDUCATION RECORD

This sample shows the features of a typical multidisciplinary patient-family education record.

INITIAL EDUCATIONAL EVALUATION

Date/Time _11/21/05   2255_

Motivational level: P = patient   F = Family

_P/F_ Asks questions   _P/F_ Eager to learn   _____ Very anxious
_____ Uninterested   _____ Denies need for education   _____ Not appropriate for education

Barrier to education: ✓ No barrier identified

_____ Visual deficit   _____ Auditory deficit   _____ Physical deficit
_____ Religious barrier   _____ Cultural barrier   _____ Dexterity deficit
_____ Language barrier   _____ Language spoken

Special learning needs _Care after surgery_

Community resources discussed:

_____ Cardiac support   _____ Twelve-step program   _____ Cancer support
_____ Hospice   _____ Achievement center   _____ Diabetic support
_____ Other _____

DATE/INITIAL	TOPIC	PT	FAM	RESPONSE CODE
11/22/05 BS	Pt. oriented to room postoperatively.————	✓	✓	2, 6
11/22/05 BS	Explained purpose of Jackson-Pratt drain.——	✓	✓	2, 6
11/22/05 BS	Instructed pt. on use of 0-to-10 pain scale.	✓		2
11/22/05 BS	Instructed pt. on coughing and deep-breathing exercises. ————————	✓	✓	1, 3, 5
11/22/05 BS	Instructed pt. on use of antiembolism stockings, turning, & getting OOB slowly. ————————	✓		5, 6
11/23/05 DR	Instructed pt. on how to empty JP drain herself.——	✓	✓	2, 6
11/23/05 DR	Instructed pt. on S&S of infection to report to MD.	✓	✓	2, 6

Response codes:

1 Received literature	4 Prior experience	7 Referral indicated
2 Communicates understanding	5 Returned demo	8 Refused/Uninterested
3 Requires reinforcement	6 Education achieved	9 Inappropriate for education

Initials	Signature - Status	Initials	Signature - Status
BS	Bridget Smith, RN		
DR	Daniella Reams, RN		

WRITING EXPECTED OUTCOMES AND OUTCOME CRITERIA

Here are two examples of how to develop patient-focused outcomes and outcome criteria based on selected nursing diagnoses.

Nursing diagnosis	Expected outcomes	Outcome criteria
Risk for infection related to incision	Patient won't develop postoperative wound infection	▪ Patient states signs and symptoms to report to MD on discharge. ▪ Patient demonstrates incision care. ▪ Patient demonstrates emptying of JP drain.
Acute pain related to effects of surgery	Pain will be reduced by time of discharge	▪ Patient rates pain as 3 or less on 0 to 10 scale, with 10 being worst pain imaginable, by discharge. ▪ Patient expresses pain relief. ▪ Patient can perform self-care activities without assistance. ▪ Patient shows no facial mask of pain. ▪ Patient doesn't guard incision site.

▪ Expected outcome statements: Expected outcomes describe the desired results of nursing actions. Be specific and use outcome criteria that are measurable, and include a target date or time. Learning outcomes focus on patient behavior that's measurable and observable. Outcomes are evaluated and problems resolved if outcomes are met. When outcomes aren't met, the plan is reevaluated. (See *Writing expected outcomes and outcome criteria.*)

Electronic health record

Electronic health record information systems can increase efficiency and accuracy in all phases of the nursing process and can help nurses meet the standards set by the American Nurses Association and the Joint Commission on Accreditation of Healthcare Organizations (JCAHO). Current computerized systems not only collect, transmit, and organize the information, but they also suggest nursing diagnoses and provide standardized patient status and nursing interventions, which you can use for care plans and progress notes. Computerized systems may even interact with you, prompting you with questions and suggestions about the information that you enter.

Computers can also be used to help you with other types of paperwork, such as nurse management reports, patient classification data, and staffing projections. In addition, they can help you identify patient education needs and supply data for nursing research and education.

Depending on your institution's software, you might use computers for these nursing processes:

■ Assessment: Admission data can be collected via computer terminals. After entering patient data, such as health status, history, reason for seeking care, and other assessment data, the computer system can flag an entry if the data are outside the acceptable range.

■ Nursing diagnosis: Most current programs list standard diagnoses with associated signs and symptoms and can suggest one for your patient. However, you still need to use clinical judgment to determine if the suggested diagnosis is right for your patient.

■ Planning: To help nurses begin writing a care plan, computer programs can display recommended expected outcomes and interventions for the selected diagnoses. You may also use a computer program to compare and track patient outcomes for a selected group of patients.

- Implementation: Use the computer to record actual interventions and patient-processing information, such as discharge or transfer instructions. Progress notes, medication administration, vital signs, and treatments can also be documented with the computer.
- Evaluation: Use the computer to record evaluation and reevaluation and your patient's response to nursing care.

The Nursing Minimum Data Set (NMDS) program attempts to standardize nursing information. It contains three categories: nursing care, patient demographics, and service elements. The NMDS allows you to collect nursing diagnosis and intervention data and identify the nursing needs of various patient populations. It also lets you track patient outcomes. This system helps establish accurate estimates for nursing service costs and provides data about nursing care that may influence health care policy and decision making. With the NMDS, you can compare nursing trends locally, regionally, and nationally using data from various clinical settings, patient populations, and geographic areas. By comparing trends, you can set realistic outcomes for an individual patient as well as formulate accurate nursing diagnoses and plan interventions. Also, NANDA assigns numerical codes to all nursing diagnoses; thus, those diagnoses can be used with the NMDS.

The Nursing Outcomes Classification (NOC) system provides the first comprehensive standardized method of measuring nursing-sensitive patient outcomes. The NOC has major implications for nursing administrative practice and the patient care delivery system. This system allows the nurse to compare her patients' outcomes to the outcomes of larger groups, according to such parameters as age, diagnosis, or health care setting.

In addition to having a mainframe computer, most health care facilities place personal computers or terminals at workstations throughout the facility so that departmental staff will have quick access to vital information. Some facilities put terminals at patients' bedsides, making data even more accessible. Depending on which type of computer and software your facility has, you may access information by using a keyboard, light pen, touch-sensitive screen, mouse, or your voice.

Voice-activated systems are most useful in hospital departments such as the operating room, which have a high volume of structured reports. These software programs use a specialized knowledge base, nursing words, phrases, and report forms in combination with automated speech recognition (ASR) technology. The ASR system requires little or no keyboard use and allows the user to record prompt and complete nursing notes by voice while speaking into a telephone handset. The system displays the text on the computer screen. These systems increase the speed of reporting and free the nurse from paperwork.

Computerized charting has several advantages:
- It makes storing and retrieving information fast and easy.
- You can store data on patient populations that can help improve the quality of nursing care.
- You can efficiently and constantly update information and help link diverse sources of patient information.
- It uses standard terminology, which improves communication among health care disciplines and promotes more accurate comparisons.
- The charting is always legible.
- You can send request slips and patient information from one terminal to another quickly and efficiently, which helps ensure confidentiality.
- It facilitates individualized patient assessments and supports the use of the nursing process.
- Charting follows facility and JCAHO standards.
- Data entry can alert nurses to take action, such as prompting that a patient needs a wound care consult or that drug levels need to be drawn when administering certain drugs.

Computerized charting also has disadvantages:
- If used incorrectly, the computer may scramble patient information.
- Computerized charting can threaten patient confidentiality if security measures are neglected.
- The use of standardized phrases and a limited vocabulary can make information inaccurate or incomplete.
- Some people have trouble adjusting to computers, thus increasing the margin of error.

- When the system is down, information is temporarily unavailable.
- Computerized charting can take extra time if too many nurses try to chart on too few terminals.
- Implementing a computerized system is expensive.
- Software that puts patient data into categories may cause important information to be omitted.

JCAHO National Patient Safety Goals

The 2006 standards for accreditation of hospitals developed by the Joint Commission on Accreditation of Healthcare Organizations (JCAHO) include the identification of goals, functions, and standards for provision of patient care. The purpose of JCAHO's National Patient Safety Goals is to promote specific improvements in patient safety. The goals highlight problematic areas in health care and describe evidence and expert-based solutions to these problems. Because JCAHO recognized that sound system design is intrinsic to the delivery of safe, high quality health care, the goals focus on system-wide solutions wherever possible.

Below is a summary of the 2006 National Patient Safety Goals.

- Improve the accuracy of patient/resident/client identification.
    - Use at least two patient/resident/client identifiers (not the room number) when giving medications or blood products, taking blood samples and other specimens for clinical testing, or providing any other treatments or procedures.
    - You must conduct a final verification process to confirm the correct patient, procedure, site, and presence of appropriate documents immediately before the start of any invasive procedure. This requires active communication. The patient's identity must be re-established if the practitioner leaves the patient's location before starting the procedure. Marking the site is required unless the practitioner is in continuous attendance from the time of the decision to do the procedure and patient consent to the time of the procedure.
- Improve the effectiveness of communication among caregivers.
    - For verbal or telephone orders, or for telephonic reporting of critical test results, verify the complete order or test by having the person receiving the information read back the complete order or test result.

– Standardize a list of abbreviations, acronyms, and symbols that aren't to be used throughout your facility.

– Measure, assess and, if appropriate, take action to improve the timeliness of reporting and the receipt of critical test results and values by the responsible licensed caregiver.

– All values defined as critical by the laboratory are reported to a responsible licensed caregiver within time frames established by the laboratory. If the patient's responsible licensed caregiver isn't available within the time frames, report the critical information to an alternative responsible caregiver.

– Implement a standardized approach to "hand off" communications, including a chance to ask and respond to questions. This includes, but is not limited to, nursing shift changes, temporary responsibility for staff leaving the unit for a short time, anesthesiologists reporting to the post-anesthesia care unit (PACU) nurse, and nursing and doctor hand off from the emergency department to inpatient units, different facilities, nursing homes, and home health care.

■ Improve the safety of using medications.

– Standardize and limit the number of drug concentrations available within the facility.

– Identify and annually review a list of look-alike/sound-alike drugs used, and take action to prevent errors by the interchange of these drugs.

– Label all medications, medication containers (syringes, medicine cups, basins), or other solutions on and off the sterile field in perioperative and other procedural settings.

■ Eliminate wrong site, wrong patient, wrong procedure surgery.

– Use a preoperative verification process to confirm that needed documents are present.

– Use a process to mark the surgical site, and involve the patient in the marking process.

■ Improve the effectiveness of clinical alarm systems.

– Initiate regular preventive maintenance and testing of alarm systems.

– Make sure that alarms are activated with appropriate settings and are sufficiently audible with respect to distances and competing noise within the unit.

- Reduce the risk of health care–associated infections.
  - Comply with the Centers for Disease Control and Prevention hand hygiene guidelines.
  - Manage as sentinel events cases of unanticipated death or major permanent loss of function associated with a health care–associated infection.
- Accurately and completely reconcile medications across the continuum of care.
  - Implement a process for obtaining and documenting a complete list of the patient's current medications on admission with the involvement of the patient. This includes a comparison of the medications that the facility provides to those on the list.
  - A complete list of the patient's medications is communicated to the next provider of service when a patient is referred or transferred to another setting, practitioner, or level of care within or outside the facility.
- Reduce the risk of patient harm resulting from falls.
  - Implement a fall reduction program and evaluate its effectiveness.
- Reduce the risk of influenza and pneumococcal disease in older adults.
  - Develop and implement a protocol for administration and documentation of the flu vaccine.
  - Develop and implement a protocol for administration and documentation of the pneumococcus vaccine.
  - Develop and implement a protocol to identify new cases of influenza and manage an outbreak.
- Reduce the risk of surgical fires.
  - Educate staff, including licensed independent practioners (LIPs) and anesthesia providers, on how to control heat sources and manage fuels, and establish guidelines to minimize oxygen concentration under drapes.
- Implement applicable National Patient Safety Goals and requirements for components and practitioner sites.
  - Inform staff and encourage implementation of the National Patient Safety Goals.

- Encourage active involvement of patients and families in the patient's care as a patient safety strategy.
  - Define and communicate methods for patients and families to report concerns about safety.
- Prevent health care–associated pressure ulcers.
  - Assess and periodically reassess each patient's risk of developing a pressure ulcer and address identified risks.

Abbreviations to avoid

To reduce the risk of medical errors, the Joint Commission on Accreditation of Healthcare Organizations (JCAHO) has created a "minimum list" of abbreviations to avoid.

Abbreviation	Potential problem	Preferred term
U (for "unit")	Mistaken as zero, four, or cc.	Write "unit."
IU (for "international unit")	Mistaken as IV (intravenous) or 10 (ten).	Write "international unit."
Q.D., Q.O.D, QD, QOD, q.d., q.o.d., qd, qod (Latin abbreviation for "once daily" and "every other day")	Mistaken for each other. The period after the "Q" can be mistaken for an "I" and the "O" can be mistaken for "I."	Write "daily" and "every other day."
Trailing zero (X.0 mg) (Note: Prohibited only for medication-related notations); lack of leading zero (.X mg)	Decimal point is missed.	Never write a zero by itself after a decimal point (X mg), and always use a zero before a decimal point (0.X mg).
MS MSO_4 $MgSO_4$	Confused for one another. Can mean "morphine sulfate" or "magnesium sulfate."	Write "morphine sulfate" or "magnesium sulfate."

In addition to JCAHO's minimum "Do Not Use" list, the following items should be considered when evaluating which abbrevations to avoid.

Abbreviation	Potential problem	Preferred term
μg (for "microgram")	Mistaken for mg (milligrams), resulting in 1,000-fold dosing overdose.	Write "mcg."
H.S. (for "half-strength" or Latin abbreviation for "at bedtime")	Mistaken for either "half-strength" or "hour of sleep" (at bedtime).	Write out "half-strength" or "at bedtime."
q.H.S.	Mistaken for "every hour." Can result in a dosing error.	
T.I.W. (for "three times a week")	Mistaken for "three times a day" or "twice weekly," resulting in an overdose.	Write "3 times weekly" or "three times weekly."
S.C or S.Q. (for "subcutaneous")	Mistaken for SL for "sublingual," or "5 every."	Write "Sub-Q", "subQ," or "subcutaneously."
D/C (for "discharge")	Interpreted as "discontinue" whatever medications follow (typically discharge meds).	Write "discharge."
c.c. (for "cubic centimeters")	Mistaken for U (units) when poorly written.	Write "ml" for milliliters.
AS, AD, AU (Latin abbreviation for "left ear," "right ear," or "both ears")	Mistaken for OS, OD, and OU.	Write "left ear," "right ear," or "both ears."

NANDA
nursing diagnoses

The 2005-2006 nursing diagnoses classified according to their domains are listed here.

DOMAIN: HEALTH PROMOTION

- Effective therapeutic regimen management
- Ineffective therapeutic regimen management
- Ineffective family therapeutic regimen management
- Ineffective community therapeutic regimen management
- Health-seeking behaviors (specify)
- Ineffective health maintenance
- Impaired home maintenance
- Readiness for enhanced management of therapeutic regimen
- Readiness for enhanced nutrition

DOMAIN: NUTRITION

- Ineffective infant feeding pattern
- Impaired swallowing
- Imbalanced nutrition: Less than body requirements
- Imbalanced nutrition: More than body requirements
- Risk for imbalanced nutrition: More than body requirements
- Deficient fluid volume
- Risk for deficient fluid volume
- Excess fluid volume
- Risk for imbalanced fluid volume
- Readiness for enhanced fluid balance

DOMAIN: ELIMINATION

- Impaired urinary elimination
- Urinary retention
- Total urinary incontinence

- Functional urinary incontinence
- Stress urinary incontinence
- Urge urinary incontinence
- Reflex urinary incontinence
- Risk for urge urinary incontinence
- Readiness for enhanced urinary elimination
- Bowel incontinence
- Diarrhea
- Constipation
- Risk for constipation
- Perceived constipation
- Impaired gas exchange

DOMAIN: ACTIVITY/REST

- Disturbed sleep pattern
- Sleep deprivation
- Readiness for enhanced sleep
- Risk for disuse syndrome
- Impaired physical mobility
- Impaired bed mobility
- Impaired wheelchair mobility
- Impaired transfer ability
- Impaired walking
- Deficient diversional activity
- Dressing or grooming self-care deficit
- Bathing or hygiene self-care deficit
- Feeding self-care deficit
- Toileting self-care deficit
- Delayed surgical recovery
- Disturbed energy field
- Fatigue
- Decreased cardiac output
- Impaired spontaneous ventilation
- Ineffective breathing pattern
- Activity intolerance
- Risk for activity intolerance
- Dysfunctional ventilatory weaning response

- Ineffective tissue perfusion (specify type: renal, cerebral, cardiopulmonary, gastrointestinal, peripheral)
- Sedentary lifestyle

DOMAIN: PERCEPTION/COGNITION

- Unilateral neglect
- Impaired environmental interpretation syndrome
- Wandering
- Disturbed sensory perception (specify: visual, auditory, kinesthetic, gustatory, tactile, olfactory)
- Impaired verbal communication
- Readiness for enhanced communication

DOMAIN: SELF-PERCEPTION

- Disturbed personal identity
- Powerlessness
- Risk for powerlessness
- Hopelessness
- Risk for loneliness
- Readiness for enhanced self-concept
- Chronic low self-esteem
- Situational low self-esteem
- Risk for situational low self-esteem
- Disturbed body image

DOMAIN: ROLE RELATIONSHIPS

- Caregiver role strain
- Risk for caregiver role strain
- Impaired parenting
- Risk for impaired parenting
- Readiness for enhanced parenting
- Interrupted family processes
- Readiness for enhanced family processes
- Dysfunctional family processes: Alcoholism
- Risk for impaired parent/infant/child attachment
- Effective breast-feeding
- Ineffective breast-feeding

- Interrupted breast-feeding
- Ineffective role performance
- Parental role conflict
- Impaired social interaction

Domain: Sexuality

- Sexual dysfunction
- Ineffective sexuality patterns

Domain: Coping/Stress tolerance

- Relocation stress syndrome
- Risk for relocation stress syndrome
- Rape-trauma syndrome
- Rape-trauma syndrome: Silent reaction
- Rape-trauma syndrome: Compound reaction
- Posttrauma syndrome
- Risk for posttrauma syndrome
- Fear
- Anxiety
- Death anxiety
- Chronic sorrow
- Ineffective denial
- Anticipatory grieving
- Dysfunctional grieving
- Impaired adjustment
- Ineffective coping
- Disabled family coping
- Compromised family coping
- Defensive coping
- Ineffective community coping
- Readiness for enhanced coping
- Readiness for enhanced family coping
- Readiness for enhanced community coping
- Autonomic dysreflexia
- Risk for autonomic dysreflexia
- Disorganized infant behavior
- Risk for disorganized infant behavior

- Readiness for enhanced organized infant behavior
- Decreased intracranial adaptive capacity
- Risk for dysfunctional grieving

Domain: Life principles

- Readiness for enhanced spiritual well-being
- Spiritual distress
- Risk for spiritual distress
- Decisional conflict (specify)
- Noncompliance (specify)
- Impaired religiosity
- Readiness for enhanced religiosity
- Risk for impaired religiosity

Domain: Safety/Protection

- Risk for infection
- Impaired oral mucous membrane
- Risk for injury
- Risk for perioperative-positioning injury
- Risk for falls
- Risk for trauma
- Impaired skin integrity
- Risk for impaired skin integrity
- Impaired tissue integrity
- Impaired dentition
- Risk for suffocation
- Risk for aspiration
- Ineffective airway clearance
- Risk for peripheral neurovascular dysfunction
- Ineffective protection
- Risk for sudden infant death syndrome
- Risk for self-mutilation
- Self-mutilation
- Risk for other-directed violence
- Risk for self-directed violence
- Risk for suicide
- Risk for poisoning
- Latex allergy response

- Risk for latex allergy response
- Risk for imbalanced body temperature
- Ineffective thermoregulation
- Hypothermia
- Hyperthermia

DOMAIN: COMFORT

- Acute pain
- Chronic pain
- Nausea
- Social isolation

DOMAIN: GROWTH/DEVELOPMENT

- Risk for disproportionate growth
- Adult failure to thrive
- Delayed growth and development
- Risk for delayed development

Selected references

Birmingham, J. "Documentation: A Guide for Case Managers," *Lippincott's Case Management* 9(3):155-57, May/June 2004.

Brous, E.A. "7 Tips on Avoiding Malpractice Claims: Careful Practice and Documentation Help Keep You Out of Court," *TravelNursing2004* 34(6):16-18, June 2004.

Carpenito-Moyet, L.J. *Nursing Care Plans and Documentation: Nursing Diagnosis and Collaborative Problems,* 4th ed. Philadelphia: Lippincott Williams & Wilkins, 2003.

Complete Guide to Documentation. Philadelphia: Lippincott Williams & Wilkins, 2003.

Cowden, S., and Johnson, L.C. "A Process for Consolidation of Redundant Documentation Forms," *CIN: Computers, Informatics, Nursing* 22(2):90-93, March/April 2004.

Devine, R. "Issues of Documentation," *Lippincott's Case Management* 9(1):52-53, January/February 2004.

Erlen, J.A. "HIPAA–Clinical and Ethical Considerations for Nurses," *Orthopaedic Nursing* 23(6):410-413, November/December 2004.

Gallagher, P.M. "Maintain Privacy with Electronic Charting," *Nursing Management* 35(2):16-17, February 2004.

Gunningberg L., and Ehrenberg A. "Accuracy and Quality in the Nursing Documentation of Pressure Ulcers: A Comparison of Record Content and Patient Examination," *Journal of Wound, Ostomy, and Continence Nursing* 31(6):328-335, November/December 2004.

Hamilton, A.V, et al. "Applied Technology Rounds Out e-Documentation," *Nursing Management* 35(9):44-47, September 2004.

Huffman, M.H., and Cowan, J.A. "Redefine Care Delivery and Documentation," *Nursing Management* 35(2):34-38, February 2004.

Hyde A., et al. "Modes of Rationality in Nursing Documentation: Biology, Biography and the 'Voice of Nursing,'" *Nursing Inquiry* 12(2):66-77, June 2005.

Kaye, W., et al. "When Minutes Count– The Fallacy of Accurate Time Documentation During In-Hospital Resuscitation," *Resuscitation* 65(3):285-290, June 2005.

Kettenbach, G. *Writing SOAP Notes: With Patient/Client Management Formats,* 3rd ed. Philadelphia: F.A. Davis, 2004.

Kroll, M. "What Were You Thinking? Charting Rules to Keep You Legally Safe," *Journal of Gerontological Nursing* 29(3):15-16, March 2003.

Langowski, C. "The Times They Are a Changing: Effects of Online Nursing Documentation Systems," *Quality Management in Health Care* 14(2): 121-125, April-June 2005.

Laughlin, J., and Van Nuil, M. "Boost Regulatory Compliance with Electronic Nursing Documentation," *Nursing Management* 34(12):51-52, December 2003.

McNabney, M.K., et al. "Nursing Documentation of Telephone Communication with Physicians in Community Nursing Homes," *Journal of the American Medical Directors Association* 5(3):180-185, May/June 2004.

Moore, K.N., and Williams, B.A. "A Year in Review: Documentation and Critical Thinking," *Journal of Wound, Ostomy & Continence Nursing* 30(6):287-288, November 2003.

"New JCAHO Documentation Guidelines Required Nationwide," *TravelNursing2004* 34(2):2, February 2004.

Owen K. "Documentation in Nursing Practice," *Nursing Standard* 19(32):48-49, April 2005.

"Quick Tips: Documentation Essentials," *Advances in Skin & Wound Care* 17(2):55, March 2004.

Smith K, et al. "Evaluating the Impact of Computerized Clinical Documentation," *CIN: Computers, Informatics, Nursing* 23(3):132-138, May/June 2005.

Smith, L.S. "Handling Documentation Errors," *Nursing2003* 33(10):73, October 2003.

Sullivan, G.H. "Does Your Charting Measure Up?" *RN* 67(3):61-65, March 2004.

Index

i refers to an illustration; t refers to a table.

i refers to an illustration; t refers to a table.

---

i refers to an illustration; t refers to a table.

i refers to an illustration; t refers to a table.

i refers to an illustration; t refers to a table.

i refers to an illustration; t refers to a table.

i refers to an illustration; t refers to a table.

i refers to an illustration; t refers to a table.

i refers to an illustration; t refers to a table.

Notes